LISTENING TO THE SILENCES
IN A WORLD OF HEARING VOICES

Roy Vincent

Roy Vincent

All rights reserved, no part of this publication may be reproduced by any means, electronic, mechanical photocopying, documentary, film or in any other format without prior written permission of the publisher.

>
> Published by
> Chipmunkapublishing
> PO Box 6872
> Brentwood
> Essex CM13 1ZT
> United Kingdom

http://www.chipmunkapublishing.com

Copyright © Roy Vincent 2008

Cover image by Douglas Wilson.

LISTENING TO THE SILENCES

CONTENTS

CHAPTER	PAGE
1. Introit.	15
2. Keep right on to the End of the Road	55
3. " When I use a word…" said Humpty Dumpty	81
4. And there were GIANTS in those days…	129
5. If you yourself have never heard discarnate voices in your mind…	175
6. Oh what a world of unseen visions..	201
7. If you have a thousand reasons for living…	245
8. Enough, if something from our hands…	297
9. The wings of the morning	355
10. I have been taught by dreams and fantasies	381
11. A message in a bottle	431
12. Still as they run they look behind	441
13. My only enemy	511
14. Seek the beginnings…	563
15. THE END, but for some, the beginning…	567
16. LOOSE ENDS AND PICTURE GALLERY	575

Roy Vincent

INTRODUCTION

...LISTENING TO THE SILENCES...
BY: ROY VINCENT

In the autumn of 1979, I began to hear voices and experience other phenomena, and have done so ever since. Thus in almost 29 years, I have never been free from intrusions that enter blatantly or subliminally into my mind and mental faculties, and forcefully or subtly into my body and senses.

I use the word 'intrusion' deliberately, for that is what they are – not the product of an aberrant mind nor of a diseased brain; not hallucinations nor yet delusions. Because of what I was doing at the outset in 1979, I have no doubt, not the slightest shadow, that what I experience is of spiritual origin. Use of the word 'spiritual' to some immediately suggests 'religion', 'spiritualism', 'theology' and the like – words that to many are off-putting, and likely to prevent them from even opening my book. Forget such preconceptions. I am an engineer and my approach and language are those of an engineer – as precise and realistic as I can be within a realm of experience that is most <u>im</u>precise and <u>un</u>realistic.

From the beginning I have kept notes, which from 1998 began to turn into coherent writing as I became computer literate. In my parallel reading from the field of mental health, I found what are called 'The First Rank Symptoms' of schizophrenia, and I realised that I had experienced them all, and recorded and written of them, albeit in my own words. Yet – and this is the most important point that I am desperately trying to make – I have never been ill from this cause, and neither have I, nor would I seek help or intervention from the world of psychiatry or that of religion. On the contrary, I write to inform those in both such worlds who endeavour to help the mentally ill and disturbed.

As fast as I wrote, my words were read avidly by friends who work in the field of psychiatry. As they read, they wanted to know about 'before' – i.e. about my life before the onset of the intrusions. I realised that I should indeed write about 'before', in order to separate it from the events of 1979 and what has followed, for apart from the fact that both sequences happened to me, they are totally unconnected.

What happened 'before' is a story in itself, and it forms the first part of my book. In 1961 I had a successful career in the nuclear industry – a career of which I was robbed through the consequences of a medical misdiagnosis, and inappropriate and unnecessary medication. What is now known to have been a Cryptosporidia infection was treated as if 'nervous', and I began a life with Librium. After two years continuous use, an addict, dependent, and showing many of the side-effects of the drug, I began a 'psychiatric' year that opened with two episodes of cold turkey, then hospitalisation for a total of twenty weeks, 23 E.C.T.s, 'experiments' with a variety of drugs such as Tryptizol, Melleril, Valium, Pertofran and assorted benzodiazepines and barbiturates, plus insulin shock 'therapy' - and that ended with a farcical second opinion from someone who went on to become a doyen in the world of psychiatry.

I retired early with my career and home wrecked, and in total, in real terms, I have lost over a half million pounds. But hard though it may be to believe, effectively I began a new life. It is a life that has been and is both fascinating and rewarding – even though after four years it included the events that then led to the spiritual intrusions. For, as I found out, not only are there the malevolent – the ones that plague the 'schizophrenic' - but there are also the benevolent.

The whole story is there in the book – of how under the tuition of renowned healer, the late Bruce Macmanaway, I found that I also had a talent to heal. It is a talent that I have used hopefully to good effect, and which has brought me many rewards in encounters with wonderful people.
My 'engineering' approach has led to a study of our interaction with the electrical environment, and an understanding of aspects of electricity and health. Becoming aware of the electrical nature of acupuncture I expanded my knowledge and experience in this field also.

I identified over thirty different ploys that are used by intruding 'entities', and describe these in detail. I also realised that channels into the minds of the vulnerable can be opened via such activities as hypnotism and hypnotherapy, past life regression, Reiki, channelling and various forms of 'divination'. There are cautions, too, for those involved in spirit release, and many of the esoteric practices that involve 'opening the mind', and references also to the possibility of such 'recreational' drugs as cannabis and mescaline having the same effect – the effect sought by the shaman figure and such. I speculate too on possible links with manic depression.

Among my heroes are such diverse individuals as Galileo, Paracelsus and Nikola Tesla, and I quote and draw conclusions from them as I do from the writing and communications of a wide variety of psychiatrists, psychologists and others in the field of mental health, such as Irving Gottesman, Julian Jaynes, Martin Roth, Kenneth McAll, A.W.Drummond, Wilson Van Dusen, Richard Mackarness - to name a few. I have also drawn from that well-known hearer of voices and seer of visions, Teresa of Avila.

I surprised myself when I found that my initial tentative writing had become a book. When I read what I have written, there are times when I feel as if I have been skinned physically, and that the raw 'me' is thereby exposed for all to see in its pulsating pain and agony. Yet I have opened myself, my life and my experiences willingly in the

LISTENING TO THE SILENCES

hope that the knowledge that I have acquired will be used by suffering individuals, or will be used for their benefit by carers and the professionals in the world of psychiatry and the caring of the mentally disturbed. As I contemplate the emergence of my text in print, I can but hope that this will be so, although, realistically, all that I can do is to put my faith in you as a reader, and join poet W.B.Yeats when he speculates –

Where My Books Go

All of the words that I utter,
And all of the words that I write
Must spread out their wings untiring
And never rest in their flight,
Until they come to where your
Sad, sad heart is.

Roy Vincent

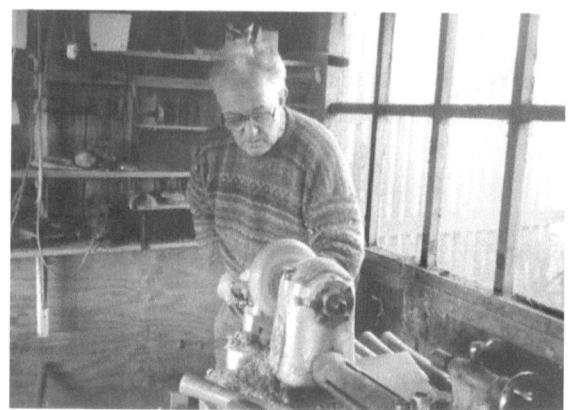

The Author at Home

LISTENING TO THE SILENCES

**Don't get annoyed
if the people coming to see you
if the people wanting to talk to you
can't manage to express
the uproar raging inside them**

**Much more important
than listening to the words
is imagining the agonies
fathoming the mystery,
...listening to the silences...**
Dom Helder Camera

Roy Vincent

Dedicated with love
To my
Daughter,
And to the
Evergreen Memory
Of deceased members
Of my Family.

Roy Vincent

LISTENING TO THE SILENCES

INTROIT...

I am probably one of the people least likely to write anything remotely autobiographical. Not that I have led an uninteresting or uneventful life. As my friends know to their cost, they have only to press the appropriate button and they will have their ears bent with anecdote and happenstance for some considerable time. Essentially I am a private person and cringe at the products of this self-revelatory, tell-all culture in which we live. Daily, hourly, by the minute, on television and radio and in the printed media, people are pouring out the dross of their lives to a gaping, prurient world, and like most trash it is soon dumped and overlaid by the next batch.

So why write anything at all? Friends persuade me that from what has happened to me, been inflicted upon me, there can be drawn that which may be of help and guidance to others; to people who find themselves overwhelmed by the problems of their minds; problems which flood their lives and threaten to submerge them, to drown them, or suck them down.

If I was to find myself trapped in quicksand, the person most calculated to be able to help me, in whom I would have most confidence, would not be an expert in sand and water mixtures, emulsions, but someone who had actually *been there*, had been mired and sucked down; someone who had actually *extricated* himself from the slough - who, even though he used the immortal words of Corporal Jones in *Dad's Army,* "Don't panic, don't panic", would say them with all of the conviction and authority of someone who knew what he was talking about, and would back-up his words with the practical rescue techniques learned in the maelstrom of personal life threatening experience.

'Life threatening'? But isn't this going to be an account of the perils that can terrorise, intimidate the mind? How can these be classed as 'life threatening'? I have twice been in these allegorical quicksands; the first time I was pushed, albeit accidentally, but over the long period in which I floundered I almost lost my 'mental life', my mind; the second, much briefer time, the one in which I strayed accidentally and innocently into a mire, I found myself in grave danger of losing my spiritual life. So, in that context, yes; life threatening. But also, and it must be faced, a point can be reached when suicide is the preferred option. So, 'life threatening'? Yes.

Unless you have been there yourself, I imagine that you will have difficulty with the concept that death and oblivion could be preferable to continued life, assuming that one had any choice. Frankly, I hope that you never find yourself in that morass. But the imagination cannot conceive of the terror that can be created in the human mind from one's own tormented soul or which can be planted there by dominating 'voices', from whatever source they may come. Perhaps a better understanding of the prospect of

LISTENING TO THE SILENCES

final submersion before the reality of which suicide is preferable, might be achieved by contemplating the dilemma of someone actually trapped and in imminent danger of being overwhelmed in real quicksand, and having in his hands the ready means of his own death and release.

Sir Peter Scott in his wildfowling book, *Morning Flight* graphically paints in words the picture of his own brother, David, facing this very situation. David had spent a day alone wildfowling and found himself towards the close of the day having shot a widgeon, but it having landed on the opposite side of a small estuary. The tide being out, he had waded across and walked along the far shore. Suddenly he found the sand to be soft; he took two more steps and it became softer. He tried to turn back and he had sunk up to his knees. At every move he sank deeper, and the sand around him had turned to a viscous pudding. His movements became desperate and he made greater and greater efforts. When he stopped, he had sunk to his waist. The more he struggled the farther he sank, until he was so much submerged that he could no longer struggle. Only his head and shoulders and arms remained above the jelly-like morass. Then he began to think carefully of his position.... In an hour the flood tide would arrive. But he would not see it come. He would not watch the water approaching inch by inch until he lost his reason. There were two cartridges in his gun...

David was within moments of taking his own life when something made him turn, and there, a dark shadow on the tide, was a small boat with three net fishermen. After desperate and hoarse shouting and waving, they saw and came near, but not near enough for a rope to reach, so two of the fishermen got out.... they were adept at moving on the surface of the quicksand without sinking in. They hopped about 'on all fours', never remaining more than a second in one place. They reached harder ground and from there threw a rope...the men gave him hope and strength, and after ten minutes of tremendous effort he felt himself gradually working up and out... It turned out that it was the first day of the smelt fishing season, and one day earlier there would have been no boat on the river.

The quicksand of the mind and the quicksand of the shore are most terrible, most vile because they are invisible, indescribable. More terrible for the victim in his mind, because he cannot shout, for who is there to hear him, if indeed he knew *what* to shout. And yet, in the fastnesses of his mind, there is a desperate call, plea, for help. The quicksands of the mind are terrible because of their loneliness. On the brightest day, in the most sparkling company, the person in depression cannot lift his eyes to beauty, nor open his ears to the laughter, life and joy around. He is in the gut-empty world of no-mind; robbed of all emotion; unable to believe in human love, nor love from *any* source. If he knew them he would echo the words of the psalmist *...you have turned my friends and neighbours against me, my one companion is darkness.*

LISTENING TO THE SILENCES

But, while darkness brings the immediate oblivion of sleep, it is a traitor. It at first hides, then treacherously opens the trap-door to the world of no-sleep; the world of the night terrors; the world of no-time between true night and day; the world of the tormenting, mocking, teasing, dominating voices - voices from where? If you read on you will find an answer. It may not be an answer which you will want to read or which you will accept, but if you don't I'm afraid that that is your problem. My answer is the answer of personal experience.

For nearly forty years, I have had experiences that I would rather not have had, experiences that could have made me exceedingly bitter. But the bitterness could further have harmed me had I let it take a hold. Instead, I have been exceedingly fortunate in being able to extract, distil from it all, much which has been, and is, enthralling and enlightening. Friends have persuaded me that others may derive benefit from my experiences and enlightenment. So, if you are yourself being engulfed in the quicksands of your mind; if you are calling for help in the silence of your mind; if you cannot silence the voices which invade your mind, dominate and torment you; if you care for someone who is struggling in the morass which their mind has become - if you are any of these I am writing for you. As someone who has been there, extricated himself, I am trying to throw you a rope; and while I do not hop around on all fours, I have learned to tread lightly, warily amongst these perils.

Roy Vincent

      I have a very good friend whose approach to a new book, no matter how devious or complex the plot, is just to dip at random each time he picks it up. I am still exceedingly baffled to know how he derives pleasure from his reading, or, indeed, apart from seeing the first and last pages, how he knows where the story begins and ends. If he ever gets to read my writings, I wonder just how he will approach them. Without trying to impose any compulsion on you, I shall be grateful if you will read what I have written in sequence, otherwise the thread, and much of my purpose in writing, will be lost.

      As I wrote at the outset, I open part of my life with reluctance, but with hope that you will benefit. Make of it what you will - each of you will see me differently. Many people quote the one well-known verse of Robbie Burns' poem *To a Louse* as if it embodies deep philosophy and wisdom; he wrote -

> *Would some power the giftie gie us*
> *to see ourselves as others see us.*

I have my medical notes covering a period of thirty years: they do not make for happy reading, particularly in respect of seeing just how one has been seen, interpreted. My advice to you is to decide for yourself just who you are, and to do all in your power to be yourself, hold on to your own identity, and strive for your own goals. It took me a long time and much hard work to recover my own life and identity after I had been robbed of them. So please, try to see me as I portray myself, and if you want to know how I lost and found myself again, well, just read on...........

"We had to destroy it to save it."

Such was the bizarre reasoning given by the U.S. Authorities to justify the annihilation of a village during that most bizarre of conflicts, the Vietnam War.

As I have begun to write, I have trawled through my own memory, and read, and come to terms with, the copious notes and correspondence that form my medical records. When you read what I shall write, I think that you may agree that the same 'justification' could be applied to the almost-achieved outcome of the treatments that were brought to bear to 'save' my malfunctioning mind. The treatments were applied with good intent, I have no doubt, by people who were established in their professions of medicine and psychiatry. In the process of being treated, my *mind* was almost annihilated. So what went wrong? Well, to start with, at the outset, there was nothing *wrong* with my mind - it was functioning well and I was in control. But *something* must have gone wrong and to describe it is the purpose of the first part of my tale. The path ahead may at times seem a little tortuous, but I am sure that you will find the journey interesting.

In the past, I have always enjoyed writing, although my authorship then had a different purpose in my professional rôle - reports, papers, proposals, were the offspring of my love of language, constrained by the accepted forms of technical writing. A fellow Welshman whose evocative use of language has never ceased to please me, is Dylan Thomas. When I listen to a recording of *Under Milk Wood*, from memories of people and places locked in my mind in my youth, I can 'see' all the exquisitely drawn characters, I can 'walk' down Cockle Row, I can 'look' through the mind's eye of blind Captain Cat. For me there is only one recording - the first made by the BBC, with Huw Gryffudd as Captain Cat; the Reverend Eli Jenkins was spoken by Philip Burton, the English master at my school, and the one who set in train my love of language. But most of all, and no matter how often I listen, guaranteed to produce the same thrill of anticipation are the opening words spoken with his unique timbre by long-ago schoolmate Richard Burton. I can do no better than to recall his voice and echo it as he speaks...

TO BEGIN AT THE BEGINNING...

A high flyer was I. Was I? I shall never know now. No self-vaunted Icarus was I, flapping higher and higher on phoney wings, only to crash to destruction when the deceit was uncovered by the harsh sun of scrutiny. No: by dint of the steady wing-beats of hard work, dedication and loyalty, I was rising and being lifted from time to time on the up draught of peer approbation. So: how did I lose my feathers? Why did I crash? Why did I have to learn to walk again?

How is it that such destruction can be visited on someone in broad daylight, in a civilised society, in his own home, in the midst of a caring family and, at work, under the gaze of a solicitous employer?

And what did I lose? I lost a home which was still being carefully built up and consolidated; I lost my wife and, effectively, my daughter; in time I couldn't sustain my job and retired prematurely; financially, in today's (2003) values, I have lost over half a million pounds, while each year I receive in pension about one third of what I could reasonably have expected. But of greater worth, a worth which can not be measured in cash, I have lost a swathe of my memory; memory of a time when life was very good; when I had a wife whom I loved and who was yet young; when work was very rewarding and successful; when my daughter was blossoming. Do you know, I cannot remember how she used to talk when she was little; the things she said; bath times; bed times; Christmas; picnics and holidays; ponies.... I can barely remember the Sunbeam-Talbot that was the family's pride, or taking my mother and in-laws for 'runs'. I am fortunate in that I have a former work colleague whom I meet from time to time, whose reminiscences remind me of the highly successful and rewarding times we had as vital players in a cutting-edge project that was a world first, otherwise *that* memory would also be lost.

So, how did I lose so much? How did I lose it uncomplainingly, trustingly? Surprisingly, and sadly, I lost it at the hands of, or perhaps more accurately, I had it all stolen by, the very people whose prime intent and professional purpose was to care for me. I lost it through the intervention of medicine and psychiatry.

There is only one way for you to understand the extent of my loss - the actual loss over the years and the potential of what might have been - and that is for me to take you sufficiently far back in my life and career to find a convenient staring point. So how about 1947? I was 21 years old, in transition between life as a Petty Officer Radar Mechanic in the Royal Navy, and life as an undergraduate electrical engineer in the University of Wales at Swansea.

LISTENING TO THE SILENCES

Three years and an Engineering Degree later saw me, in 1950, make what was for me a very desirable move to the Lake District in Cumbria - scene of several pre-war family holidays - to work in the embryonic nuclear industry. My radar training and experience, combined with my degree, fitted me for the very fascinating and often novel world of measurement. I was becoming an Instrument Engineer. First promotion, and 1953, and I was part of the team destined to run the world's first nuclear power station, Calder Hall - which at the time that I joined was just a large hole in the ground! An exciting time of very hard but fascinating and rewarding work, and of personal change - of marriage in 1955, and parenthood in 1956, and a second promotion.

The Works developed and expanded, as did the science and technology, and my responsibility - which led to a further promotion at the end of 1960. Thus, in what turned out to be an exceedingly crucial year, 1961, at age 35 I had the grade of 'Principal', and a salary (2003 equivalent) of £50, 000. I had been to France as an advisor during the commissioning of their first power reactor, and to Stockholm to address an international conference. I had a career, a home and a family, and the probability of more children. And with a further thirty years of potential employment, who knows how my future might have blossomed?

Roy Vincent

To mention 'diarrhoea' in the context in which I am writing may seem an unnecessary and unpleasant irrelevance: unfortunately, it became very relevant. We lived in Seascale, and in the late summer of almost every year the notorious 'Seascale Bug' would strike, bringing stomach upsets, sickness and diarrhoea to the populace at random. When, thus, in 1961, I started with my episode of the 'runs' it just seemed as if I was one of that year's unfortunates. But this was no ordinary visitation of the 'Seascale Bug'. Soon it seemed as if the whole of my inside had turned to fluid - the mediaeval term 'the flux' was probably very appropriate. Day after day after day it continued, defying all the usual nostrums and quick-setting cements that were commonly effective. My 'samples' yielded no known bacteria. My weight dropped by over a stone; the lavatory pan was my boon companion.

Then, one day, a visit to my G.P. produced something new, something different. My medical certificate sported the letters C.A.N. in place of the usual 'enteritis', and a prescription which, when dispensed at the local pharmacy, produced a bottle of black and green capsules coyly hiding behind the label bearing the legend 'Librium'. Now, remember, this was 1961; Librium was brand, spanking new; the word 'tranquilliser' was not in common parlance. No warning bells rang in my mind - and why should they have? Like most people, I believed implicitly in the medical profession, in what they said was wrong with me, in the ways in which it should be put right. The average layperson has no base from which to query or dispute the medical opinion; one's view is often met with the slightly tolerant smile that seems to say, " The patient has an opinion, humour him and it will go away".

I promise you this: there had been no discussion concerning my nervous state, nor was anything said about Librium, its purpose or its side effects. I had to deduce, yes *deduce,* that C.A.N. meant 'chronic anxiety neurosis', and that I was 'on' a tranquilliser. You may wonder at the lack of communication. All I can say is that I was very debilitated and unsure of myself, and that the doctor in question was very reserved, almost taciturn, and did not open himself to discussion. One former colleague at work even now reminds me of the response that *he* got when suggesting an alternative to *his* continuing treatment; whatever he was then told was prefaced with the put-down "We in the *learned* profession...". (I must emphasise that I am not recounting this to denigrate in any way the doctor in question, who was immensely appreciated in the community both as a person and G.P., but simply to emphasise something to which I will no doubt return many times in this account and the other parts of my 'story', namely this communication gulf between medical professional and lay-person).

So, dutifully, I took my Librium in complete and blissful ignorance of the most common side effects - of confusion, drowsiness and inability to control voluntary muscular movements - and *physical dependence*! How, I wonder, would my employers have reacted had *they* known, for the Department at work of which I was head was responsible for every one of the measuring and safety devices in the whole nuclear power station of four reactors and eight turbines?

No doubt everyone has those events in their lives over which they groan internally and long to extinguish the event and its consequences; this is one of my most desperate, as must be that of anyone who has started to take an addictive substance. How many clocks would be put back if given the chance? My anguish is made all the greater with the 20/20 vision with which all hind sight is blessed, and the knowledge, gained some 25 years after the events, of a newly identified parasite that can inhabit the lower gut and produce uncontrollable but *self-limiting* diarrhoea. Such a parasite one can acquire from polluted water or milk, or from animals - a route that the family hobby of riding and horse-work made readily available. *Cryptosporidium* is the name of what it is now believed was the cause of my illness - one of a group of parasitic protozoa.

Looking back at the events covered by the next two years, much of what I did, felt and suffered can now be understood and many things fall into place. First, there was the growing addiction. My very first act on waking was to pop a pill. If I didn't get my noon 'fix' on time I started to get the shakes. It was while I was doing this one day at work that I received my one piece of cautionary advice. It came from a former G.P.

LISTENING TO THE SILENCES

who had given up medical practice to found a firm which made endoscopes; he was visiting to supervise the installation of one of his industrial size 'scopes. When he saw the pill going in, he advised me instead to unwind at home each evening with a glass of sherry. Kind man that he was, on his next visit he handed me a brown wrapped bottle - "Special varnish" he said, "Don't open it here in daylight". I still think of rich, dark port wine as 'special varnish'. How I wish that I had been able to take his advice, but by now I *believed* that I had a C.A.N. How else could I explain the shakes that were cured by my next 'fix'? How else to account for the drowsiness that was besetting me in my office, the 'numbness' which enveloped my midriff and radiated outwards, the confusion or slowness in understanding the developments in computing, which specialist members of my department were engaged with? How else could I explain to myself the frequent malaises that had all the hallmarks of 'flu without the temperature?

Life at work was getting difficult, particularly the drowsiness - but how can you explain to your next senior something that you didn't understand yourself, and which he didn't confront directly? (The problems contained in that one sentence, and all the other examples that emerge of the inability to address or articulate a difficulty or problem, of the impossibility of admitting or communicating to one's partner, friends, colleagues, medical advisers, more than an inkling of the gut-wrenching, mind-warping fears and fantasies which emerge, are topics to which I must return somewhere in the discourse if I am to draw meaningful conclusions and offer advice to others on ways to cope or support; but how difficult it is!).

In the main, I was still doing a good job; no catastrophes, and many innovations at which I was particularly good. I remember, too, delivering a lecture to the Engineering Society on the subject of computers in general, and the ones in particular that we were then incorporating into the plant - the last major, positive event at work for some time to come. Such changes as were happening to my life and demeanour were yet acceptable and bearable compared with what was to come as 1963 was settling into autumn.

The G.P. who had made the original diagnosis and prescription had moved back to his beloved Scotland, and to his replacement I remember saying "You have inherited my chronic anxiety neurosis" - me still accepting what I had been told, and he having no reason to question it. Socially we got on very well and his wife and mine became firm friends. However, his professional visits to the home began to cause him some concern and in time, he expressed the view that what I was experiencing was psychosomatic. He advised that I should see a psychiatrist and arranged for me to do so. After the encounter with Librium, the meeting with the psychiatrist has become another of my life's great 'I wish it hadn't happened ' moments.

LISTENING TO THE SILENCES

From this point on, I have copies of all my medical notes for the next thirty years - both those of the consultant and those of the local practice. The reason why I acquired them is revealed much later in my saga. Reading the notes - not an easy experience to cope with - it is revealing to see oneself as a 'he', a third person, almost a specimen with a label. To me, as an engineer, the most glaring difference between my profession and that of the psychiatrist, is the latter's lack of certainty, of objectivity. I was used to dealing with a reality - my whole purpose in my work was measurement - the complete delineation of the state of being of a piece of plant or an operation as it was *then,* at that moment. I had seen my devices - the nerves of the plant - put in place (nearly 50 years on, I have the personal and professional satisfaction of knowing that many of them, those completely inaccessible inside the nuclear reactors, are still there, still functioning). Their characteristics were known, for we had calibrated them; they told the operator exactly what was going on in the remote reaches of his plant; if anything broke down outside the reactor I had to know exactly why it had failed, and could only replace it with apparatus that had been thoroughly tested and calibrated.

My Consultant (MC) appeared to be thorough, no question of that. We talked, he arranged tests, e.g. was hypoglycaemia a possibility? But to the outsider, there appear to be no certainties in psychiatry, only opinions and educated guesses based upon the personal experience and training of the one particular practitioner; possibly even the 'school' of psychiatry to which he subscribes; no precise measurements or standards. Labels are put on 'bottles' of symptoms - but the contents of the bottles seem to change at the whim of one school of research or another. Take for instance Alzheimer's disease. I can read the standard, original definition of a 'pre-senile dementia', which, when originally identified and defined by Alzheimer himself, applied essentially to persons under the age of 55. Yet in a recent paper describing research into the prevalence of Alzheimer's disease amongst professional footballers, the author states that the condition is rarely experienced in persons under the age of 60!

It is only in later years and being outside the maelstrom that I was then in, and fully in charge of my life and mind, that I can look back and be critical. But let me emphasise again, as I do through all that I write, that apart from those whose reasoning and lack of perception I condemn, and who will emerge later, I am not critical of the *intent* of any individual: I appreciate most deeply the care and concern which were lavished upon me by *all* the people whom I encountered. But I am a professional in my own right; my training and experience were on a par with most of the medical practitioners in *their* profession, and so I justify my own right to be critical of analysis and results. All this, of course, looking back with the benefit of the records in my possession, to let me see into the thought processes of those who were examining and analysing *mine.*

My perception of the lack of objectivity begins in the letter to GP2 sent after my first consultation. I was seen effectively as a 'garrulous, bespectacled, Welsh hypochondriac'. Welsh and bespectacled were irrelevancies that I couldn't alter, but who would *not* be a garrulous hypochondriac after two years on a continuous and substantial intake of Librium (which modern professional medical opinion now recognises as having been totally inappropriate and unnecessary!)? The fact that he rated me as of above average intelligence mollifies the personal affront to my self-image, which itself pales into insignificance before the recollection of what else appeared in the letter, and its immediate effect. After two years continuous use, at 10mg tds, my Librium was stopped forthwith and replaced by Tryptizol.

Oh Boy! Does anyone want to know what 'cold turkey' is like? My advice: don't try it! Recollect - I had been taking Librium in substantial dosage for over two years. Information readily available and unequivocal says that it is for *short-term* use. There is also full information about withdrawal after use - in my case after such dosage for so long my withdrawal might have taken *over one year*! Mine was overnight! The bizarre reactions and symptoms that I experienced are only partially recorded in my notes, but it was enough that when food was put in my mouth I lost contact with it, for I had no taste, no feeling down my throat. My stomach might not have existed for there was no sensation when I pressed that region, and I had no pressure sensation in my bladder. It was as if everything from my mouth to my fork no longer existed. The symptoms which I was experiencing were in fact so 'global' that in the correspondence between MC and GP2, they were referred to as '..this remarkable set of symptoms' and 'multi-various physical symptoms'. The possibility that they might be the effects of the instantaneous withdrawal from Librium was just not considered; everything I was experiencing was put down to a never-before-recorded idiosyncratic reaction to Tryptizol.

Time off work and a return to Librium produced a measure of stability. 'Stability'? Huh! Work was becoming a daily nightmare, if that isn't too paradoxical, while what was going on in the minds of my wife and daughter, I would not like to examine even after all this time.

If you don't succeed in flattening him at the first go, why, just have another. A couple of days on Stelazine - immediate disaster - then a second bash, this time with Melleril. Same result; bizarre symptoms; brief flirtation with Nardil; reduced to quivering jelly. Hospital? Yes please. Refuge. I could, with relief and without feeling guilty, put aside my responsibilities at home and work.

LISTENING TO THE SILENCES

E.C.T.? If you say so. "Sign here" - as a voluntary patient. Bang! The next assault on my precious mind began.

Isn't it amazing how docile we are? Or maybe then we were more docile, accepting, than people are now. Perhaps people nowadays are better informed, or demand more information; also there are patients' support groups, and others active in attempts to outlaw E.C.T - it is, after all, a bizarre and dangerous 'treatment'. Whatever the analysis, there I was, good little Indian, ready to accept what the kind gentleman said because it would make me better. I am sure that you want to know all about it, for it is done in your hospitals, and by people who, indirectly, you employ.

Three times a week the Ward went into its well-rehearsed routine. You wake and get up as usual, but have no breakfast. Shortly, you have an injection of a belladonna (deadly nightshade) derivative whose purpose is to dry the mouth and prevent you choking on your saliva. Meanwhile the nurses are playing trains with the beds, pushing them end-to-end in the corridor outside the treatment room. Next, as your turn approaches, a second injection, this time of a curare derivative. Curare, as you probably know, is the poison that South American Indians put on their blow-darts; the object of its use in this situation being to cause complete muscle relaxation and minimise the risk of vertebral fractures (after all it *is* electro *convulsive* therapy) -

no mention of the possibility of *these* when I gave my 'informed' consent!

Let me quote from *The Oxford Companion to the Mind*:

"E.C.T: *Applying a voltage with surface electrodes on the head across the brain. This is done under anaesthesia or muscle relaxant, as it produces convulsions which can be dangerous.*
E.C.T is extensively used as a convenient and quick treatment for depression, though there is no theoretical basis to justify it.
There is considerable criticism of its extensive use because it may produce permanent brain damage, especially losses of memory and intelligence, though the evidence is not entirely clear."

I want you to take particular note of the last sentence for reasons that will become pertinent later.

You lie on the bed, shoes off and tucked under the mattress end. Chug - chug, the train moves on and your 'carriage' is manoeuvred into the treatment room. Dentures out and into a glass. An anaesthetist tries to find a suitable vein in your arm and, when successful, dribbles in Pentathol, or a similar anaesthetic. Gentle bliss and oblivion. Next, electrodes are placed on your temples and a burst of electricity is switched into your lovely, delicate, unsuspecting brain. You don't know this, of course; what next you are

LISTENING TO THE SILENCES

aware of is gradual reawakening, bemused, head not present, an aching void in its place and sticky jelly clagged in your side hair. You gingerly get up, reclaim your shoes and teeth, and emerge into a pointless day. Nothing has *really* gone away - although it is at this point, and from now on, that your memory starts to be eroded, never fully to return.

The staff were all immensely kind. I joined occupational therapy and became adept at basket making ("*In front of two, behind one*" was the oft repeated cry!), washed the dishes, and whiled away the evening in the quiet room. Then welcome bed, sans teeth, sans mind, and with hope of oblivion. Of course, there were sleeping pills - Soneryl, Sonergan, Seconal, Amytal, Mogadon - all have gone down my throat. But they were never effective at the time when *I* wanted them to be. Three in the morning. Someone once said that 3 a.m. should never have been invented; how I and many others would fervently agree. Wide awake, and staring into the void of my mind - not a place for exploration - torch flash on face as the 'night watch' passes. Finally, and inevitably, get up for a pee (do all hospital ward toilets have such an unpleasant odour?). Lovely, kind Nancy, wife of Keith, a foreman at work, sitting in the night-station; brief chat; *Sorry, I can't give you another sleeping tablet; here, try a Paracetemol*; back to bed, maybe fitful sleep until the dreaded, but welcome day dawned again.

Roy Vincent

I do not want to remember too much detail of such a drab time in my life. Nor, I suppose, will you want to read about it - but you should, for I am sure that unless it is to visit a close relative, or as a patient, you won't enter a Psychiatric Ward. You won't see the uncontrolled misery and loneliness in faces; you won't see the eyes glazed with drugs or E.C.T; you won't see the hopelessness of a person cut off and isolated from a welter of problems that will still be there on discharge. But like you, no one will want to visit. People can't cope, don't know what to say (Except, perhaps, "It'll be all right if you pull yourself together - yes, that's it - pull yourself together"). Great original thought; how many times did I hear it being said - often by husbands to wives, or wives to husbands, themselves full of woe at the disaster that had befallen their lives and homes.

My own wife was magnificent. Never missed a visit; even later, when attending an evening class to prepare for employment should I become incapable of returning to work, she made sure that she came during the day. But she was the only one in a total of about twenty weeks in hospital. Nor were there visitors to the home when I was there and recuperating, apart, that is from a good friend and colleague from work and our Parish Priest. Not one.

When, later, I became involved in complementary cancer care, I heard the same story; very few people, even close relatives, will chat. Most go out of their way to avoid even

LISTENING TO THE SILENCES

simple contact, conversation. There seemed then - I'm not sure about now - to be a stigma attached to someone with mental health problems, and a reaction that almost seemed to say that it was the fault of the ill person. (Many times have I heard people say, and I have said it myself, "I wish I had a crutch or a leg in plaster so that folk can *see* that there *is* something the matter!").

But don't you think that you have a duty to learn more, to be compassionate, to understand, to be able to *talk* to people about their problems? For, after all, people are now being discharged to 'Care in the Community'. Well, for God's sake, you *are* the bloody community; they are there with you - in *your* care, not conveniently isolated, socially sanitised in some distant Victorian pile. The only time *you* want to know is when someone has an intractable 'personality problem' i.e. someone who might be a sexual deviant, a paedophile. Then, Geronimo!, get out the vigilantes; hound them out of the community; castrate the buggers; lock them away even though they haven't committed a crime. They used to *burn* witches and social undesirables, didn't they? Not much really changes; the hysteria is still there. It is *your duty* to 'get real', to understand fact and not mob panic. After all, not every schizophrenic is an axe-wielding maniac; most of them are very sensitive, isolated people. Statistically, *you* are just as likely as the next person to succumb to a nervous condition, a mental illness; if you learn more about it now perhaps it will never happen, you'll recognise the warning signs!

In writing this account, I have started what has become, for me, a very interesting process. I have, until now, only read my medical notes in a very tentative way, just enough, really, to be able to compile a coherent account for my lawsuit. What little I read disturbed me and brought back such painful memories, un-bottled such nasty genies, that I hastily put the stopper back in the bottle. But as I now have a worthwhile reason for analysing that past, I am delving further and further in as I search for actual dates, actual events, actual drugs and treatments, actual dosages. Memories of events, sequences, dates and people are emerging, but, apart from the recollection of some individuals who did their utmost for me, I am finding much to cause me serious disquiet, and some to make me so very angry - even after so much time has passed. So angry that I can't yet begin to write about it, but shall confront it later when I finally summarise.

In total I had ten E.C.T.s as an in-patient and, after the greater part of eight weeks in hospital, I was discharged home 'much better', <u>still</u> taking Librium and Seconal. I am not a pharmacologist, but I *can* read, also I have or have had a number of friends in medicine and some in psychiatry, so an appreciation of drugs and their effects, alone or in combination, is not beyond me. While I intend to summarise and comment upon my various 'therapies' during my conclusion, it is worth noting a few facts as I go along. Thus, Seconal is a barbiturate from which there can be severe withdrawal effects similar to those seen in alcohol abstinence. Librium, on the other hand, is a benzodiazepine, which *also* can cause dependence and withdrawal symptoms, and is prescribed for the *short term* (2 to 4 weeks only) relief of anxiety; its use should be reviewed regularly and should be discontinued as soon as possible - and other cautions and side effects too numerous to list here – except that benzodiazepines and barbiturates should not be taken simultaneously! At this point in my story, I had been taking Librium for *thirty months.*

For some reason the notes and correspondence in my file are a bit sketchy over this period, don't ask me why. What I next see recorded, is that I had thirteen E.C.Ts as an outpatient between 14th April and 24th May 1964. I look at the copy of the form that I signed indemnifying the hospital against any injury that I might suffer in treatment, and at the form listing each session - the voltages and duration etc. - and memories come back of the breakfast-less journey to the hospital, crammed in a Social Services car, and the return journey, zombified. And I weep inside now, as I must have done openly then.

Thus fortified, I finally got back to work. While I had been off there had been some logical organisational and staff structural changes. Calder Hall had become just another power station. The cutting edge of technology had transferred to the up-and-coming Advanced Gas Reactor, and staff of my grade were being dispersed, some to AGR and, in my case, to create a brand new department. Because of my innovative skills in the field of measurement that had come to the fore during the commissioning and experimental phases of the Calder reactors and plant, I was to be involved with experimental instrumentation.

        But where had I put my mind, my technical knowledge and expertise? Who were these people? I couldn't put names to faces or faces to names. I was isolated - physically in an office high in a new, tall building, and mentally because I had no base from which to think. At work I paced the office, bemused and feeling trapped. I couldn't express what I was feeling to anyone at work, for apart from the fact that you feel ashamed of your own lack of purpose, lack of achievement, people get embarrassed when you talk about personal, particularly nervous, suffering. (It was only later when I was competent again and people saw me working and coping with the aftermath of what I had been through, that their confidences came pouring out, because they knew that I had been 'somewhere' - somewhere akin to where they were in their heads and lives. Gradually, I began to learn that behind practically every second door in this peculiar artificial village in which we lived, there was a little hell, disguised from the world by the special face that was kept by the door and put on when going out).

LISTENING TO THE SILENCES

When your mind is empty, incapable of constructive thought, it is very wide open to all the anxieties, doubts, and uncertainties concerning your present and future. What future? You can't even face the present, this day. Night is awful. Whilst bed is so desirable, such a refuge, the effects of the sleeping pill soon wear off, and you lie there sweating, almost seeing the entire board of management in censorious array like vultures on the bed-end.

One reason why there was not a lot written and my notes are so sketchy at this time, is because I wasn't talking about what was actually *in* my mind, what I was planning to do. I was planning to take my own life. But I couldn't talk about it - it had to appear to be an accident, and if I showed premeditation, I thought, my insurance policies would not pay out; but I couldn't ask anyone if they *would* pay out because that might show premeditation and my insurance policies might not pay out. My planned method was electrocution, but that is difficult to stage in the home in such a way as to appear to be accidental, and my ingenious mind just was not functioning.

As I walked to the train each morning, I used to look at the wheels of the school buses and wonder if I could find the courage to stumble under one; or, on the platform, whether I could contrive a fall in front of the train as it came in. At night I used to wish fervently that I had been killed along with the thirty-five friends and shipmates who had been fragmented or incinerated within feet of me when the destroyer,

Roy Vincent

HMS *Saumarez,* in which we were serving, was mined. Obviously, I did not succeed or even attempt, (though it has only struck me as I write that in the Seconal at home I had the ideal 'remedy' - easy to overdose, but in my state of mind I couldn't even see *that* possibility). There is, however, something that I can tell you without fear of contradiction: there is no place on earth more lonely than the mind of someone who wants to die, to achieve *oblivion* (unless it be the mind of someone facing execution). The most isolated Siberian tundra or Gobi desert wastes would provide more solace than the domain of your mind.

Before I contrived my 'accident' or otherwise achieved my own destruction, I was saved by Pentathol. Have you lost the plot? Let's get up to date. We are now at the end of July 1964, and a new strategy was being proposed. I may not be giving them enough credit, but MC, GP2, and the medical staff at work were individually and collectively concerned about my state of mind and future, and discussing ways and means. The Pentathol strategy applied the relaxing anaesthetising properties of the drug to achieve within me total bodily relaxation, in the hope that my mind would respond as well. (In case you have forgotten, I still had no mind). So, three times a week I was driven to the hospital in a Works' car and had Pentathol dribbled into me as I slowly 'blissed out', as my Buddhist friends would say. There was one Indian registrar who could dribble it in *very* slowly and actually inject *two*

LISTENING TO THE SILENCES

syringe-fulls - oh! the ecstasy (and the agony - for nothing goes away, and the let-down on waking is so bleak).

But fear not, dear reader, (sound of bugle, yet far off) help is on the way. MC has been to a conference, and come back bursting with new ideas. For me there had been a paper in which excellent results had been achieved in some creatures - possibly wild dogs - in which large doses of Valium (or Librium, I am trying to recall a memory) had been used to good effect. Well done! You've caught up with the plot! *I* would have large doses of Librium (or Valium). There is nothing that I can find in the notes that relate to this particular trick, but like some other 'special' memories that have stayed with me, this one is particularly vivid, as is the memory of the reaction of GP2. He visited me at home almost every day, in my darkened room from which I wouldn't stir. After several days, he stared into my eyes, realised where I was (or wasn't) and said "You're drugged out of your mind!". Before you can say 'benzodiazepine', I was back in hospital.

All of my files, notes and correspondence were obtained by my Solicitors as we sought to make a case to sue the makers of these drugs, an abortive venture, as it turned out, so fickle is blindfold Justice. In making the case, I had a long session with a Consultant Psychiatrist who was retained by the various law firms. He started interviewing me in the usual manner, but as my story unfolded he just sat there, silent, a sad, sympathetic little smile on his face, his head sometimes shaking from side to side in sheer disbelief that so much could have been visited on one person.

But don't go away, psychiatry has so *much* to offer. The time has come to introduce you to yet another form of shock treatment - insulin shock treatment, or, as it now is, *modified* insulin treatment (it was modified so that there is now a smaller chance of killing you). This form of shock treatment relies on the injection of increasingly large doses of insulin with the object of reducing the blood sugar level and bringing on a coma. This is how the modified form works: you are woken at about 5 am and given an injection of insulin. You continue to lie in bed for a couple of hours and soon start to sweat and shake uncontrollably, then, while still in bed, you get placed in front of you a tray with a dish of corn flakes heaped, and I mean *heaped,* with glucose powder, and a full fried breakfast plus toast. No problem eating it, you are ravenous. A little while longer in bed then get up and have a shower (compulsory). I became so inert and depressed that I couldn't even bother to shower, sweaty and niffy though I was – sometimes I just used to shut myself in and pretend.

I had in all twenty-six such episodes that, at five a week, took me into the sixth week. How depressed I got, so very, very depressed. I used to pace the corridors feeling utterly lost, pointless and empty; sometimes I went into the next-door geriatric ward just to see people who had less mind than I had. I craved exercise, but when I asked if I could go to the older, former hospital not far away where I knew there was a rehab gym, I was fobbed off and got no help - "Just go for a walk". Where? In the wet, featureless lanes with their potholes and puddles, just behind the hospital, in the autumn? So drab, so weary, so empty - the name 'Sneckyeat Road' does as little for me now as it did then! One day, MC said to me "You were referred originally with an anxiety state, now you have a full blown clinical depression". Well, we were making progress, that's something.

When it looked as if I was in for a long haul, the occupational therapist suggested something that I had always wanted to do. Weaving. There was a table loom as yet untried. Great! I'd have a go. What to make? " Why not place mats?" said my wife who occasionally came in to OT. So off she went, and came back with some bright orangey Courtelle, and I started. Things that I had only read about before began to become realities - making the warp, the poree cross, and whatever the other one is called; heddles, shuttle, and beater all became realities. Then, entering the warp. That could have been difficult, but one of the nurses had worked at Coates' thread factory where she had been involved with just such a task in making up thread samples for display and advertising. So, with one at one end and the other at the other end of the loom we were soon 'entered' and I was away.

Roy Vincent

While my days weren't 'swifter than the weaver's shuttle', they nevertheless received a boost from this particular shuttle. I had to overcome some difficulties of technique, but eventually I created six place mats, a centrepiece and a tray cloth. I still have them, a little worse for wear.

One hears so much these days in our new 'consciousness', our new awareness, of 'body, mind and spirit' - the totality of being human. My body was still there, recoiling from the many attacks made upon it; my mind had a certain ephemeral quality, though, on reflection, it had the reaction of a lead balloon showing sudden half-hearted attempts to lift off. My spirit? Now there's a thought; if I ever had a spirit, where was it now?

Becoming a Catholic when I married I had become a very diligent follower of my new 'brand' of Christianity, but in my depressed state, where indeed *was* my spirit? Had I just been going through the motions? Had I ever had anything of the sort? Must find out. The church not far away was manned by Benedictine monks, and so, remembering one whose words one Sunday at Mass had impressed me, I rang. With not a moment's hesitation, he jumped on his Noddy bike and put-putted over to see me. I still have a little book which he gave me (Funny, his name was Father *Little;* the book - *They Speak by Silences* was a series of meditative thoughts by an anonymous monk of the silent Carthusian order and is one that I still, more than thirty-five years later, use for 'provocative' meditation) in the hope

LISTENING TO THE SILENCES

that I would find solace in its words, and to this day I am grateful for his earnest attention and compassion. But in spite of his help, what I now know as 'spirit' never materialised in me, and never did until I experienced the events that I write about elsewhere.

Here is a thought, though; if you want to know what it is like to be in deep depression (no, it is not just being 'fed up'!), read Psalm 88 - at least that is its number in the *Jerusalem Bible.* I'll quote briefly, but do read it all for you may get some insight. It is called 'Lament': as he cries out to his God...

...hear my cries for help;
for my soul is all troubled.
my life is on the brink of the Underworld;
I am numbered among those who go down to the Pit,
a man bereft of strength;
a man alone, down among the dead,
among the slaughtered in their graves,
among those you have forgotten....
...You have turned my friends and neighbours against me,
now my one companion is darkness.

But soft! What is happening? MC is beginning to have self-doubts. Would I like a second opinion? - He would. So 'twas arranged, and one November morning I was driven with others who had a variety of appointments, to the ultimate seat of learning; me to see a Big Wheel (BW), one who went on to become a Very Big Wheel, at the mention of whose name a young psychiatrist, to whom I quoted it many years later, visibly genuflected.

But no, such is the way that things work, protocol etc., I did not immediately see BW; instead, at first, I was taken to his Registrar or Little Wheel (LW). For about half an hour, possibly forty minutes, he interviewed me as if it was my very first encounter with a psychiatrist. Now, there is an unkind saying in education that "those who can, 'do'; those who can't 'do', teach; those who can't teach, teach others to teach; while those who can't teach others to teach become either education administrators or researchers". I feel that there must be an equivalent gradation in psychiatry. I don't know what had brought LW into the profession, and into research in particular, but it certainly wasn't his human interplay. He exhibited not one glimmer of concern or sympathy for my condition or experiences; he had about as much empathy towards me as a gardener has towards a green fly. He was hostile, sarcastic and belittling. Just one example will suffice: I tried to explain the depths of my desire to die, to commit suicide. Had I, as one does, gone to a high place to throw myself off? No? Well, I couldn't have been all that serious, could I? It may not sound a very great put-down, but in the context of the others, the sarcasms and negations of what I was telling him, it was.

LISTENING TO THE SILENCES

However, he had been well primed in his negativity. The letter from MC itself was so negative, but not only that, he seemed to go out of his *way* to be negative. Take, for instance, his comments about the state of our marriage: he records that both my wife and I said that we were happily married; however, *he* knew better, *he* had got a snippet (apparently from GP2) which cast doubt upon *our* understanding of the situation, doubts that he reinforced, but did not specify from a source that he didn't identify. One wonders *why* he had to put in yet another negative, unsubstantiated, keyhole-peering remark. *Why* did he not rely on what my wife and I said? After all, we were the main players. Throughout this period, she could not have been more devoted, more caring; 'TLC' might have been coined to describe her attitude.

In our wider life, and with our daughter, we were fortunate to have a family interest - almost obsession - in riding and horses. We rode whenever possible, had riding holidays, took a deep and intelligent interest in improving our riding skills, mixed with like-minded people and made many friends outside the works environment, outside the peculiar Seascale society. Many of these friends we still have. Yes, *we!* For although, as I shall describe, we ultimately parted and divorced, we have remained excellent friends, a friendship manifested in a variety of ways that are not here relevant.

Before my life was so bludgeoned, I frequently rode a particular horse that was being looked after by some friends. Smokey. Such an eager, willing horse; black; not very big; but he took me everywhere, from the miles of beach to the fell-tops, and along all the many bridle-paths with which this area is blessed. He was a boon companion and I can still recall his moving body under the saddle. When I was recuperating after the first spell in hospital, my wife told me what she had been keeping from me - Smokey was dead, killed by lightning in his field. She also told me that she had been saving up to buy him for me. *That* reflects the marriage that I knew at that time, not the almost evil representations or half-hints that the letter contains.

I have tried since, indeed, I am trying now, to deduce why things were being said about our marriage that at the time were patently untrue. Since we are in the domain of Sigmund Freud perhaps we can get a little Freudian. I have observed in many men, probably in myself also, the in-built, virtually unconscious belief held by each that he is the one who can take over this female's life, protect her, sort her problems, give her better sex than she is currently getting. To do which, as in nature, he has to expose the weaknesses, real or invented, in her current husband, partner, boyfriend; particularly if the latter is in any way vulnerable. I see a manifestation of this occurring among the fifteen or so rams that are sometimes held in my field in the autumn. If one has any defect, first one ram and then all the rest in turn or together, will butt

LISTENING TO THE SILENCES

and harry him persistently, all, no doubt, responding to the in-built behaviour of their evolution. We are the sum total of *our* evolution, nothing lost, nothing taken away, and we have it within ourselves to behave just like the rams.

I am not in the remotest way suggesting that anything improper was even *thought*, but my wife was a very attractive woman, not only in her looks, but also in her vivacity and openness of speech, and the marriages of GP2 and MC were under stress. Remarks made to me by GP2 during his consultations showed a certain disillusion, while MC in a short time parted from his wife and they ultimately divorced. In my analysis, I am suggesting their own personal situations were unconsciously being played out in mine, and in my 'vulnerable' state I was the ram being 'butted' - and once one starts everyone joins in. A bit convoluted, but *I* know what I mean.

You may think that I am being selective, or that I have an agenda of vindictiveness against the people whom I perceive as having perpetrated wrongs upon me in the past. I can tell you this; if anyone has proper credentials and a legitimate reason for wanting to see the letters and reports, they can come here and I will willingly show them and put them in context. What I find hard to reconcile are the two images that I now have of MC - the man who sat, as I shall describe, urbane and friendly, tying salmon flies in a little hand-held vice, while I had my fortnightly 'psychotherapy', and the man who wrote the letters and reports that contain *nothing* to indicate that I had any achievement or standing. In fact the reverse; his whole thrust seemed to say that I never had any potential and never would. I know that he had only seen me from the outset under the influence of Librium; I know that when first seen I had a label around my neck which said 'Anxiety State', but I would have thought that he would have had some discernment, and would have realised that I wouldn't have got where I had without talent. We were roughly of an age, and had reached about the same level, each in our own profession, and, indeed, I had reached at thirty-five a grade that many engineers in public service didn't reach in their whole careers. As I wrote earlier, I had represented the Company in France and Stockholm, and, big disappointment, I was told when I was making recovery that it had been intended that I should be seconded to Japan during the commissioning of some of the Japanese nuclear reactors, but that my illness had scotched the move. So perhaps you can understand my perturbation and inability to comprehend the behaviour of someone in whom I confided much and perceived as a friend and confidant. However, now I realise as I read deeper and deeper in my files that what I thought were personal confidences were, in fact, incorporated into the next progress report to my GP, and retained in my personal file where they remain yet, colouring the view of me of every subsequent GP who has read them.

LISTENING TO THE SILENCES

When LW had completed his interview, he went to see BW and was confined with him for about twenty minutes, after which I was invited in. Neither sat; I don't remember whether or not I did. I was not put at my ease, nor made to feel welcome - I felt I was an irrelevance. I still had my raincoat folded over my arm; such was the extent of the courtesy offered to me. I remained in the room for no more than ten minutes, and can only remember one question or remark. This was to be asked what my greatest concern was, to which I replied that my memory had been so affected that I feared it would not fully return. I was assured that it would - and that was that. Back to the hospital and await the verdict. When it came, I was told that Pertofran and Valium had been recommended, and that the recommendation would be accepted. So began the next phase of my drug regime. I was eventually to take Pertofran for ten years and Valium for twelve.

I don't know whether MC knew, or even guessed, that the letter that he received analysing my consultation had not been written by his Guru. I know now, having read it several times, that it may have been *signed* by BW but was definitely drafted entirely by LW. There is virtually every undermining remark, put-down or sarcasm that he had spoken to me appearing in black and white. This letter, too, has its niche in my surgery file. Therefore, MC was, in reality, relying upon the analysis and opinion of someone effectively of lower standing, and one presumes, less experience than himself.

      I recollect when, early in my career, I attended a junior management-training course. One of our group exercises was to conduct a court of enquiry into a site accident. We were given the 'official reports', witness statements and other corroborations that we studied, and then we called and interviewed every one of the parties, admirably role-played by staff of the Training Department. We questioned and re-questioned and then we deliberated and finally reached our conclusion. But where had we gone wrong? What had we missed? Well, I'll tell you. The accident had happened on a day late in November, at 4 pm. It had been *dark*! So obvious when you see it, but it had eluded some eight or so budding young managers. So what relevance does this bit of philosophy have here? Well it concerns the analysis essentially by all three, BW, LW and MC, of the reasons for my loss of memory and my great concern about it. I won't rehearse the reasons given other than to say that the word 'hysterical' appears. Now, can you recollect that earlier, after the description of E.C.T and the definition quoted from my reference book, I asked you to note a particular sentence? Hands up who can remember. Read: learn: memorise:- *There is considerable criticism of E.C.T because it may produce permanent brain damage, especially losses of memory and intelligence.* How many

LISTENING TO THE SILENCES

E.C.Ts had I had? Well done, that's it:- *twenty-three.* I rest my case.

No, I *do not* rest my case. Just where had they come from, these three 'soothsayers' who, each like an ancient Etruscan haruspex, were picking over the entrails of my life and mind? I have related how it came to pass that *I* was suffering this 'disembowelling' process, but how was it that *they* came to have such jurisdiction over my mind, my precious mind? Were they part of a self-selecting, self-perpetuating 'priesthood'?

The next time that Stephen Hawking appears on your television screen, pause a while and reflect upon that contorted body, the twisted face and head; read some of what he has written, and reflect further that this is one of the most brilliant minds of our time contained there in that pathetic shell. When you have done that, see whether you can disagree that one's mind is the most precious of one's possessions. I was in grave danger of losing mine, of having it destroyed; I *know* how precious it is and I defy you to disagree!

Some years after the time of which I am writing and, as I shall relate, I made my way back up the recovery ladder, I was, for a time, in charge of training for the whole of the Sellafield complex. As part of my self-education in this post, I took myself off to a conference at Cambridge organised by a research team who looked at aspects of industrial training. One of the discourses involved someone from the Bristol University Dental School. The school had a problem. Aspiring dentists proceeded into their training for several years before they actually came to grips with a tooth in a mouth. At this stage, it was found that some were so lacking in manual dexterity that they were forced to abandon dentistry and transfer to normal medicine on a parallel course. To minimise the waste involved in this abortive training, the Dental School were working with the researchers to try to devise a simple test of manual competence that could be used to assess aspirants *before* they embarked upon a course for which they were obviously not suited.

Is there, one wonders, an assessment process for aspiring psychiatrists, one that seeks to determine whether *they* have the necessary skills and talents to be allowed access to the most precious possession that anyone can have? Do not treat this as an irrelevance, a hypothetical question, for statistically you are as likely as the next person to have the 'entrails' of *your* mind picked over, to have *your* brain corrupted by some mind-altering drug, potentially with side-effects far worse than many 'conventional' illnesses. I have only, within the last few days, noticed a small letter 'hiding' in one of the files of my records. It is the letter written by MC to BW following receipt of his advice with respect to my further treatment. He thanks BW for his advice and taking the trouble, then goes on:

LISTENING TO THE SILENCES

'I must both thank you and apologise to you for the trouble you have gone to with the cases I have referred to you during the year I have been over here. They have, I am afraid, run to this sort of pattern and you will appreciate that this is the result both of the difficulties that they present and, I fear, lacunae in my own training.'

Yes, I have looked it up, just to confirm what I believed the definition to be: a *lacuna* is a gap, omission, hiatus; *lacunae* obviously are these in plural. Imagine what would have been my thoughts had I been aware at the time. I had been a patient for just one year and was, therefore, one of the first patients of the consultancy; there had been other second opinions; had we, by any chance, each fallen through a lacuna?

Let me recap at the end of this 'formative' year in my life. When it began, I had already been taking Librium for two years; I continued for virtually the whole of the year, with a mid-point interval at a double dose rate, before changing to Valium. There had been brief interludes with Tryptizol, Melleril, Nardil and Stelazine; there had been Soneryl, Sonergan, Seconal, Amytal and lastly Mogadon to pacify my nights. I had suffered twenty-three sessions of E.C.T and twenty-six episodes of modified insulin shock treatment. In total, I had received forty-three injections of Pentathol, plus twenty-three each of belladonna and curare derivatives, and now I was going to start on a regimen of Pertofran,

Roy Vincent

Valium and Mogadon. (Dare I ask you to remember that at the very outset, I had no episode or history of nervous or psychiatric ailments - I had uncontrollable diarrhoea, nothing else?).

In time, all good things come to an end and I left hospital and recuperation, and started back at work. My employers were very supportive, and placed me with congenial people in work that was quite undemanding. So slowly I settled. The gradual restructuring of my life began and the building of confidence was real. After a time I was asked to take over Engineering Training and, eventually, the Training Department covering the whole of the establishment. At one time, had I been taken to a high place and, with all of the possible jobs in the Works laid out before me, asked to pick one, the last, the very last choice would have been Training! However, I was more grateful than I could say to the Works' management for the way in which I had been reintegrated into work, and, anyway, it is said that in every Welshman there is a latent preacher or teacher, so maybe I had met my destiny. Many interesting developments were taking place in the world of industrial training and I was soon absorbed.

At home, I found in time that my wife had carried the burden of my condition for too long, and she herself became ill. There came a time when it felt as if we were two drowning people clutching at the same straw. MC, who was aware of what was developing, urged me most

LISTENING TO THE SILENCES

strongly one day - "For God's sake, get out - go and camp somewhere, but get out". And so I did. I took a flat in a converted farmhouse - and by one of those quirks for which fate is so famous, the flat below me was taken simultaneously by the Clinical Psychologist from MC's department.

Once one has separated, it seems to be virtually impossible to reunite and rebuild what had been before, and so, inevitably, my wife and I divorced. In time, I was lucky in finding this house with its land suitable for horses, moved here in 1971 and have lived here ever since. Again, giving the lie to what MC had said about our marriage, it was my former wife who actually was instrumental in my finding it in the first place.

Almost without a break until about 1970 I continued with psychotherapy, although, at the time I wasn't aware that that is what it was, so little did the 'medicine of the mind' figure in one's everyday considerations; all I knew was that it was 'good to talk'. However, coping with a solitary life and the increasing demands of work (ironically, because I became enthusiastic and could see the potential of the new moves in industrial training *I was placing the demands on myself*), because of these factors I found myself 'going backwards' at work. Whereas I had had much support following my initial return to work, and when I took up my role as Training Manager, now I found that patience seemed to have run out, and my absences were seen in a different light. It was not realised, probably wasn't even addressed, that the continuous drug regime was taking a devastating toll of my faculties. I was even now taking Pertofran and Valium, and had recourse to Mogadon at night, so you may perhaps judge that the start of each day was a little uncertain. I had a most marvellous Girl Friday at work, Val, who could look at my eyes first-thing and then decide if she should stall callers until after 10 am. In time, the constant struggle became unbearable, and one day, in late summer 1976, I set out for work and didn't arrive. Instead, I turned off my normal route and took refuge with a friend with whom I holed-up for two days. That, essentially, was the end of my working career. In time I was pensioned off at fifty-two and then a new phase in my life - indeed, a new *life* - began.

But what sort of new life? The very state of not going to work was in itself a new life, and I knew within myself that I had had enough; nothing was worth the growing loss of ability and status, and the struggle to do well things that previously I could have done in my sleep. If I had known how this new life was going to unfold, what would I have thought, what would I have done? But I wasn't yet in the state of mind to ask myself "What am I going to do with this freedom now that I have made my escape?". I was rather more like the survivor of a shipwreck who has only just made it to a shore - he didn't *care* what shore - all he knew was that he wasn't fighting something alien anymore. When I look back at that time, it is quite startling to recall how a new life developed almost by spontaneous combustion. I marvel at the expansion - expansion of my circle of friends, expansion in the range of my activities; activities and contacts that opened up an entirely new world - a world that I hadn't previously explored or even thought much about.

And my spirit? I had never, not since I posed the question in hospital twelve or so years previously, found an answer - never really given it much further thought. Just five more years down the line and I was to have some enlightenment. It was as if in me there was taking place the metamorphosis of a former caterpillar, now in its cocoon, waiting to emerge to make its destined flight. But I knew as little of what was involved in flying as did the caterpillar when it started to spin the silk of its cocoon. All of this lay ahead. I still don't know whether I would have taken a different path - too often in life we never have the option to choose, or never realise that there *is* a choice, until we have committed ourselves. As you read further, perhaps you will have an opinion; for myself, I shall leave the analysis until I reach it in the logic of the narrative. At this moment, I have just been cast up on the shore and I am so grateful that I have survived.

Roy Vincent

CHAPTER 2

Keep right on

to the end

of

the road,,,

Roy Vincent

LISTENING TO THE SILENCES

,,,keep right on round the bend.

Sir Harry Lauder was one of my mother's favourite performers and we had most of his records at home, although, when he sang about 'keeping on round the bend', we didn't then see a potential meaning that now is so obvious. The thrust of the words of the song, the going forward in spite of everything, the taking charge of your life in spite of everything, were an instinctive part of the philosophy of the home. Our parents, my brother and I agree, could not, with the resources at their disposal, have done more for us as children. When we hear or read of the awful things that can happen to kids, even in their own homes, by members of their own families, we look back with gratitude at a childhood where everything was positive, free from abuse (apart, that is, from having a piece of soap pushed up your bum if you were seriously constipated - whatever would Mr. Jung have made of that?)

We were encouraged to achieve our best in everything we did - "Hitch your wagon to a star my son" would say our father. On the wall, hanging below the clock, was a pokerwork motto:

Life's battles don't always go
To the strongest or fastest man,
But soon or late the man who wins
Is the man who thinks he can.

While on another wall the 'Maxims of the late King George V' daily exhorted us to a life of high standards and caring for others; sentiments reinforced by regular attendance at Sunday School. And thus, by encouragement, example and osmosis, we adopted our parents' standards. So there was no question but that, by whatever means I had, I would go forward. 'Excelsior' my father had sung - the moving tale of the young alpine traveller - onward and upward! Although I must admit that I wasn't consciously thinking along these lines; my main need at that time, an unexpressed need, for I was living alone, was to have my 'wounds' bound up after treatment with a soothing salve, and compassion and understanding - yes, those especially.

How many Western movies have you seen where the hero finds himself well and truly put through the mincer? He gets pistol-whipped from behind; he has someone's fist elbow deep in his middle; several boots are planted in his anatomy; he is dragged by a rope through rocks and cactus and has umpteen bar-room chairs disintegrated over his head; he finally ends up abandoned in a corner, a dribble of blood at the corner of his mouth. But it's only halfway through the film - surely? Of course, the lovely heroine is suddenly there, or the bar-room girl with a heart of gold, full of compassion, who turning modestly away, lifts a skirt and tears strips from a snowy-white underskirt, and with great tenderness cleans and binds up his wounds. Then before you can

LISTENING TO THE SILENCES

say, "Swear in a posse", he's on his feet and buckling up his gun belt; the rest you know. Mind you, he never marries the bar-room girl - and the men in black hats always get their come-uppance! But there's always that moment of tenderness, compassion, which softens the plot and tugs at the heartstrings.

Off the silver screen the damage and the hurt are real and intense - yes, I've actually done the one where you are unconscious, trapped by flames in a small cabin in the interior of a blazing ship that is in some danger of sinking or drifting onto a hostile shore. I have no idea what brought me round, but consciousness presented its own problems. Whereas, I recollected, there had been *four* of us in that cabin, now I was alone, and, strange, the door was a mass of flames lighting up the eerie orange brown smoke which comes from exploding cordite. But this wasn't part of the plot; what had happened to 'before'? *Before*, we four had been at our Action Stations in the radar cabin; three to operate the radar and me to repair anything which became faulty. *We*, i.e. the British Navy, had been about to exert the right of free passage through an international channel - the Corfu Channel - that was being threatened by the Albanians. The *who*? Earlier in the summer, they had had the temerity to open fire with light weapons on a British cruiser as it passed along this Channel, and such things definitely do *not* go down well in Whitehall.

But this was 1946 - *peacetime* for God's sake! Ah, but the Cold War had begun and the Albanians were working off a different script. *They* said that the ships sailed too close to their territory. But Whitehall doesn't negotiate with a barefoot republic, a bunch of Commies. No: if the buggers dared to open fire - well, we were at Action Stations! 'Nuff said. But the politicians had underestimated the cunning of these Balkan peasants. With the aid of their neighbours, the Yugoslavs, they had laid some mines in a channel that our minesweepers had not long before cleared of wartime mines, and they had got us! One of the magazines and one of the boilers exploded, and many were killed, while many others were burned or scalded.

      I must have been made unconscious by the initial explosion that had been just beneath the radar cabin, but on coming round, I was in no state even to guess what had happened. When later I was able to talk to my colleagues, I found that, being nearer the open cabin door, they had caught the power of the successive explosions and been burned and scalded and concussed. In their confused state, they had thought that I was following. All of which was purely academic as I rapidly came to understand my predicament. You don't think, you just *go*. While visual scenes are flash-bulbed on my memory, the physical getting out is/was a blur. I was out on deck, but there was yet another fire blocking the way. The *sea* was on fire as well. I thought I was totally alone, until I looked up and saw the Jimmy and the Bo'sun on an upper walkway - a sight that brought me to my senses. And so I painfully skirted the fire, and

LISTENING TO THE SILENCES

made my way aft towards the Sick Bay, not realising how many had been hurt - many much worse than me - and how many had been killed.

More vivid in my memory now than much of what went before, is the recollection of other people's acts of sympathy, of immediate care, which came in spite of the main concern of putting out the fires and stopping the ship from drifting ashore or sinking. The socks that were found and eased over my flayed hands and forearms; the immediate brandy, and later, rum; the hug of a young matelot when the pain was unbearable. Finally the morphine, and a space on the deck, head cushioned on a dead Maltese steward. Then it started to rain.

Evening brought transfer in ships' boats (*please* mind my hands!) to an aircraft carrier in which a friend, David, was serving. More compassion and practical care from him - better attempt at dressings, attention to my face and a bucket held to receive the rum and brandy on their return. Then, next day, taken on board a hospital ship, saying goodbye to my friend whom I didn't meet again for another thirty-seven years, and then in the oddest circumstances.

The hospital ship provides many, many memories. One, thankfully now just a rueful recollection, is of the three-hourly penicillin injections - for two hours you were getting over the discomfort of the last one, then there was an hour to anticipate the *next* - for all of six days (and at night, when you were wakened, desperately trying to remember which cheek of your bum had received the previous one)! The most potent and recalled memory is of the temporary dressings being removed and new ones applied. Sedated I lay, arms immersed in warm saline solution, while the old dressings were being gently teased away. What fills the picture are the faces of the surgeon and nursing sister, one on each side, bright in their working lights, faces that radiated concern, gentleness, tenderness and a *humour* which bound them all together - a total compassion so real that I could have reached out and touched it. Even now, more than fifty years on, if I am feeling bruised by life I can recall their faces and delicate touch, and derive comfort from the memory.

But, in the sequence of my narrative, I have reached 1976, thirty years on almost to the day from when the ship was mined. My life and work have been 'wrecked', devastated, albeit in different ways from when I was at sea, but nevertheless, there is equally the crying need for help and compassion and the gentle touch. Looking back at that time from the vantage point of today, I can see how my need was met; not dramatically, immediately as in the Navy, but imperceptibly like a reservoir being refilled after a drought. The people who met my need were many and varied, and I doubt whether at the time they knew what they were accomplishing - it might even come as a complete surprise to them if ever they should chance to read this. Most helped me by simply being themselves, absorbing me into parts of their lives - or continuing to share what it

LISTENING TO THE SILENCES

was that they had that was special, for some had been friends for many years.

Probably the most obvious and direct help came from my then G.P. - if we are still numbering and counting he was about six or seven. I came into his patch when I moved this house, and, as happens in our slower moving rural lives, friendship developed. Sandy had a more open approach to medicine than many, and we explored widely the possible causes and factors contributing to a depression, and mine in particular, for that is what we still believed ailed me. The first achievement was getting rid of Valium, which we managed surprisingly smoothly, particularly so when one considers the length of time for which I had been taking it. Slowly, almost by stealth, we arrived at a day when I could truly say that I was a drug free zone! Had I known then what I know now, namely that, totally and completely, prescribed drugs and other clinical interventions had been the cause of my trauma and personal tragedy, I would have decked the house with flags and called for a national holiday to celebrate a famous victory. But we took it in our stride, and continued working at the strategy that previously we had only discussed in theory.

We had both come under the influence of Dr. Richard Mackarness and his book *Not All In The Mind*. Mackarness, a psychiatrist, had achieved quite dramatic and well-documented cures in patients with seemingly intractable conditions, and had done so entirely through diet. Specifically, he had identified foods or food additives which, when removed from the diet, had resulted in the immediate improvement and ultimate cure of the individual. (I have deliberately avoided use of *allergy* because I believe that it has developed a blanket and unspecific meaning). Mackarness required a five-day spring water fast. I didn't do this, but adopted a very limited diet of foods which consensus said were those least likely to have any adverse effects. It is my belief that the eliminating and cleansing effect of the limited diet, together with my own natural water supply, and the support of Sandy himself, were the prime reasons why coming off the drugs was so comparatively painless.

Apart from a very short period when events were occurring that I shall relate in sequence, and during a very brief emotional crisis, I have never again taken any drug of any sort.

As is the case with most people, I had grown up eating what was the normal, conventional, accepted diet of our time and situation. It was more a matter of eating what one enjoyed, rather than eating with an analytical mind that sought to ensure that all the natural substances that were needed by the body and brain, were ingested in the quantities and proportions which evolution said were necessary. The germ of thought implanted by Dr. Mackarness' book, and the realisation that diet could so affect behaviour and mood, have both influenced my thinking and dietary practice ever since. I have, or have had, several GPs as friends, and have discussed diet and its influences with them on numerous occasions; they have all agreed that far too little time in their training was allocated to the subject - sixteen hours in a five year course, said one. It was as if diet and nutrition were hived off into someone else's speciality, and that was that. The myth of the 'Balanced British Diet' and its ability to provide all necessary nutrients in correct proportions seems to have held sway. Unfortunately, and for example, the level of vitamin C expected from the BBD was just that which would prevent scurvy; levels far too low, as many authorities now agree. While the intake recommended by Linus Pauling would overwhelm many people, my own inclination has been to aim more for *his* levels rather than those derived from the mythical BBD. However, I must move on, though I am sure that diet and its influence will appear again.

Sandy and I also conversed widely on topics such as organic gardening and alternative energy sources, and we each in our own way was heading along the path of healthy unadulterated living. Part of my future eating was in one of my fields in the shape of my beef-on-the-bone bullock, Bert - or Berk, as young Toby would have it. Now Toby would gladden anybody's heart. He and Ben were sons of Carole and Des, who had entered my life in my response to an advert for a piano (somehow I seemed to have a surplus). Before I knew it, I was fully absorbed into the family - and, totally unplanned or by conscious intent, received more of the balm that I so desperately needed. But, in that curious way which life has, we became mutually supportive, for my new friends were experiencing a personal disaster following a vicious redundancy.

A wooden pole, by itself, has limited strength and usefulness; however, take *three* poles and make them into a tripod or sheer-legs and you have a combined strength and potential use *greater* than that of the three as individuals. And so it was, as is testified by the inscription on the flyleaf of a bird recognition book that I possess - 'To one prop from two props, with love'.

Two others who were always 'there for me' were Tricci and Peter. Farmers, I had originally met them through my riding activities. To extol them in the manner that they deserve would, I am sure, embarrass them, so what can I say? Two more naturally caring and generous people would be difficult to find, and their home has been a haven on so many occasions. Tricci's profession of physiotherapist in a way completes a circle, for almost daily she gave postural drainage to another of my 'carers'. Val, also my Girl Friday at work, was herself a victim of unjust life. Pneumonia in childhood had left her with one (incomplete) lung and she needed help with its clearance, but yet, with her limited capacity, or *in spite of* her limited capacity, she put more into, and got more out of life then most people with all of their physical resources. Hers was yet another home where, with her parents, I was always trebly welcome. How tragic was her early death.

Take any road from beside my house and in a very short distance, you go down a

LISTENING TO THE SILENCES

hill. At the bottom of the hill to the north, the road brings you to the home and workshop of Klaus and Brenda. Klaus is an 'émigré' from the Black Forest area of Germany, and is a wizard with metal - whatever you want he will make it. Brenda comes from a village very near by here and derives great satisfaction from their smallholding, and her Jersey cows, fowls and garden. They both come into their own later as I shall relate, but also at this time there was always a gentle welcome and wide ranging discussion. And then there was Number-One Son, Patrick, who came one Saturday to 'Bob-a-Job'. He worked with such gusto that would put many adults to shame, that immediately I asked his parents if he could become a regular. And so began an enduring friendship, based initially on our intention to garden, but often devolving into peripatetic philosophy of which Aristotle would have been proud. Patrick normally works all hours now, but when he can spare the time and call, the resulting breadth of discourse is to be marvelled at, and mulled over for several days.

Go down the hill to the west, and you arrive at the cottage where lived someone who gave me so much in unassuming friendship. Bob had, with his smile, given me the freedom of the Parish when I first arrived. A complete book would not do justice to his life, and one of my great regrets is that I never recorded him talking, telling the most wonderful anecdotes of life in this parish where he had always lived. Another home into which I was always welcome and where the 'crack' was always good and fascinating, and where Maggie his wife was always glad to be part of it, in spite of her speech limitations following a stroke (even if she *did* think that I talked posh! - what me, with a Welsh accent?). Bob was probably one of the best friends I have ever had, and from him, by 'infusion', I achieved so much in confidence as to be able to set to work on my house and make it the place that I desired it to be. I had little or no DIY skills, but simply by seeing him at work, and realising that he, in turn, had learned by 'doing', was largely self taught, made me realise that, within reason, I was capable of doing, achieving anything that I chose. From the window beside me, I can see the churchyard where Bob and Maggie lie, though 'Rest in Peace' would be totally inappropriate for Bob, for he just could not stand being idle - knowing him, he has probably re-roofed Heaven and fettled all the down-spouts since he arrived. And wouldn't it be wonderful to think of long-suffering Maggie, released from the crippling effects of her stroke and wandering freely, picking her favourite snowdrops that are so prolific at this moment?

Having said all this, it is quite probable that not much of what was happening inside me was visible to the outside observer, and, from what my friends have implied since, some were beginning to despair a little of my ever regaining full control. Next time you see a chrysalis, why don't you spend a little longer in looking at it, and try to imagine what is happening inside? I doubt whether anyone, not even myself,

LISTENING TO THE SILENCES

was aware of my restructuring, and what was about to burst forth. All will be revealed if you are patient, but first please bear with me as I explore some concepts that the process of telling my tale has forced me to consider.

Roy Vincent

CHAPTER 3

"When *I* use a word", said Humpty Dumpty, "it means just what I choose it to mean,,, neither more nor less."

Roy Vincent

"The question is," said Alice, "whether you can make words mean different things."

In my narrative I have already taken you back to 1946. In the interest of exploring some further ideas I am sure you won't mind going the extra mile to arrive at 1939, and the beginning of World War 2. When the utter seriousness of the situation became so starkly visible, the great majority of people of all ages were determined 'to do their bit'. For teenagers like me, there was salvage collection 'for the war effort', fire watching, and in my case, at weekends and in the holidays, farm work and a forestry camp; then, later on, joining one of the cadet forces. My father was too old to take up again his rifle and bayonet put down at the end of WW1, so he became a Special Constable.

      The combination of wartime diet and many miles of beat pounding produced a leaner, fitter Dad than we had seen for a number of years, while 'The Law' took on a different image when its face was that of your own father. Of the few accoutrements that he brought home, one was his police whistle, surreptitiously tried out, and another was his police manual or handbook, which defined just about everything. It provided fascinating reading to a fourteen-year-old, particularly the descriptions or definitions of deviant or sexual crimes. One phrase that stood out was 'unlawful carnal knowledge'. *Any* sort of carnal knowledge was eagerly sought, but the *unlawful* sort was wide-eyed imagination stuff.

Quite recently, a friend has suggested that when someone was arrested 'for unlawful carnal knowledge' the initial letters became the standard abbreviation in police notes, and, in turn, became the word which many people still abhor and never ever use - in spite of being told by 'alternative' comedians and TV programme makers that it is an adult world. Humpty Dumpty would have a field day with modern TV 'thinkspeak'.

It was an even more reprehensible word in 1939; and so, picture the dilemma of many of the young men joining the forces from then on, and finding themselves in a totally alien culture and vocabulary. I served on the lower-deck of the Navy and encountered such a variety of words - genital, copulatory and excretory words - used alone or in such 'poetic' combinations - largely to try to give some colour and emphasis to an otherwise very limited vocabulary. The dilemma that presented itself was, essentially, how to appear manly, one of the lads, without resorting to the all-pervading obscenities. Some found the answer in back-slang - i.e. the reversal of the offending word. Thus "Chuff it!" - "Oh dear, I have

LISTENING TO THE SILENCES

hit my finger"; "Chuff off!" - "Please go away"; "Chuff me!" or "Well, I'm chuffed!" - "Gosh, how surprised I am!".

The euphemisms and service slang returned to Civvy Street as we all became ex-servicemen - though we continued to hear them in context in 'The Navy Lark' and 'Much Binding in the Marsh' et al. But gradually Kilroy wasn't everywhere and Chad no longer demanded "Wot no....?" - totally meaningless concepts to most readers I am sure. Individuals continued to use their service slang, however, and gradually origins were lost and meanings changed as they were taken up by wives, girlfriends, work mates. And so it was that 'chuffed' was demobbed and achieved a different connotation - one of approbation. Thus, to be "Dead chuffed" is to be highly pleased - although I still get an odd reaction when an attractive young woman tells me that she had been "very chuffed"!

How many times and in how many ways do words and ideas undergo such metamorphosis without any serious help from Humpty Dumpty? Words that have a legitimate and specific meaning in their original creation and context are taken up and fed into the common vocabulary because they may 'sound right' or appear to give verve to an unimaginative vocabulary. Take a simple sounding expression such as 'negative feedback' - as originally coined in the terminology of electronic and control theory there was a specific meaning, namely that of taking a small part of the output from an electronic circuit or a control system, reversing it and feeding it back to the input end of the circuit or system and as a result, producing stability. Because it sounded meaningful in the instant-speak of the media or the City, the expression was taken up, lost its original meaning, and became yet another easy-come-easy-go bit of jargon. Just as 'black box' emerged also from the world of electronics design, where it is applied almost without exception to any innovative electronic device. Thus, when aircraft flight recorders were first used in planes, the boffins, when talking to the media, inevitably used the jargon and referred to the recorders as 'black boxes'. Not knowing any better, the media people assumed that the device was indeed a Black Box, and some even to this day refer to it as such - even Black Box Flight Recorder - which is rather like continuing to say "Gee-gee horse" when you've actually grown up. Someone even purported to have located the Professor Black who had invented the Black Box!

       How often has history been re-written or myth created because someone who wasn't even there, who only knows half the story, or wants to impress with his instant 'knowledge', or, having good access to the media of the day, wants to 'say his piece'? Constantly, for example, so-called 'documentaries' are shown on television where someone is putting an entirely new slant on the last war - rubbishing the accepted version of events, denigrating the leaders or Service heads of the time, calling into question decisions, plans.

LISTENING TO THE SILENCES

Obviously much information was kept back or propaganda disseminated, either to fool the enemy or to encourage domestic morale. But how can someone today, reading from the records, possibly think that they can construct the actual situation as it then was? I can say, without fear of contradiction, that they can never recapture the ethos of the time, a feeling or mood or determination that has to be experienced to be understood. When you look at newsreel of London on VE night, how can anyone who wasn't there, capture the thrill and the joy and the exuberance of that day and night? And yet, I can look at the scenes in front of Buckingham Palace or in Whitehall as Winston Churchill addressed the crowds, and still recall with a shiver, and know that I was somewhere in those seething rejoicing masses. But how could I convey to anyone that thrilling mood, the laughter, singing and dancing? Impossible! How can any history be truly written to represent the totality of an event, occasion? Having lived through some events and seen how they are now, even less than sixty years after their happening, depicted and analysed, I despair at finding *any* history of *any* time or event with much more than an outline or sketch of the actuality or truth. Everything is subjective in the eyes of the participants, and even more so in those of the subsequent analysts. When, as often happens, a history is deliberately rewritten or misrepresented, where is truth?

Take one Naval event that has gone down into popular perception - part myth, part history - the Mutiny on the Bounty. Unless you have been living with the pygmies in the deepest Amazon forest, you cannot fail to have seen on television at least one of the many re-runs of the film featuring Charles Laughton and Clark Gable. I saw it in 1938, the year of its first release, and like everyone else, I have lived with the belief, yes, *belief,* that Cap'n Bligh was a vile, cruel tyrannical man who drove his crew to mutiny by ceaseless flogging, keel-hauling and other nastiness. *Mea culpa!* How wrong I had been. Total character assassination in the interest of popular writing and cinema box-office. The film was based upon a book by Nordhoff and Hall, who seized, like many authors, upon the unhealthy and prurient fascinations that physical and capital punishment have for many people. Thus, what an opportunity to dwell at great length on the detail of flogging, the making of the cat o' nine tails, the way the man was triced up, flogging round the fleet, keel-hauling and the rest, not to mention the Press Gang! And what good cinema it made - the repulsive Laughton as the vile Bligh, and the handsome, plausible Gable as *Mister Christian!*

Sorry to disappoint you. There was no Press Gang, no flogging round the Fleet, no keelhauling. In the whole of the twenty-seven thousand miles of the voyage to Tahiti, there had been, and reputable historians accept this, just *two* floggings, the normal punishment at that time for the offences committed. HMS Bounty was not a man o' war, she was an armed transport, purchased for the express purpose of taking

LISTENING TO THE SILENCES

breadfruit plants from Tahiti to the West Indies. Lieutenant William Bligh had sailed twice before to the South Seas as Sailing Master under Captain James Cook. His character would have been totally known, and he was recommended by Joseph Banks the botanist and explorer who had voyaged with Cook. Thus, unlike Cook who carried a party of marines on board for protection, Bligh had none, for no trouble was anticipated. Following a practice introduced by Cook and learned from him, Bligh, in fact, took considerable care over the health and well being of his crew. Amongst the enlightened practices were the feeding of the men with anti-scorbutic foods such as sauerkraut and a type of marmalade; below decks, he introduced a form of fumigation and 'sweetening' by burning charcoal in iron pots. His big mistake was to allow the men total laxity in Tahiti, many of them taking native 'wives', and it was the enforced leaving of these and the idyllic island life that were the chief causes of the mutiny.

Bligh had been chosen to command the voyage because of his exceptional reputation as a navigator, surveyor, cartographer and naturalist, and his skills as a navigator were tested to extremes when he was cast adrift with eighteen others in an open boat just twenty-three feet long. (The very same size as the boat in which I, myself, learned to sail). Sailing principally from memory, with no friendly land near, he successfully navigated a mainly unexplored ocean, covering over 3,600 miles - much further than Southampton to New York - and reaching Timor in forty-seven days, without the loss of a man, placing it high in the list of epic small boat voyages - and *mapped and surveyed as he went.* I do not class him as a personal hero, but I admire his courage and skill, and was glad to read his own account in a re-issue of his log and narrative to mark the bi-centenary of the voyage.

This is just one, and probably a minor one, of the many instances of truth being stood on its head and history being re-written, for financial gain, personal power, national pride - it is happening all the time. As communication is so rapid and wide-ranging nowadays, the fabrication is often seen and exposed in a very short time, but it does not *undo* the harm already done, and people are very slow to eliminate the misunderstanding, the misconception, the *lie* from their minds. (I'll bet that you will have the greatest difficulty in accepting that Bligh was not tyrannical and cruel; Hardy, Nelson's Captain at Trafalgar is recorded as inflicting far more severe and frequent punishments than Bligh ever did). If you use or are in touch with scientific literature and other people's research, you must be aware of many cases where results have been 'massaged' or even falsified to achieve the outcome that the researcher wanted in order to promote an idea or enhance a personal reputation. The problem can be that, even when the falsification is exposed, there will still be people who will have taken on board and continue to accept as true, the originally published conclusions - as in the case of cot deaths. There are still some who accept that a

LISTENING TO THE SILENCES

proportion of deaths are due to 'breathing apnoea', in spite of the fact that it is now known that the five siblings upon whom the research conclusions were based, had all been murdered by their mother. Not, however, deliberately falsified results, but incredible naïveté on the part of the researcher, and only brought to light 25 years later by a very perceptive District Attorney, the mother then confessing.

Unless a whole concept is indelibly carved in stone, or defined with a nicety that defies alteration, you can bet your last penny that *some* wiseacre, know all, will come along with "what it *really* means is...". Even when a definition *has* been given, that does not stop an idea being hi-jacked and a concept being totally altered from that intended by its progenitor. Take a simple notion such as 'Ley Lines'. Simple? Not any more. Someone who comes to the concept now will find a mishmash of conflicting ideas ranging from sacred ways linking mysterious sites of ancient significance to lines of earthly power and energy, and *black* ley-lines and *white* ley-lines, ideas that are guaranteed to produce apoplexy in most archaeologists today. If these same archaeologists were to use the 'ley-line' concept of Alfred Watkins properly, they would find in their hands a tool with which they could open up much relating to human activity stretching back three or four thousand years. "Who on earth," do you ask "is Alfred Watkins, and what did he do?" Well, he is only the bloke who *coined* the term 'ley-lines', and, if you are interested, you will find all about it in his book *The Old straight Track*. I shall give details in an addendum. Watkins' ley-lines are a fact, a reality, and I get immense pleasure as, with map and compass, I identify and follow them over the never-ploughed, never-developed terrain with which this area abounds. There are wonderful moments of serendipity as I come across a totally isolated and abandoned little bridge or stepping stones, or see the shadow of a long abandoned track when the sun slants across a slope, or a light fall of snow reveals it. Likewise, the 'earth currents' are a reality, as anyone who wants to read can find out (Encyclopaedia Britannica is a good starting place, and knowledge of them can provide an understanding of the causation of certain serious illnesses, but, as with Watkins' lines, I'll provide more information for the enquiring mind in the addenda or appendices). An interesting reflection is that I find that many people who have come to 'ley-lines' in their mystical, 'earth energy' form are just not interested in the truth of their origin, and indeed, would rather have their mystery than the truth.

But don't you find this to be the case in whatever area of activity or human knowledge that you care to choose? 'Don't give me facts, I've made up my mind'. 'When I've made up my mind nothing will shift me'.

I have related how I came to join the Training Department as a stage in my rehabilitation at work. One of my first tasks in my

LISTENING TO THE SILENCES

new post was to become familiar with the newly adopted Système International d'Unities, the SI System, or International System of Measurements, and then, having become familiar, to assess the impact within the Works and produce publicity. Why should this be of such great, or any, significance? Well, the world, i.e. the complete scientific, technological, commercial, industrial community, embracing the whole planet, had agreed upon the exact definition of every function capable of being measured. Thus, a metre is the same in Novaya Zemlya as it is in Wagga Wagga, and likewise, from degrees Celsius to teslas or sieverts, anywhere in the world they are the same. This is the world of the engineer, the scientist, of practicality. If you buy a car, you expect that all the wheels will be round, and of the same diameter, and that the pistons will slide effortlessly in their cylinders whether the car is made in Taiwan or Toulouse. If you tune your radio to a designated frequency of transmission, you will receive your programme whether you use the most sophisticated hi-fi system in your home or a wind-up clockwork radio in the African bush. Would that other realms of human activity were as precise and predictable!

"But", you may say, "what about the world of imagination, of fantasy, of the spirit, even; are they not suppressed, stifled, by your desire for order, definition, predictability; are you not creating a world of automata, robots, without any individuality - removing the ability of individuals to choose for themselves?" Not at all. Does not our society, civilisation, depend upon universally accepted laws, laws which if broken have defined consequences? Is it not obvious to all, that children, to take an example, are far happier, grow more assuredly, when their world is certain, regulated? Whether one likes it or not, the 'natural' laws exist, apply, whether or not one accepts them. Ignore them at your peril. If you disagree, try jumping off a cliff and see whether you can suspend the laws of gravity. But an understanding, recognition of the laws of physical existence can be liberating and certainly do not stifle the imagination, the sheer *magic* of living.

Running over the fell-side behind my house is a narrow mountain road that I take when heading out of the area. This road at its summit goes through a pass of sorts. One morning some years ago I took the road just before daybreak; a beautiful morning with a strong following breeze blowing in from the sea, and over the pass. When I arrived at the summit and looked over, I just had to stop and gaze in awe and wonder at the literally breathtaking sight that met my eyes. *There* was the magic. Tendrils and streamers of mist flowed down from the pass, wreathing around the scattered trees and junipers. Every blade of grass, every twig, every frond, had its dewdrop, every hollow its little pool - and every single drop of water held its own personal rainbow. The ridges of the hills and mountains ranged east to the distant Pennines, over which the sun had just emerged, and every ridge was a line of opalescence, of pearl. What it was to be faced with a sea of rubies, diamonds, amethysts, and a backdrop of mother-of-pearl! I simply sat *entranced*. Yet, in my stillness, the logical 'me' knew that the air coming from the sea was moisture laden, saturated, and that as it was funnelled through the 'venturi' of the pass, it was speeded up and compressed, only to expand and cool on the down slope, just as the gas circulating in a refrigerator system is compressed, expands and cools. The cooler air could not hold the moisture and it settled on all available surfaces, forming drops which then refracted the incident light - and so on. Does that deny or remove the beauty, the magic? Not for me, for I can find a different kind of magic in the order, the functioning of natural phenomena, natural laws.

On an even grander, more immense, scale, who can look at the pictures received from the Hubble Space Telescope and not be amazed? One that I remember in particular is of a gas cloud trillions upon trillions of light-years in length, in *one corner* of which a completely new *galaxy* was forming. Yet even here, in this immensity, one can marvel at the skill of the astronomer-scientists who can, by the application of universal and natural laws, identify and quantify the component gases and measure, for instance, the speed of movement of surrounding stars. But, and more amazingly, in the face of that immeasurable immensity of uncertain origin, a neuroscientist at a very recent international conference on research into the human brain could say that, with its billion, trillion connections, the human brain is the most complex unit in the whole Universe!

But more than that, and here is the awesome thought, every brain is contained in a unique human being, and each being is at the centre of its own universe. A universe made up of the material composition and the - what? Whatever it takes to make that individual unique. Whatever it takes to make me gaze transfixed at the beauty of a mountain dawn, while around me the sheep continue grazing or ruminating, completely unmoved. I will not even *begin* to *try* to take the thought any further, but think instead of the dedicated work of the brain-scientists, the neuroscientists as they struggle to understand the totality of this 'universe within a universe', the human brain. With my own experience in the world of measurement, I can marvel at the skill and ingenuity of the measuring techniques, devices, without necessarily understanding the complexity of what it is that is being studied, measured; just as these same scientists might have equivalent difficulty in appreciating the complexity of measurement within a nuclear reactor.

On the other hand, why should we not, just for a little while, pause and consider this wonder of wonders, the human brain, and the unique vehicle, the human body in which it finds itself? Unique in that its fingerprints have no duplicate worldwide, neither is there matching DNA anywhere on the planet, so we are told - six thousand million and still counting and expanding exponentially. And yet this brain, this body, are in one gigantic lottery. How else can you explain, for instance, to a cretinous dwarf in Bangladesh that if someone had provided a modicum of iodine to replace that which his native soil lacked, he would have a mind which functioned properly and a body which grew to a normal size? Or what about these brains, which are not going to live more than a year or so because they are in diseased or starving children 'living' in what is so easily written off as the 'Third World'? Or these that will be programmed from birth to carry on a warring, family or religious feud whether in Afghanistan, Sicily, Northern Ireland or wherever? Happy and fortunate these brains, which are being nourished physically and lovingly fed knowledge, in what are going to be well rounded people. Most *un*happy and *un*fortunate these brains, which started off so well and hopefully, but which became polluted and destroyed by alcohol and drugs; or equally unfortunate these others which, because they or their owners show some aberration, difference from the accepted norm, are destined to be invaded and possibly warped by prescribed drugs, some of whose very *side*-effects can be so alarming just to *read* about, or, Heaven forbid, shocked into submission by a bizarre 'therapy', that is not understood and is administered by practitioners, some of whom are not fully trained in its application and who would not submit to it themselves.

Many people, if they consider it at all, are happy to let the lottery be administered by God or Allah. Believers in reincarnation put it all down to past lives and the carry-over of karma there from. Others believe that they arrive back into the new brain-body combination complete with a worked out plan of action. David Icke, in one of his books, when considering the tragedy of cot-death, suggests that maybe the infant had just to go through the birth process to finish off its overall development as a well-rounded spirit, or that the parents had to go through the trauma of bereavement to complete *their* full development.

Astrologers have *their* own way of looking at the origins and future of each unique brain-body-spirit combination. But in which, oh where, in what system do I find my own raison d'être? Do I join the other five hundred million people worldwide who are Sagittarians, or do I throw in my lot with the slightly smaller number who are, to use Chinese astrology, Wind Buffaloes? My date and time of birth, according to the Mayan calendar, are so auspicious as to make me a possible candidate for some celestial high office; so do I settle for that? If I should read my 'horoscope', courtesy of some newspaper or magazine, do I reflect upon the idea that in Ulan Bator or on the shores of Hudson Bay, other Sagittarians are having, have had or are going to have a similar day to mine?

It is into this gigantic lottery, with the dice forever being thrown, the wheels forever being spun, through this minefield of human beliefs and practices, that the mainly white, middle-class males who make up the bulk of practising psychiatrists and psychologists must make their way. It is the minds that are the products of these origins, beliefs and life-styles, minds that are not behaving as their owners or the society in which they live would have them behave, which have to be regulated, mended. But first, they have to be categorised, and here we enter an entirely different and additional lottery, a lottery with so many possible variables, variables that are as numerous as the practitioners. The practitioners are as varied as their own origins, upbringing, the school of psychiatry or psychology in which they were trained, or to which they adhere -, schools that may spawn closed minds and tunnel-visionaries equally with the brilliant, the caring; practitioners who find it necessary to use an esoteric language that might give Humpty-Dumpty some problems, so subjective are its interpretations. One psychiatrist, for instance, writes of the 'private language and idiosyncratic narratives glorifying or obfuscating disorders of the mind'. Well, he wrote it; who am I to disagree?

I wrote earlier of the definitions and standards that governed the work and communication of my own profession. Would that there were similar standards and points of reference in the professions of the mind. But, on what scale and from what point zero do you place, for instance, an individual who is 'manic depressive'? The Clinical Psychologist who became my neighbour when I took up residence in a farmhouse flat after leaving my home, had analysed herself and concluded that *she* was manic-depressive. Over a period of four years we became friends, and I can promise you that she demonstrated nothing other than the expected and frequently observed mood swings of her gender. I sometimes wonder just how she would have characterised Harry (obviously not his real name) who used to come and stay with me from time to time, seeking the sort of sanctuary that my house and surroundings provide. Now Harry *was* a manic-depressive! Did he not have a total of nineteen months, and still counting, of 'voluntary' incarceration to his credit? He was a general practitioner who could no longer practice, but who had many insights into what had happened, was being done to himself. He wrote a diatribe against psychiatry and the prostitution, as he saw it, of true medicine, by doctors who engaged in psychiatry. He could not get his essay published, so, having the only copy extant, I shall include it in my writings should they ever see the light of public day. Posthumously as it turns out, for Harry died young from the accumulation of all that he had received or inflicted on himself.

It is perhaps not surprising that one of Harry's heroes was Philippus Aureolus Theophrastus Bombastus von Hohenheim, who preferred to be known, and who can blame him, as Paracelsus. Having read the account of the latter's life and work in *Encyclopaedia Britannica,* he could definitely become one of my heroes.

LISTENING TO THE SILENCES

Beginning his education in the Bergschule in Austria, the young Paracelsus was being trained to become an overseer and analyst for mining operations in gold, tin and mercury and other metals and ores, gaining knowledge and experience that laid some of the foundations of his later discoveries in the field of chemotherapy, which, for someone born when Columbus was discovering the New World, was most remarkable. He attended the Universities of Basel, Tübingen, Wittenberg, Vienna, Leipzig and Heidelberg and along the way graduated in medicine. But, in spite of, or because of this experience, he rejected much of the, then, traditional education and medicine - which is perhaps the rebel spirit with which Harry identified. Paracelsus wrote "The universities do not teach all things, so a doctor must seek out old wives, gypsies, sorcerers, wandering tribes, old robbers and such outlaws and take lessons from them. A doctor must be a traveller… Knowledge is experience." We are a bit short on sorcerers, wandering tribes and outlaws these days, but in spite of that I find much in the *spirit* of Paracelsus to which I warm, and I would far rather find my own remedies in natural herbs and substances than in neatly packaged capsules in a bottle. It is interesting to reflect that many of these self-same capsules will contain in refined form the very remedies that had been used and dispensed during numerous past centuries by the old wives, gypsies and sorcerers. In the refining, much will have been lost, for often within a plant and discarded in the refining are the buffers and catalysts that aided the process of healing and minimised adverse side effects.

It is all too easy to conjure up in one's mind pictures of a Golden Age of caring, of dedicated nuns, monks and friars issuing forth from their monasteries and priories, dispensing unqualified love and tinctures and salves made from the herbs and simples grown in the physick garden, with no thought other than the physical and spiritual well-being of the sick, the mentally afflicted, the halt and the lame, the paupers (although William Cobbet insists that pauperism did not exist before the dissolution of the monasteries - provocative thought!). Doubtless such an Age never existed as such, but isn't it a lovely concept to reflect upon, particularly in respect of the mentally disturbed? It is *so* difficult to understand and tolerate, let alone to care for (and *love(?)* someone whose mind is out of kilter. In some cultures, such are seen as being precious to God; the practising Christian will try to see the suffering Christ in each one; others will reach out in care through such organisations as the Samaritans. As I write elsewhere, one longs for the actual concept of 'asylum' - not the *buildings* but the 'benevolent affording of shelter and support to some class of the afflicted, the unfortunate' - as an attitude, a reality, not the reality of the medico-commercial industry, which seems to direct, control, dominate and profit from, make a career structure from, the treatment and management of the misfortunes of the nervously disturbed and mentally ill.

LISTENING TO THE SILENCES

My own Consultant, MC, appears, from my notes, to be very glib at allocating classifications. For example, he categorised my then wife as 'dominant'. How sterile! You might as well try to classify a will-o-the-wisp! Born in India to a doting father and a mother who should never have had children; partly raised by an ayah and 'bearer', and then dispatched to the vastly different world of England at five years old into the care of a kind but very firm and vigorously disciplining aunt, whose prescription of senna and Mass on Sundays purified both body and soul. Rebel? Yes. Individual? Yes. An intelligent and sensitive horse-woman; an artist manqué as her later exquisite and innovative pottery demonstrated, she should have gone to art-school or university not to a teacher training college run by nuns. Different? Yes. Dominant? Just what the hell does that mean apart from being a meaningless bit of shrink-speak? The same classification was applied by him to another lady who subsequently, and for a short time in the 'seventies, graced my nuptial couch. Now it would be most difficult, if not impossible, to find two such different women. Apart from each having the usual complement of female accoutrements, furniture and fittings, they just could not have been more different! The second lady defined herself as 'bloody minded'. Who could disagree with her?

You may sense as you read that there is a developing, growing anger. It is not an all-consuming anger that is gnawing away at my inner man and possibly harming me. No; but it is an anger that has grown steadily since I first took a tentative look into my medical notes some eleven or so years ago. As I write elsewhere, I could not at first read the notes in their entirety because of what was stirred up by my reading, but what I did read began a change in my perception of the people who had had virtual control of a period in my life, a period in which my then life was shattered - but from the shards of which, fortunately, I have been able to create an entirely new one, one which in itself is immensely satisfying. Until I started to read the notes I looked back and acknowledged what had been attempted on my behalf and the time that had been allocated to me, and, at least twice, I had written to MC to thank him for his concern and the hours that he had spent with me. With the reading has come the revelation, the realisation that there were at least two sides to the man that were now becoming apparent. There had been the urbane friendly chap who sat tying salmon flies as we chatted and he gave me my fortnightly psychotherapeutic 'fix', that contrasted totally with the man who had written these letters and notes. With each reading I experience a deeper sense of betrayal. From our very first encounter I had, as I recall, tried to convey openly all that was passing through my life at that time and before. But where were my achievements, the successes, the things that I was proud of? They figured not at all. On the contrary, anything, any event that had a negative component, any past goal not achieved, these were all listed and psychiatric 'conclusions' drawn. These 'insights', together with an unnecessary amount of personal and family detail, were then relayed in correspondence to my G.P. and, as I note elsewhere, into my Practice records, where they remain, colouring the perception of me by any subsequent doctor who has read them.

Why, then, am I continuing to read and write about these times, these people? Why not just put them back where they had been for all those years? I ask myself these and other relevant questions frequently at the time when anything likely to disturb my peace of mind surfaces; I ask them mostly during the 3 a.m. stint. Yes, often I wake still at about that time. I am much more aware now than I was in times past of the reasons for waking, and I have devised several strategies aimed at countering them or the consequences of being awake. In spite of these insights, I still meet the occasions when it is virtually impossible to still my mind and its content of the tragic memories that the reading and writing are bringing back to the surface. How they flood in and keep recycling - perceptions of losses, real and virtual, the 'what if?' and 'if only' - and pictures of faces harrowed by misery, despair and tears. And I curse myself profoundly for having been so stupid as to begin the process of remembering, analysing and writing, and of wasting time during the day pounding this keyboard, when I would far rather have a chisel or gouge in my hands, carving or wood-turning, or be doing something out-of-doors. By which time I have usually abandoned any thoughts that I may have had of an immediate return to sleep, and am downstairs making a cup of tea. Reality and healthy recollection soon return, and with them somehow a remembrance of when, a few years ago, I had a profound and focused prayer life. I used, in fact, to welcome my frequent waking at six bells in the middle watch, because in reality it did become a 'watch'.

As I take up my narrative in a little while I shall relate how I entered into a more determined way of living spiritually. I had learned the strategy of 'offering' a particular period of time, a specific activity or a difficult or unpleasant task, for the benefit of some group or individual. Thus, and for example, if I had a particular prisoner of conscience in mind I would 'offer', say, the cleaning of the kitchen floor tiles on his behalf. This meant that I held him in focus and performed the work for his benefit; which in turn meant that I could not let him down and tried to produce an immaculate result from my work, and the work in its turn became a form of prayer.

In my own middle-watches, memories were wont to return of my past nights of desperate despair and anguish, and I started to 'offer' the time of wakefulness. I used to think of and pray for people currently in psychiatric wards, and for the staff attending them, and also for the physical prisoners, locked and isolated in the meanest of accommodation in our jails. In particular I prayed for the innocent people in

LISTENING TO THE SILENCES

prison, of whom, we are more and more beginning to realise, there must be many. In time, I found that I had no problem with being awake at these times and in fact came to value and look forward to this very private and personal time.

*By the grace You grant me of silence without
loneliness, grant me the
right to plead, <u>to clamour</u> for my brothers
imprisoned in a loneliness
without silence!*

The emphasis of my spiritual life has changed over more recent years, and in many ways I regret my move away from that particular form of prayer. On the other hand, what has happened may be the result of the activities of that time. The practical, pragmatic 'me' has always taken the view that it is not sufficient to project prayers heaven-ward in the pious hope that 'something will be done'. In the reality of life I reckon that you have to be prepared to add action to supplication, and rather than asking "please will *you* do so-and-so?" asking instead "please help *me* to do so-and-so." And so it might be that in this remembering, analysing and writing I am creating my own answer to my original prayer and doing something *practical* for the benefit of the ones for whom I had originally prayed.

I found a parallel to my line of thinking recently when listening to a man on television describing his own experiences. I had switched on briefly mid-morning while having my tea break to find this man recounting the horror of his twenty-five innocent years in prison. When, in his late teens and describing himself as "withdrawn and inadequate", a young woman was murdered in his neighbourhood, the man had a very vivid dream in which he clearly saw the face of a woman and the circumstances of a murder. What he saw in the dream was of such clarity that he himself believed that he could only have known such things if he had actually been involved. On going to the police, more to get clarification than anything else, the young man found himself taken in as the only suspect, all other investigation was dropped, and his feet never touched the ground until he was locked up for life. After three years in prison, he realised that he was innocent and just could not have committed the crime, and has spent the remaining time trying to get his case re-heard and securing his ultimate release.

During the interview the man was asked why, having lived through such traumatic times, he was still continuing to be involved with the processes of law and the prisons. His reply was that if he could prevent anything similar from happening to only one other person, he would willingly keep exposing himself to the publicity and the agony. It is in this respect that I see some parallels to my own circumstances. I had been in a form of prison of someone else's making for nearly seventeen years, although I didn't in fact know that I had been 'innocent' until some time after my release. My sole motivation in writing and opening up my past to scrutiny is just the

LISTENING TO THE SILENCES

same, namely to try to 'release' even one other person, or to prevent someone from being entrapped in the first place. If I can do this, I shall consider the time to have been well spent.

Sitting on the same sofa was the psychologist who frequently appeared on the particular programme, and he just seemed unable to contain himself as he waited to get in with the psycho-gobble about dreams, causes and interpretations thereof. There seems to be nothing that cannot be explained courtesy of Messrs Freud and Jung! But he found himself totally out of his depth, and fortunately shut up when the man described the overwhelming and disabling emotion which swept over himself, and which, often with only the slightest trigger, caused him to curl into himself so tightly and weep uncontrollably. I have never been so drastically affected, but I recognise the times past when, metaphorically and internally, I have 'curled up and wept' at the memory and actuality of the pain and loss and humiliation experienced by myself and those whom I formerly held so close and dear. The psychologist started to develop an instant explanation of 'panic attacks' but was promptly and completely silenced by the man himself.

Why do these psychologists and psychiatrists who appear so widely and frequently on television and radio, have to believe that they have an instant and complete answer to every human situation and problem that crosses their orbit? Can they never be persuaded to say " I don't know" or "That is outside my experience"? Yes - *out side my experience.* It should be patently obvious that, except in a rare few instances, very few of the practitioners of these 'arts' have experienced the mental conditions that they are trying to define and correct in the people before them. It is purely hypothesis and theory that is being put into practice, often at the expense of people's minds and lives. A surgeon has a particular task before him, and if he gets it wrong and cuts off the wrong bit, or has an unacceptable number of fatalities to his credit, then eventually someone notices and steps are taken. Likewise, if a drug therapy results in numbers of babies being born with vestigial development, that, too, becomes obvious. But who is there to blow the whistle on a psychiatrist? If patients deteriorate, well it's just a continued manifestation of the original 'syndrome' (how they love that word!) and a more advanced drug regime is called for. Is there not a crying need for a less interventionist approach to people's distressful inability to cope? Less a need for invasive action, but rather a system of support, of 'cocooning' people until their crisis is past, and they and their partners, friends, develop a greater understanding of causes and practical remedies. Often understanding, communication and support are all that many people need. From many sources, it is obvious that the first and often only response is the latest in-vogue and well-marketed tranquilliser or anti-depressant.

LISTENING TO THE SILENCES

During another morning tea break switch-on, I happened upon the same sofa psychologist presiding over a phone-in on 'control freaks'. Women, some of whom were obviously in great distress, were describing their situations in which husband or partner was exercising such a degree of control over most aspects of their lives and activities as to make their lives intolerable. I understand and sympathise greatly with the callers and their desperate need for help, but what disturbed me about the programme response was that, without having met or heard from the partners in the marriage or relationship, the men were, without exception, labelled 'control freaks' by the psychologist and presenter, who was just as bad with his glib, 'know-all' categorisations, and then of course, having stuck on a label, 'they' all come into a common category - 'they' all behave like this; 'they' all do that and the other. This facile and often stupid labelling (bearing in mind that the current Prime Minister is also designated a 'control freak!), creates great dangers in its wake, bringing back to mind my own sad decline, which began with the application without consultation or justification of the 'chronic anxiety neurosis' label.

I make no apology for revisiting this part of my story. I am not doing so in order to extract the maximum of hand-wringing sympathy from you, nor to take up my cudgel, metaphorically to beat the heads of the psychiatrists and doctors who were sequentially participants in the original drama. No, I want to analyse in more detail what was written and, equally importantly, what was *not* written in the hope of exposing the vulnerability of the individual caught in the toils of 'the system'.

Just suppose that I had been suspected of having committed some major crime, and that BW had been retained by the prosecution as an expert witness in order to provide a psychiatric assessment of me. So great is his status in his field, that his name on an adverse report would mean that it would be accepted without question by judge and jury alike. If my crime had been murder, the chances are that, virtually on his assessment alone, I could have been found guilty and be on a one-way ticket to Broadmoor or some similar establishment.

I regard myself as intelligent and articulate, yet what happened to me did happen in spite of that, largely because, in effect, I had yielded control to those whom society places in authority, and whose competence we are not in a position to question. Just imagine the situation of someone who is less articulate, possibly with the difficulties of communication experienced between people of different ethnic or social backgrounds, or someone who may be withdrawn or, for whatever reason, disturbed, being arrested for some crime or misdemeanour and held in custody, possibly allocated the duty solicitor and, if necessary, the duty psychiatrist, each of whom may simply be doing a job and not have the true well-being of the prisoner at heart. Such people are easily misunderstood, and easily influenced and vulnerable, and, as we are aware, dire things can happen to them. I recall the case of a young man from New Zealand who had been arrested for shoplifting in London. He was held for psychiatric assessment and then ordered by the court to be deported. However, the psychiatrist who had examined him wanted to study him further for her own purposes and arranged for him to be held and not immediately released. In his despair and isolation, the young man took his shirt, tied one end to a bed leg, rolled the rest tightly around his neck - and strangled himself.

Nothing as dire happened to me, although I came perilously close to suicide - and all because of a label and inadequate communication between people with preformed minds, people with limited experience of the way of life of many of those who come before them as patients. Try as they will, it is nigh on impossible for them to identify, or even understand the problems and stresses. I have mentioned already the artificial community, Seascale, in which I lived. When I was in hospital, I was struck by the fact that, in proportion to its population against that of the rest of the hospital catchment area, Seascale was over-represented, particularly by its womenfolk.

It was an artificial and peculiar community in many ways. The original Seascale had been created in the latter half of the nineteenth century to give some purpose to the newly laid Furness Railway. Conceived as a select watering place, it had a core of basic shops, two hotels and several boarding houses, two private schools and a golf course. It was run by long-standing residents, and there seemed to be a general resentment against this hoard of 'off-comers', many very well paid by the standards then prevailing locally. The purpose of the addition to the village was to house staff brought in to create and run the new nuclear complex of Windscale and the later Calder Hall power station. Virtually every house had its graduate, possibly two, for wives were often as well qualified as their husbands. That was part of the problem - the educated mind with very little outlet. Cars had not yet become readily available or affordable in the years following the war. Children poured out of the woodwork, for, for many, it was the first home of the young after demobilisation and graduation.

Men had their work that was, in the main, revolutionarily new, and all-absorbing, often requiring long hours at work, trips to headquarters and to contractors' works, and, of course, it was secret. Even if we wanted to talk about our work and associates at home, it was difficult because of the unusual nature of what we were doing. Then there was the shared camaraderie of war service that isolated the men from their women. In other men's reminiscences I was in the cockpit of a Lancaster bomber over Germany; trying to establish radio communication in the desert; in Changi jail in Singapore - or wherever the world-wide conflict had taken me and my colleagues. The women were isolated - intellectually as well as physically. They went 'home' (i.e. back to mother)

LISTENING TO THE SILENCES

to have babies or at every opportunity; they pushed prams in the teeth of the winds that rushed in from the Irish Sea; they had the 'hierarchical' coffee morning! Everyone's grades, and hence salary, were known, and houses were allocated by size of family and by grade. Thus, when I reached the grade of Principal, we moved into an 'A' type house, i.e. four bedrooms plus garage. These were the ladies who found their way to the newly opened psychiatric wing of the now-being-constructed hospital and the newly appointed consultant MC, who, in turn, sent some for a second opinion to BW. With the best will in the world, how could these specialists really understand the home life, social background of many of their patients? Of the three psychiatrists whom I saw, not one had been in the armed forces; none had been in industry or saw many people outside their profession other than patients. Thus it was that LW and BW, on the basis of forty and ten minutes contact with me, respectively, presumed to analyse, categorise and prescribe.

As with many of my colleagues at work, I had at first lived in a nearby hostel for unmarried or unhoused staff. I lived there for four years and many friendships were formed. We got to know each other's girl friends who later became wives, and our children grew up in the influence of these groupings. I still have a number of on-going friendships from those days, ones that were formed nearly fifty years ago. Of some partnerships only a widower or widow remains, and in a haphazard way our paths sometimes cross, and we reminisce. On two separate occasions, I had virtually identical conversations with two of the widows. Both of the husbands had been friends of mine and aspects of the past were being discussed, and both widows used exactly the same words - "I never really knew him". Now this had been after thirty-five to forty years of marriage, and, in one case, the upbringing of three children. "I never really knew him". If this was the case after such a long period of shared life, how possibly could a psychiatrist in one short interview do more than scratch deeper than one micron into the surface of the individual before him?

My label of 'chronic anxiety neurosis' was applied to me when all else had failed in the ongoing battle against my enteritis, not as the result of thoughtful consultation and analysis, and the Librium prescription was the medicine of last resort. My second GP (GP2) accepted the diagnosis and continuing prescription seemingly without question. But where were the cautions, the restrictions? With so many 'Home Doctor' programmes available on CD in our computers, it is now so easy to access the information that was presumably made available to medical practitioners with the launch of new drugs. One does not have to be well qualified in medicine or psychiatry, but only to be able to read - yes *read.* Thus benzodiazepine - for the *short-term* relief of *severe* anxiety. But they have paradoxical side effects - thus *increased anxiety*, and *perceptual*

LISTENING TO THE SILENCES

disorders, which, coupled with the *drowsiness* and *light-headedness*, were the likely cause of the apparently psychosomatic disorders that ultimately led to my referral to MC. But this was after *two years* of prescription. Where lies the responsibility to assess continuously the results of medication?

Should not MC have carried out an audit when I was first referred? He classed me effectively as 'garrulous, giving a wealth of hypochondriac detail', yet another of the paradoxical side effects is *talkativeness*! My referral letter records the fact that I had been taking Librium for two years - where was his awareness of the oft stated caution that withdrawal should be *very slow* after such a long period of usage? He should surely have been aware that *abrupt withdrawal* might produce *confusion, toxic psychosis, convulsions or a condition resembling delirium tremens.* As I have recorded elsewhere, my withdrawal was *immediate*, with the consequences that I have noted. Yet no alarm bells seem to have rung and caused him to review the medication - only puzzlement at the presumed and never before recorded idiosyncratic reaction to the new drug that he had prescribed. But, as his notes record, I was having problems also with *micturation* and *libido*, standard and well recorded side effects of benzodiazepine. Well?

When I became an in-patient in his ward, MC prescribed various *barbiturates* to help me sleep. Now, there are cautions listed advising against using the two types of drug together, which it would be tedious for me to include. One side effect of barbiturates is the *suppression of breathing*, yet when one day on the ward I commented that my breathing was very restricted, I was told that as my lips had not yet turned blue I had no cause for alarm - all very jocular, but not very perceptive. I later recorded *numbness of my scalp and part of my face, tinnitus.* At one time, my *vision* was disturbed - at times blurred, and, for a period, I lost *peripheral vision.*

Remember, all this medication was gratuitous; I had never had the conditions for which the drugs were compounded, although in all the literature, I have not been able to find any comments relating to the effects of *unnecessary* prescription. Remember also that benzodiazepine are classed as *minor* tranquillisers; God help you if you get on the wrong side of the *major* ones, the *anti-psychotic* drugs. I don't suppose that you will be aware, though, your mind will probably have gone into orbit! In the wide world of industry and agriculture, people have to be tested and licensed and re-tested periodically to ensure that they are, and continue to be, fit to handle noxious and potentially lethal or harmful substances. Surely these drugs should be placed in a similar sort of legal 'containment', and practitioners should be re-tested at periodic intervals?

You are being very patient if you have read this far; I hope that you are not finding it all too tedious. As we are yet in the Wonderland of Alice, perhaps we have strayed into the Caucus race. "What on earth is the Caucus race?" said Alice. "Why", said the Dodo, "the best way to explain it is to do it" - no start, no finish, just keep running in a circle until you feel like stopping, and everyone is a winner - that is what it feels like to me at times as I revisit my past. The people who have read this far tell me that they want to know the full story, so you can blame them not me; I'm still running in my circle, how about you?

The letter written by MC to BW in which he asked for a second opinion gave no account of the drug regime of the previous three years, but simply mentioned the brief high dose of Librium within the sequence of E.C.T and insulin therapies that he listed. My own reaction on first reading it was one of total surprise and dismay at the absence of real fact and the sheer negativeness of his narrative. He records, for instance, that I had failed my Higher School Certificate (today's A-level). There were reasons, such as having to take subjects that were not my first choice because of limitations in the availability of staff, war service having claimed several, and other reasons, which it would be tedious to relate. Why did he not say, for instance, that I had been Head Boy, Head Prefect and School Captain, that I had for several seasons played rugby with the First XV and had represented the School at throwing the javelin, or that I had taken major roles in school plays (Richard Burton was a contemporary and fellow thespian), or that I had delivered the valedictory address to a long-serving, and now departing, headmaster?

This disappointment, and the one of not attaining a commission, plus any other of life's seeming catastrophes that he could include, were seized upon by LW in the letter which he wrote for BW to sign, as examples of my inability to cope with failures. How little he knew! Within a fortnight of getting my exam results, I had volunteered for the Royal Navy, and was accepted for a University Short Course with the hope of ultimately being commissioned. In a further short time I was at Glasgow University being trained in aspects of seamanship, signalling and sailing, and learning the practice of coastal navigation, while academically I was studying Natural Philosophy and Geography. Disappointed? Like hell! I was revelling in it all. I cannot convey to you the joy in my life in at last being in a boat and learning to sail under expert tuition, nor of being taught the intricacies of knotting and cordage by a Chief Petty Officer who, at *seventy,* had returned for service - someone who had actually served in *sail*. My cup of happiness was very full. I passed with distinction, fourth out of a course of about eighty. My academic subjects were also passed well and there was the prospect of a return to Glasgow on demob.

Those of us who had chosen to try for a seagoing commission joined, next, a formal training establishment, where we learned more seamanship, gunnery and so on, and were tested in our 'power of command' and our ingenuity in

LISTENING TO THE SILENCES

trying to cross a crocodile infested river using only a length of rope and two short planks. The hoped for commission did not materialise, which disappointment is another which LW in his analysis said I had difficulty in coming to terms with. Oh! Get a life! If he had probed further he would have learned that, out of the whole group, less than 15% succeeded, and he would have learned also the prime reason, namely that on D-Day, and after, the anticipated losses of landing craft commanders had fortunately not happened - and it was for such jobs that we were principally being prepared, and were therefore not needed. We 'rejects' didn't sit around moping, fat chance anyway, and at eighteen one is nothing if not resilient. Within a very short time, several of us had chosen to be trained as Radar Mechanics, and away we went into a fascinating new world, a world that had only been created in the previous three years, and an entirely new track, which fundamentally altered the course of my life.

In this short interview, LW had me dissected and sorted, or so he thought. Oh, the arrogance of the man! Take this point: at sixteen I had had a severe gastric upset which had resulted in a barium meal, abdominal X-ray and the conclusion of our family doctor that "I had nearly had an ulcer". LW's contempt was palpable - "You can't *nearly* have an ulcer, it must have been dyspepsia" - end of story. What sheer bloody arrogance! The family doctor had been a *family* doctor. He had delivered me in our home and had tended all my growing-up illnesses, as well as removing my adenoids. Which of these two men is most likely to have been able to assess the causes of my gastric ailment? But this is what one is up against, and the consequences, and not just for me, are enormous. When you contemplate the 'armoury' that is at the disposal of psychiatrists, you should quail, not only have they powers of incarceration but they have, in the shape of drugs, prisons without bars and shackles without chains. And yet, as my case shows, conclusions can be reached and decisions and actions taken on the basis of the most cursory analysis and arrogant self-belief.

There is so much in these two letters that could be subjected to *my* analysis and comment, but no great purpose would be served; I think that I have made a sufficiently valid point. I must also acknowledge, though, that LW and BW had not been given a full picture in that details of the drug regime and symptoms had not been included in the referral letter; facts that might have alerted them and inspired a deeper examination. On the other hand, to be sent for examination having been preceded by a comment such as MC had made, namely that I 'presented a puzzling mixture of anxiety and depression, with, at times, an ominous schizoid flavour' does not allow one much scope to demonstrate that one is not actually doolally.

I know that in concentrating upon my own experiences at the hands of three individuals

LISTENING TO THE SILENCES

I am presenting an unfair picture of the whole profession. There are undoubtedly many dedicated and competent psychiatrists in practice, and I know that I would not like to do their work, and I acknowledge their commitment and caring. I know, too, that it will be said that my own experiences are unusual and a-typical. I sincerely hope that they are, but that being said, there are elements that one learns are still being repeated in the lives of other people, and will continue to be repeated as long as humans have human failings both as patients and practitioners. Essentially, all the latter really have to do, and yet it is most difficult, is to listen with a mind which is not preformed, and to make judgments that are not instant but which are open to further scrutiny, and which can be revisited, revised and reversed, and do not result in the compounding of one symptom by one drug, which creates another symptom or side effect, which has to be treated by another drug, which creates another side effect which... Do I exaggerate? I have a friend who was having problems sleeping. She was given sleeping pills (designed for the *short term* - ha bloody ha - relief of insomnia), which have the adverse effect of creating nausea and vomiting; so now she has a gut problem and more medication. The pills also interfere with the heart and circulation, so more medication, and they cause anxiety, so she has an anxiolytic drug, which also can produce depression, which requires an anti-depressant. No, I do not exaggerate - this is real. But listen, yes, if they would only listen. I had a venerable friend who was chuntering away one day when I called. He had painful arthritis in his shoulder and had been to a consultant, but "...they don't *listen*... they never listen, in spite of what you have to tell them...and as for N (naming his GP) *she* tells you what you've got and then you have to *pretend* to have it!"

I am fast approaching the point where I shall leave my medical records behind, although MC will briefly tread the stage later in the saga. Before I finally quit them, two further points from the notes, if you don't mind. One fills me with dread at what finally might have happened to my mind, for I see that after twenty-three E.C.T.s and the insulin jamboree, MC had been considering *further* E.C.T! Fortunately, as he records, I firmly rejected the idea. I speculate with horror that my poor innocent mind might not have survived yet further assault.

The other entry concerns a later time when I was divorced and living alone, but in regular contact with my daughter and former wife. We had decided that our daughter should move on from ponies to a small horse, and together went to a recommended dealer who found for us a delightful little mare, an Irish hunter of about fifteen hands and which had already been hunted by a girl of roughly my daughter's age. We put her through all the tests for steadiness and suitability that we could devise - from standing by the roadside while lorries with flapping tarpaulins thundered by, to having a car rev-up and its horn sounded under her nose, and a shot-gun being fired behind a hedge. She, whom we called King's Courier, or KC for short, came to stay with me, and my daughter would come from school at weekends to ride. One Saturday it was raining, and she wore a police cape that covered herself and the saddle, but, unfortunately, something that I hadn't anticipated happened. The cape flapped in a breeze and startled KC, which caused the cape to flap more and startled her further. The mare took off on a road beside a river that was in full spate, soon came to a skew bridge, leapt the parapet, and broke her neck as she hit the water. Fortunately, my daughter was flung clear and I bless forever her keenness in swimming, for, heavily clad though she was, she got to the bank and came and found me.

MC comments upon the episode in the next letter to my GP and goes on to write, "...I think that Roy is more distressed at the loss of the horse than at what might have befallen his daughter".

I was once acquainted with two men, one at work and the other through the church. The first had two sons and the elder went to university to study geology. On the first weekend visit home, brand new geologist's hammer, family trip to Wasdale, two boys dash up Yewbarrow, eldest jumps over a rock, hammer in hand - never seen alive again. He wasn't found until next morning, for he had immediately lost his footing and crashed down some way to his death.

The second man also had a son, and the lad had reached the magic age that allowed him to ride a motorbike. The longed for day arrived as did the gleaming machine, bigger than youngsters are allowed today. They lived just a short distance from the 'Irton Straight', where everyone of my acquaintance who owned a bike used to go to test it after adjustment. The lad must have dreamed so many times and lived it all in his mind, as I had lived my sailing. The bike roared into action. He went around the corner heading for the Irton Straight, and they never saw him alive again.

I used to see both men frequently. I never ever saw them smile. Their eyes showed that they were locked in a world of perpetual misery and possibly self-condemnation. I looked briefly into that abyss and came away quickly. You don't dwell on it; you don't think about it. If you do, ever so briefly, you don't share your thoughts with anyone - certainly not with a psychiatrist, no matter how friendly he then appeared to be. Since reading what he wrote, and remembering all that he had caused to happen to me, I have feelings now that would cause me to use the language of the lower-deck. But what's the point?

LISTENING TO THE SILENCES

Come, let us move on....

But where, oh where shall we go?

Let's send Alice to enquire, shall we?

Strange, where did that Cheshire cat appear from? Perhaps he knows...

" Alice, will you enquire directions for us, please?"

"Would you tell me, please," said Alice, " which way I ought to go from here?"

"That depends," said the Cheshire Cat, "on where you want to get to.

Over there… lives a Hatter,……… and over there … lives a March Hare.

Visit either you like: they're both mad."

"But I don't want to go among mad people," Alice remarked.

"Oh, you can't help that," said the Cat: "we're all mad here. I'm mad,

you're mad."

"How do you know I'm mad?" said Alice.

Roy Vincent

"You must be," said the Cat, "or you wouldn't have come here".

Which seems to be where we came in.

Perhaps we should emulate the

Cheshire Cat

and

j u s t   d i   s   a   p
        p   e   a
           r

CHAPTER 4

And

there were

G
I
A
N
T
S

in those days.

Roy Vincent

The moving finger writes....

When I first began to describe my experiences, I had no plan to write what you have read so far. Initially I wrote in order to try to help individuals who had begun to 'hear voices' and who were also experiencing some or all of the other phenomena generally associated with what is commonly called schizophrenia. As fast as I wrote, my screen was avidly read by friends who currently work in branches of psychiatry. As my account unfolded – an account of events that began in 1979 – my friends wanted to know about 'before'.

You have just read about 'before', which ended in or about 1976. As I wrote of those times I became concerned that someone reading about the events of 1979 et sec might conclude that they arose as a result of my earlier experiences, and might write them off as the experiences of a 'damaged' mind. I am as certain as I can ever be about anything that the only connection between the two parts of my history is that they occurred to and in me. In order to try to create a break in thinking and any consequential linking, I wrote the section just ended ('When I use a word...') and the next one ('And there were Giants in those days'). The former enabled me to philosophise a little about my relationship with psychiatrists and psychiatry. The next section, while providing a break, will also enable me to introduce some information and speculation that are both necessary when I come to what will be the penultimate part of my work.

Because I know where the writing is taking me, I know that the information will be necessary for a full understanding. However, I know from the comments of some who have already read the next section that I might be in danger of losing you as a reader. I ask you most strongly to *try* to stick with it even though as you read you may wonder how any of it can *possibly* be of relevance in the field of mental health and the care of the disturbed. All that I can say now is that I ask you to ponder the fact that we as humans are the product of all that has gone before in our evolution, and that every aspect of our physical, mental and spiritual life and previous development, impact upon our current state of being. Thus something as mundane as diet, or as esoteric as our interaction with our total environment – physical and electrical – can dictate how we react physically and mentally. Everything reacts with everything else – and we are piggy in the middle!

An understanding of our precarious place in evolution can help us to mould our lives in such a way that we minimise our chances of ill health, or can help us to recover from any distressful state into which we have succumbed. So as you read remember that this is my goal. If you can't cope or fail to see the relevance, just skip, although unfortunately much of what comes later when I am providing information about survival strategies might be lost on you. I'll leave it to you…

And having writ moves on....

LISTENING TO THE SILENCES

> He who is born in imagination discovers the latent forces of **NATURE**. Besides the stars that are established there is yet another **IMAGINATION** that begets a new star and a new heaven.
>
> Paracelsus

For as long as I can possibly remember, I have been fascinated by water. Not, in spite of my mother's exhortations, the sort that would have removed the tide-mark from around my neck, but the sort that harboured fishes; that provided a home and food supply for wildfowl; but, most of all, the sort on which boats plied, on which ships sailed. Given the chance, I would have spent my days in a boat. I sailed and tried to build model yachts, and read about them, and drooled over catalogues of fittings - *goosenecks* and *deadeyes* and the rest - whose use on *real* vessels I could only guess at. I read, read, and lived it all -the voyages of *Lightning, Flying Cloud, Thermopylae, Cutty Sark -The Fight of the Firecrest* - the voyages of Joshua Slocum. So much did I absorb and live what I read that, when I first took the tiller of a small boat, I *knew* what the feel of a weather helm would be, where the wind would be on my cheek and how the luff of the sail would lightly shiver as we sailed close-hauled. What a day of memories in the making! What a day. The Naval

Division at Glasgow University had acquired sailing facilities on a loch just north of Glasgow and, as well as sailing dinghies on loan, had 'won' a whaler - an open sea-boat of about 21 feet long, and built on the lines of the Viking vessels - high bow and stern and swept lines. It was a bright, scudding April day: blue sky and clouds - and the *feel* of a boat under sail. What can I say? I have sailed in many small boats since, and in many places - Famagusta, Haifa, around Britain - yet nothing can override or extinguish the memories of that first time. And to cap it all, the setting. The loch was in a hollow as the land rose around it, and on the brae beside the water, the field was being worked with horses, while a man scattered seed two-handed - the Lutterell Psalter come to life. Oh, how I loved it all!

But as well as the ships and the sailing, I had an equally passionate love, and that was for navigation. From a second-hand bookstall in our local market I had bought a book on coastal navigation and, again, read and read and absorbed. When, then, the war gave me the chance to do what I had always wanted, to go to sea, and I joined the Navy, with the hope of getting a commission as I have related, I found before me another chance to bring to life my daydreams and imaginings, and to add them to the sailing, for part of the early training involved chart-work. I revelled in the struggle with tides and currents, compass deviation and variation and the like, and in the feel of parallel rulers and dividers as the courses were laid off. As you have seen, I didn't achieve the hoped for commission but, instead, transferred to what was later to influence the course of my life and choice of career.

Radar is an important adjunct to navigation and as such has to be equally reliable, precise. Thus the coast as shown on the radar screen has to be *exactly* as represented - twenty miles and bearing such and such, not give or take a mile or so; or plus or minus so many degrees. In that training and work with radar was born what has become in essence a way of life, of being in touch with reality, of having to be accurate, precise and reliable - the very qualities that were essential in, and pervaded, my whole working life in measurement and safety.

From my love of navigation stemmed another and essentially parallel one - a love of maps and charts, and, by extension, a great interest in mapmakers, navigators and the early explorers. Travelling back in time for two millennia, one of the key centres for the study of all of the sciences and of astronomy and navigation, was Alexandria - centre also for exploration and trade. From the Alexandria of AD 150, came a map and a science that were to influence thought, travel and exploration for the next fifteen hundred years. Claudius Ptolomaeus - Ptolemy - was primarily an astronomer and mathematician, but also a geographer and cartographer. "He stands a Colossus astride the ancient world and his influence is even felt today", says one modern writer. With access to the extensive libraries of Alexandria, and with contact with the mariners who traded to the east and west of this hub of human activity, Ptolemy was in a position to map the known world. Into the accumulated data he was able to introduce an order or system that has since been followed by geographers in all ages; it was he who introduced the method and names of latitude and longitude.

However, in certain very important elements, Ptolemy was in serious error. By his method of measurement, and choice of the Canary Islands for his prime meridian, he greatly overestimated the length of land eastward from this line, and consequently reduced the gap, presumed water, between Europe and Asia. Moreover, whereas the early Greeks had been content to leave blanks in their maps where knowledge ceased, Ptolemy filled in the blanks with theoretical concepts. Such actions would not have mattered so much in a lesser man, but so great was the reputation of Ptolemy that his theories assumed equal validity with his undoubted facts, and were not seriously questioned for 1,500 years. His reputation allowed him to influence a debate whose outcome and repercussions were to reverberate down the centuries. Ptolemy placed the earth at the centre of the universe, and there it stayed, in spite of the arguments of great minds, until the force of observation and truth prevailed.

Will you not weep inside if not openly as Galileo must have done when he was forced to write:

LISTENING TO THE SILENCES

'...but because I have been enjoined, by this Holy Office, altogether to abandon the false opinion which maintains that the Sun is the centre and immovable, and forbidden to hold, defend, or teach, the said false doctrine in any manner........I abjure, curse and detest the said errors and heresies, and generally every other error and sect contrary to the said
Holy Church...'

Galileo Galilei

And will you not spare a thought for the predicament of Christopher Columbus as he sailed westward in the mistaken belief that the globe was as small as Ptolemy had indicated? And after sailing as far as your calculations deemed necessary, how do you come to terms with the fact that you have *not* reached Japan or the Indies as planned - but *where?* "Dammit", "Shiver me timbers" and other such vile nautical oaths, "It *must* be the Indies". And so, dear children, that is how the *West* Indies got their name, for that, in fact, is where Columbus had arrived - blame it all on Ptolemy.

But, is it not the same in many walks of life and in many professions, that someone who has a certain expertise in a particular field, possibly even a very narrow field, is, nevertheless, assumed to be expert in a whole range of related, or even possibly totally *un*related topics?

Television and the other media constantly expose us to such 'instant gurus'. It seems to be a form of psychological conditioning created by the endless chat shows and interviews, where pop-stars, sportsmen and sports-women, so-called 'celebrities', and a whole host of others who fall into no particular category, are treated as if they are fountains of all knowledge and experience under the sun. Likewise the politicians, newspaper columnists and 'agony aunts', who are always so readily and instantly available, and who are trotted out to comment and give an 'informed' opinion on all that is passing across the face of the planet at that moment; or who are expected to be wise beyond their years, experience and knowledge; or to be ready with deep, psychological insights into all that ails the world.

I have related how I came to take charge of the Training Department at the Sellafield establishment. From Day One, I was expected to have total knowledge of the field of industrial training. I was in post. I had a title. It was as if I had been initiated, inducted, empowered by Divine touch. The mantle had descended upon me, and, like a priest at his first celebration, a doctor at his first consultation, I was deemed capable of delivering all the 'magic', an informed opinion.

It requires a high degree of discernment to be able to decide, in real life, just *who* really know what they are talking about and just *who* are delivering whole loads of 'flannel'.

Someone who would not qualify for the epithet 'instant guru' was Sigmund Freud. He emerges from the field of mind exploration, mind mapping, like a latter-day Ptolemy. From both the popular and professional perceptions of his work, and the extent to which its influences thread our lives, Freud might also be classed as a Colossus, a modern one no less, standing astride the gateway to the mind. His thoughts and theories are all pervasive, extending into a world far beyond the confines of psychology and psychoanalysis, from the 'Freudian slip' in speech to the ever-present sexual motivation, which he believed fuelled a person's thoughts, actions and relationships. From him have come concepts of the human mind and behaviour that have dominated thinking and practice in the 'management' of the deviant mind and aberrant behaviour for a large part of the century that has just ended.

In as much as it is necessary to try to understand some of Freud's reasoning and conclusions in the areas of thought and action that I felt might impinge upon my life, I have read and tried to comprehend with remarkable lack of success. There are thoughts and reasonings that I find so irrelevant to my life and my relationships with others, and inferred motivations which I reject so completely, that I wonder what was awry with the life and thought processes of the one who conceived them and gave them birth.

I have a number of friends who are Buddhist and who have as their focus a centre near where I live, where their guru, a lama, resides. The lama is a prolific writer and, some would say, aims to out-rival the Dalai Lama as leader of the Tibetan Buddhists outside Tibet. I have read and tried to understand and see the relevance to my life - to anybody's life - of some of his writings. Mentally, I end up with a feeling that my brain is about to boil and that steam will come screaming out of my nostrils and ears.

In some ways this is analogous to the reaction that I get when I read even simplified versions of Freud's works. They seem to have as much relevance to my thinking and the way in which I conduct my life, as have the tantric and metaphysical convolutions that come from the mind and pen of the lama. I reflect to myself that, having significantly passed my seventieth birthday, I have, somehow, managed to live a life that, while it has been eventful, and while it has contained episodes and moments that I would dearly like to go back and wipe out or change, has nevertheless been one in which I have experienced much happiness and achieved such a lot that I consider to have been worthwhile - but from which I shall have no problems about departing in due course. I further reflect that, somehow, I have managed this life without it being necessary to come to terms with the mysteries of the Tantra, or the equally deep and devious mysteries of the mind of the psychoanalyst and his interpretations of one's motives.

Can it be that Freud's world, like that of Ptolemy, had a limited horizon? Ptolemy knew that his world was round, but he obviously did not know how big it was. He was certainly a brilliant

LISTENING TO THE SILENCES

thinker and innovator, but with such a lot of knowledge not available to him, he assumed too much and interpolated too much - with what disastrous results to those who came after him we cannot know. We shall never know, for instance, how many people disappeared off the edge of the known world simply because they had assumed that Ptolemy's configurations and distances were correct. If, for instance, you provision for a voyage according to Ptolemy's stated distances, and find that in reality you are travelling half as far again, the chances are that food will become short and you just might not return. Or you may simply disappear into the 'terrae incognito', the 'aut- *or* aust-landes', - the unknown, out- or east-lands, beloved of early mapmakers. (Who knows but that the *autlandes* may in fact be the origins of *Atlantis* - say it quickly out loud and see what I mean!)

I wonder how many human minds have just disappeared off the edge of the unknown 'world of the mind' since Freud tried to map it and set its limits? He obviously knew the extent of the physical world, for it had undoubtedly been well mapped before his life-time, but his intellectual world was very restricted, its bounds being the hospitals and consulting rooms, and the mainly Central European capitals. The conflicts of his world derived from artificial 'territories' and potentially opposing loyalties. Thus were his theories accepted by some or rejected by others because he was an Austrian; because he was Jewish; because he was or was not a Freemason;

because he had served under *this* professor, or was a product of *that* school of thinking; because he espoused and then rejected mesmerism? Who knows? But as he worked developing his early career, there were becoming known aspects of knowledge of the *real* world around him, realities which, did he but know of them, had always had the ability to influence the minds and physical health and behaviour of people. Disturbed behaviour in individuals had long been observed and, depending upon the culture prevailing, had been ascribed to a wide variety of causes. However, these external influences that were now beginning to be revealed, have only been seen in comparatively recent years as having this potential to upset people and influence their behaviour. Even if he had been aware of what was being unfolded, I wonder how much relevance Freud would have given to it within the context of his own work and research, for it would require an element of scientific and technical understanding that many, even to this day, do not bother to acquire.

About to step centre stage is a man who did much to provide the means and methods by which knowledge of the realities of this all pervading, all surrounding world could be exposed and defined. And what a man! One of my heroes: at whose funeral three Nobel Laureates would address their tributes to "one of the outstanding intellects of the world, who paved the way for many of the technological developments of modern times": whose notebooks are still being

LISTENING TO THE SILENCES

studied by engineers who are looking to see if there are, even now, brainchildren of his inventive mind waiting to have life breathed into them: whose name you should bless each time you switch on a light, a television or radio, or, additionally, any electrical appliance that has a motor in it: a man who discovered much about the electrical nature of the air around us and the earth on which we live, and who, even, has a unit for the measurement of magnetism named after him: one who in a colourful life experimented with techniques that were the forerunners of today's 'Star Wars' techniques, aimed at disabling enemy aircraft before they could drop their bombs.

Born in Croatia not many miles south of Freud's birthplace; born in the same year as the Austrian, and surviving him by just four years, Nikola Tesla produced much of note, both in Europe and in the United States of America, where he eventually settled. It was Tesla who devised the concept of alternating current, which is now universal in the generation and supply of electricity, and who invented the induction motor, a type that powers just about everything that rotates by electrical means today. The scope of his work and his many patents are widely described in numerous books, but I intend to confine myself only to two areas of influence in our lives that are of relevance to my story.

The first branch of knowledge that Tesla uncovered, and which is relevant to my tale, relates to various aspects of the electrical nature of the air around us and of the earth upon which we live. It was knowledge that allowed others to make further discoveries, and to open wide the doors that he had unlocked. For example, from an understanding of the behaviour of air in certain naturally occurring electrical situations, it can be derived that molecules of the air divide into two parts called ions, one positive and one negative. This can happen during thunderstorms and heavy rainstorms; through exposure to ultra-violet light and cosmic rays; beside waterfalls, or on a surf-washed shore, and in other locations and situations. In our original evolutionary state, there were very many more ions created in those earlier times than now, because of the naturally occurring radioactivity, which has subsequently been decreasing with time. We *need* a natural balance, with preferably an excess of negative over positive ions. Much research has been, and continues to be done into this topic, particularly, for example, when designing the living environment of astronauts or nuclear sub-mariners, but also where it impinges upon the wider field of human, animal and plant health.

The relevance of this knowledge to the topics of which I am writing can be seen when one considers the consequences to humans and other forms of life of a gross imbalance between the types of ions. From the human point of view, a significant excess of positive ions can have a calamitous effect. (I should point out that individual people vary greatly in their response to the conditions that I shall outline - about forty percent are particularly sensitive). The *specific*

LISTENING TO THE SILENCES

relevance to the 'world' that Freud was in the process of analysing and mapping, the human mind and human behaviour, can be seen in the fact that the region of Europe in which he lived is in the path of the Föhn wind (as also is the region where Jung lived in Switzerland). It is now fully appreciated and understood that this wind, together with a number of other well known ones world wide - the Sharav, Chinook, Santa Anna, Sirocco for example - produces a severe excess of positive ions, a fact that now gives an actual explanation for effects which have long since been recognised and have passed into folklore.

There is well researched and documented evidence that says that sensitive people, and other people whose response is perhaps less obvious, can be severely influenced, to the extent that sleeplessness, depression, suicide, aggravations of unknown origin, can all increase dramatically when these winds blow - or even in many cases, as the weather system is approaching and is yet some way off. In Switzerland and Southern Germany, people blame almost everything unusual on the Föhn wind - fights at home, suicides, murders, traffic accidents, depressive states. One can read that in Munich and many other parts of Central Europe north of the Alps, surgeons actually postpone major operations if a Föhn is forecast, because of problems with blood clotting.

An American, Fred Soyka, experienced at first hand the effects of the Föhn wind, and wrote about them in his book *The Ion Effect*, which begins…

"The search for information that led to this book actually began in 1970 as an attempt to prove to myself that I was neither a manic-depressive nor a hypochondriac. For ten years I had lived and worked in Geneva, and almost from the moment I moved there from New York I suffered totally inexplicable fits of anxiety, depression, physical illness, and the kind of bottomless despair that at times even led me to flirt with the idea of suicide. Neither doctors nor a psychiatrist could explain what was happening to me, but when one said vaguely that it might be "something electrical" in the air of Geneva I seized upon it as a possible explanation and spent five years travelling through Europe, the Middle East, and North America meeting scientists and amassing an awesome pile of scientific literature.

I made three discoveries. The first was that in certain places at certain times – in Geneva, in a large part of Central Europe, in southern California, alongside the Rocky Mountains and in at least a dozen other parts of the world – the air becomes sick not because of the pollution we all know about, but because of imbalances in the natural electrical charge of the air."

What, then, I am suggesting is that many of the patients who were being seen by Freud and his Central European contemporaries

LISTENING TO THE SILENCES

were, in fact, suffering from conditions whose cause originated outside themselves. Unable to explain these 'neuroses', it was perhaps logical that subjective causes should be examined, or that analysts should look for explanations within the often limited or circumscribed experiences of their own lives - possibly imbuing their patients with their own personal deficiencies and quirks. It must also be borne in mind that analysts and associates of patients could also be sensitive and react to the influences of the air imbalance, or that staff in hospitals for the disturbed could become aggravated and provocative, sparking off confrontations that would be laid, naturally, at the doors of the inmates, who, after all, were the ones assumed to be need in need of treatment.

I shall write more about these and other relevant matters in later sections, relevant to us in Britain for, although we do not have named winds to blame, nevertheless we have identifiable patterns of air flow which, by their electrical nature, produce effects comparable to those of the Föhn and similar winds. In the meantime, I shall lightly skim over those of Tesla's discoveries that are relevant to my theme. He discovered, and demonstrated, that electricity can be transmitted through the air, and that the earth itself is an electrical conductor; and he had wonderful ideas for using the earth to distribute electrical energy without the need for cables. To digress briefly, I never fail to laugh when I read of the consequences of one phase of his experiments.

Roy Vincent

"Tesla's Colorado Springs tests were well remembered by local residents. With a 200-foot pole topped by a large copper sphere rising above his laboratory, he generated electrical potentials that discharged lightning bolts up to 135 feet long. Thunder from the released energy could be heard 15 miles away in Cripple Creek. People walking along the street were amazed to see sparks jumping between their feet and the ground, and flames of electricity would spring from the taps when anyone turned them on for a drink of water. Light bulbs within 100 feet of the tower glowed when they were turned off. Horses at the livery stable received shocks through their metal shoes and bolted from the stalls. Even insects were affected: butterflies became electrified and helplessly swirled in circles, their wings sprouting blue halos of St. Elmo's Fire." To cap it all, during one high-powered test, he completely destroyed the generator at the local power station. Not *such* a good day!

The concept of the earth as a conductor of electricity may seem to be a long way from human mental health problems: not so. Many people are aware of the state of unease that can be produced by an approaching electrical storm. Part of the cause of the unease will undoubtedly be the increasing concentration of positive ions - a concentration released when lightning flashes. (Recollect the calming internal feelings that one experiences when a much-heralded storm has discharged its 'wrath' and one

LISTENING TO THE SILENCES

is now surrounded by negative ions). Another component may be due to what are called 'standing waves' that Tesla identified; these are peaks and troughs of energy propagated in circles like ripples on a pond when a pebble is dropped in. The waves centre on the storm and move with it, and can be measured at distances in excess of 300 miles. They can be shown to produce unease in people who would themselves be totally unaware of a cause that was so far away. (The disturbance in the behaviour of animals while a storm is yet far off is often noticed and demonstrates that they are reacting to something that is real and not subjective.) Internal disturbance produced by an event as obvious as a thunderstorm can be understood and accepted; similar effects resulting from something unseen such as a *distant* storm may induce significant unease in a sensitive person sufficiently to affect temporarily their mental balance.

Staying with the natural world, and also with the earth as a conductor, we return to central Europe - Bavaria perhaps, and to the work of a number of people, of whom the one who has described it in an available book is Count Gustav von Pohl. Von Pohl's book, *Earth Currents: Causative Factor of Cancer and Other Diseases*, makes interesting reading, particularly in the context of my writing, because some of the 'other diseases' may be classed as 'nervous', psychiatric.

Earth currents are a reality, as are the *ley-lines* of Alfred Watkins to which I referred earlier. It is an immensely great pity that the two have become merged into one concept. The amalgamation is now what many people refer to as ley-lines. It is a pity because the 'Watkins' lines, as he himself described them, should be of value to anyone interested in the movement and communication of people in times as far past as pre-Roman, whereas knowledge and understanding of earth currents and their potential to influence adversely people's health, should be at the disposal of, and accepted by everyone concerned with human and animal well being.

It is unfortunate that a significant number of people have little or no scientific and technological knowledge, and are 'switched off' at the prospect of having to try to understand anything electrical. This is doubly unfortunate because every living thing is a construct of electro-chemical and bio-electronic processes. Furthermore, the planet on which these life processes take place is itself a gigantic electrical machine. The molten iron core behaves like a huge self-exciting dynamo that effectively creates a bar-magnet whose poles produce the earth's north and south magnetic poles. Consequent upon this are the lines of magnetic force associated with all magnets. The lines are conventionally accepted as flowing from the north to the south poles, and have an average strength of 50 micro-teslas. At the latitude of the British Isles, they emerge from the ground at an angle of about eighty degrees to the horizontal, then pass the equator parallel to the surface, re-entering the ground at a similar angle at the latitude of Patagonia, with varying angles of emergence or descent at other latitudes. The presence of a constant and homogeneous magnetic field is necessary for healthy life, for this is one of the background conditions of evolution. When I discuss this concept in more detail in later sections, I shall draw attention to experiments and speculations concerned with the effect on life forms of an absent or modified field.

Taking the reality of the earth as a gigantic rotating electrical machine a step further, one is faced with the fact that all such machines produce attendant lines of electro-magnetic force. In general, these lines form regular matrixes over the surface of the globe, and have been classified as 'Hartmann' and 'Curry' grids respectively. Where one grid interacts with the other, local 'electro'-stresses are produced that can have the effect in life forms of producing what has come to be known as 'geopathic stress'. Many people are sensitive to these locations and cannot bear to remain in them; others are unaware, but nevertheless react internally, and in time may become ill. If, as might easily happen, it is suggested that such illnesses are of psychosomatic origin, it is well to remember that animals and plants also react and may suffer.

If the earth was completely homogeneous, that might be the end of the story as far as the currents that originate locally are concerned, but as it is not, other processes prevail. As an example, consider the situation in which of two different types of rock abut against each other - possibly granite against limestone. In the presence of water, the effect of an electrical battery would be created, and, if a suitable conductor existed, a current would flow. Such a conductor could be an underground aquifer, which, when a current flowed, would be capable of producing its own local 'stream' of geopathic forces. Any forces produced would add to the effects of the previously mentioned Curry and Hartmann grids that might cross its path. In a similar manner, underground fault lines and ore deposits provide conducting paths that, again, would create variations in the grid-induced stresses.

However, the earth is not alone; our parent sun exerts a wide range of electrical effects upon us, apart from giving us light and heat. The sun generates ultraviolet rays that have the effect of ionising the gases in our attendant space. The ions so created are whisked along at colossal speed in the jet streams of the upper atmosphere. Where there exists a flow of charged particles, there exists an electrical current. Essentially, the jet streams create very large currents (at times, as much as 500,000 amperes at local noon) flowing at high speed parallel to the surface of the earth, and which, in turn, have a number of significant consequences. The first and most influential result is the creation of currents within the ground by a process known as 'induction', and which, in a similar manner to the 'battery' currents, seek the path of least resistance. (The path of least

LISTENING TO THE SILENCES

resistance was dramatically demonstrated in 1989, when a huge burst of solar electrical energy hit Canada in a region where there are vast tracts of granite, itself a very poor conductor of electricity. Taking the line of least resistance, the solar electricity burst down the main electrical distribution system and blew all the protection equipment, depriving eight million homes of their power supply for up to a week.)

The charged particles created by ultraviolet rays in our stratosphere recombine when the sun goes down and the currents from this source cease. The jet streams themselves are also a variable phenomenon, and move back and forth across the latitudes with the seasons, producing passing reactions at ground level that may be a component in the ailments that affect many people at different seasons of the year. In the latitudes of the British Isles, the jet streams flow roughly from southwest to northeast, which is also the direction of flow of many of our weather systems and winds. The parallel flowing of the two masses of air, one high and, effectively, an electrical current, the other low and near the surface, causes the latter to adopt particular electrical characteristics derived from the former, reminiscent of, but not the same as, the Föhn wind. The surface air movement from the southwest forms one of the winds that I mentioned earlier, within which people who are sensitive experience specific reactions that I shall describe in detail in the appropriate later section.

Roy Vincent

As I write, and then review what I have written, I am consciously aware that many who will read my words will find themselves in strange territory. Many will query the relevance of what I am writing to mental health, and ultimately, to the understanding of voice hearing and allied phenomena. Perhaps some may feel that they are in danger of becoming lost in an intellectual maze. I am aware also that I have studied and discussed these topics for over twenty years, and live in daily familiarity with my studies and observations. To you who find yourselves in a mental maze, let me say that, just as Theseus was able to move through the maze of Minos by following the thread provided by Ariadne, so also is there a thread running through all that I am writing in this particular section. The thread is this: many individuals who are deemed to be mentally ill are not *intrinsically* ill, but are reacting with a greater or lesser sensitivity to external phenomena. I can only really hint in this part of my narrative at the extent and all-pervasiveness of these various phenomena, and as I read and study even more deeply myself, I realise that there is so much yet to comprehend. I shall try to present a more detailed analysis in later sections, but hope that I am succeeding now in showing that, outside ourselves, and totally outside our control, there are major sources of influence upon our physical and mental well-being and behaviour. I have been asked many times by individuals to whom I have introduced this topic, "What is the point of even considering, let alone trying to

LISTENING TO THE SILENCES

understand these phenomena when they are effectively outside one's control?" The answer is given by those who suffer acutely from the induced effects, and who then realise that *they themselves* are not intrinsically ill, but are reacting to external stimuli that have a *limited duration.* There is no longer the recourse to the bottle, whether of tranquillisers or alcohol, but, instead, the realisation and acceptance that in a few hours, or a day or so, depending upon the particular phenomenon, the symptoms will pass and normality will return. Seeing a life re-emerge after being in a state of inexplicable suppression, makes worthwhile for me the many hours spent in observation and study.

Before passing on from these 'extra-terrestrial' influences, mention of 1989 and the huge burst of solar energy in Canada, reminds me of that year and the two following. These years were at the peak of a sunspot cycle. At such times, many people are grossly affected, and not just as individuals but in the mass. Thus, experts in the field of study would say, the extraordinarily powerful display of the aurora borealis early in 1989 (itself the result of the solar energy) was just a preliminary to the events that followed in such places as Tienaman Square, Strangeways prison (riots), the Persian Gulf (war) and in the disintegration of the Communist Bloc. Individually, I met many who were inexplicably disturbed, and I remember full well that in the spring of 1989 I went for five weeks without a single night of restful or complete sleep. Someone perhaps better known than me is Vincent van Gogh, whose 'religious mania' and suicide both occurred in years of sunspot peaks. The reason that I am including more on this topic than I might otherwise need to do in order to make my point, is that the next peak (years 1999 to and including 2001) produced a comparable range of events, the consequences of which are still unfolding as I write.

The Chinese, an enlightened and pragmatic people, once had an understanding of some of the effects I have described, even if they did not have our modern comprehension of causes. Thus I have no doubt that a component of their natural energy, *chi* or *Qi*, is formed by the 'air electricity', while their 'dragon lines' could be our 'earth currents'. The Chinese, as with many other cultures who were aware of effects without knowing causes, used to enclose sheep on a plot where it was intended to build a house, relying on the animals to show, by their avoidance, the unhealthy locations. Western study of another eastern area of discovery, acupuncture meridians, reveals these to be a form of electrical circuitry of the body and one of the paths of entry or influence of negative ions. In Britain Dr.Julian Kenyon is one who has studied extensively the electrical nature of acupuncture and his books on the subject are well worth reading. In the United States, Dr. Robert O. Becker has written fully from his own research and does much to confirm the truth of these studies. Later I hope to make

LISTENING TO THE SILENCES

significant the reason why I am mentioning acupuncture now.

Whether Sigmund Freud, at whose door I am probably laying much undeserved blame - whether he would have taken note of these effects and phenomena of which he would be largely unaware, is open to question. Questionable because it is apparent that many who have followed, and continue currently to follow, the path that he and his contemporaries opened up, are either still ignorant of, or *choose to ignore*, the causes and effects that I have described so far and to which I will add briefly if you will bear with me.

While the one giant was defining human mental aberrations, and arriving at conclusions that I speculate are flawed because he was not in possession of all the facts, my other giant, Tesla, together with other of his well-known contemporaries, was causing great benefits to be introduced into our lives, together with a then unforeseen, and now continually expanding, range of problems. The great benefits are those resulting from the 'domestication' of electricity. The problems result from the adverse effects upon human physical and mental health of all the means of distribution of electricity and all the appliances and processes that we gladly embrace - and which add to the 'pollution' of our homes, workplaces and general environment. Just as life without motor vehicles would now be unthinkable so likewise would be life without electricity.

However, whereas the majority of life- and limb-threatening problems associated with the former have been identified and tackled, many of the problems that derive from the latter are ignored or frankly denied.

Just as the tobacco manufacturers and their apologists go through a weird process of truth manipulation in the casuistry of denial of health risks, so equally do the spokes-people for the electrical utilities and their retained researchers. However, you have a personal computer, you have access to the Internet; there are hosts of entries under such topics as 'electro-magnetic fields', 'electricity and health' - use your ingenuity - go surf! If you are unwilling or unable to read and explore yourself, just observe. Does an overhead fluorescent tube give you a headache or make you feel confused? How do you feel in bed with an electric under- or over-blanket switched on? If you stand close to your microwave oven when it is running, do you get an odd feeling in your head or central chest? I am not writing this to *alarm* you, but to *alert* you. If you *understand* a little about the potential hazards, and learn how to use the benefits and minimise the risks, all will be well. Can you do without your bedside radio-alarm? That unexplained early morning headache or depression might vanish. Have you developed night-time breathing problems, asthma even? Consider removing that television and/or computer from the bedroom. If you are pregnant, whatever you do, do not use an electric blanket through the night; use it to warm the bed then remove it totally

Every effort is made to deny that there are problems with overhead cables and distribution in general, but the electrical fields generated can be measured or computed, and certainly cannot be wished away nor denied. Rationality and reason should take over, particularly amongst those who study mental health and when considering, for instance, the inexplicable decline of certain people. Take the case of someone living on the ground floor of a tower block in a flat adjacent to where the main electrical feed enters. The field generated by the current supplying all of the flats can be huge, and is known to affect individuals and cause conditions such as depression, or others resembling M.E. If the flats, for example, have under floor electric heating, this is switched on and off, on and off, on and off... through the night as thermostats and demand dictate, and a switched field is often worse than one in a steady state. I keep referring to the fact that I am very sensitive to my electrical environment, and I know from experience that I would find such a location intolerable.

It was my own acute sensitivity that alerted me to consider a possible cause of the death from motor neurone disease (mnd) of my friend and former G.P., Sandy. My visits to my local health centre are infrequent, but each time that I went I became aware of internal feelings that, over time, I have come to associate with electricity or geopathic stressors. The feelings are such that I prefer not to use the patients' waiting room and remain in my car or sit on a bench near by. It was while I was using the bench that my eyes were opened to the source of my disquiet. An electricity distribution pole stands near the corner of the building. One cable runs down the pole, under the consulting room and eventually feeds a small housing estate. Another feeder passes overhead parallel with the roof of the building and supplies more local houses. The *voltage* presents no problem, being simply that of normal domestic supply. It is the *current* that is carried by a cable that creates the harmful electromagnetic (em) field.

Where Sandy sat, he had an electrical feeder approximately two metres to one side, which then turned and went below him at a distance of about one metre. The overhead line ran at a distance of about two metres from his head. I have an instrument that detects em fields and it shows that where he sat was in a centre of high intensity. Sandy was very generous with his time in the consulting room – time that would inevitably be extended during winter months, when the electrical demand would be greatest and the current (and hence the em field) strongest. I have subsequently learned anecdotally of three others who had died from mnd and who worked or slept in locations where the em field would have been high. Two had operated electrical woodworking machines, and had stood close to powerful motors, while the third had lived in a bungalow that had under floor electrical heating.

LISTENING TO THE SILENCES

I wrote to the MND Foundation with my observations and received a polite reply, but was told that they were following entirely different lines of research, and did not have the resources to investigate mine. If my analysis is correct and the electrical field did serious and ultimately fatal damage via the nerves of the physical body, is it not reasonable to deduce that such a field would have a strongly adverse effect upon the brain and mental processes of an individual who spent time in it?

What I am trying to do, and hope that I am succeeding in my attempts, is to demonstrate that there have always been natural phenomena external to humans which, when they have operated, have caused unquantifiable disturbances in human behaviour. The existence of an external cause being unknown, people have been treated as if they were inherently out of control or even mad. From the mid-nineteenth century onwards, other developments have caused to be introduced into industrialised human life, artificial, man-made additions to the natural phenomena, introductions that have resulted in much more serious disturbance, and a vast increase in apparent mental illness. It is so very unfortunate that the serious analysis of the aberrant human mind, that also began roughly in the mid-nineteenth century, has developed and has continued without a knowledge of, or subsequent recognition of, the contribution to mental disruption of many of the adverse external influences.

I have noted above, and will describe more fully later, some of the direct results and possible harmful effects of the introduction of electricity into our lives and homes. My intention now is to illustrate some of the *indirect* consequences of the wide availability and greater use of electricity in all sorts of situations and processes, with a potential to cause harm that I am certain that Tesla and his contemporaries could never have envisaged.

The development of steam-powered pumps had already begun the process of bringing piped water into towns and homes. The increasing availability of electrically operated pumps did much to speed up the spread of such a desirable innovation. Unfortunately, every benevolent advance seems to have a downside, and one of the negatives of this progressive leap was the introduction of lead into people's lives via the domestic water pipe. Brought into use in the latter half of the nineteenth century and only, in Britain, phased out in the equivalent half of the twentieth century, lead pipes created an unwelcome and potentially harmful addition to the 'diet'. The effect of gross lead poisoning was already well known, but what the civic engineers and medical watchdogs were unaware of were the harmful effects of chronic low-level exposure i.e. at a level insufficient to produce 'classical' lead poisoning. There are a number of medical problems, such as stillbirths and heart disease

LISTENING TO THE SILENCES

that have been shown to be caused by low-level lead poisoning. In the context in which I am writing, the interaction of lead within the nervous system is very significant, creating, as it does, learning and behavioural deficits, as, also, is its implication in the generation of delinquent and criminal behaviour - themselves often the result of poor mental development.

'General malaise' - a portmanteau and convenient term standing for the vague symptoms of depression, muscle aches and pains, lethargy and frequent infections - together with immune dysfunction, can all be laid at the door of low-level lead poisoning. When one considers that acid rain, increasing in volume over the century, has leached increasing amounts of lead out of domestic pipes, is it any wonder that more and more people have consulted their doctors with such a catalogue of vague symptoms as those listed, and, there being no obvious cause, have then gone away with a so called 'happy pill'? Lead levels in people have increased and continue to increase, for, additionally, lead has been well and truly introduced into the atmosphere, and atmospheric lead knows no boundaries. Does it surprise you that, in industrial nations, our body lead levels have increased to between 500 and 1000 times those of our ancestors? Does it surprise you that so many people, exhibiting all of these vague symptoms that could be laid at the door of lead, end up being treated for that catch-all condition 'depression'? Does it surprise you that so many people become addicted to their resultant anti-depressants and never dare to relinquish them?

Lead ingestion is not the only downside of municipal water. In earlier days, water was obtained from springs and wells – from deep in the ground, where it had had a chance to capture some of the minerals that are so necessary for a healthy life. Gradually the wells and springs were abandoned in favour of the piped water, and, in many ways, health improved with the eradication of waterborne disease. Unfortunately, in many new catchment areas the water was unable to acquire the desirable minerals, resulting in depletion that may have contributed insidiously to deterioration in health in other ways, and in mental health in particular. I have drawn attention to Seascale, the village in which I lived for a time. Until 1976, it, and the surrounding area, derived a water supply from Wastwater, the not far distant lake. In the period when Calder Hall Nuclear Power Station was being designed, I had access to an analysis of this water, for it was to be used as the boiler feed-water in the process of steam generation. To my astonishment, I found that it was almost totally devoid of minerals. The rain ran quickly over insoluble rock, and stayed locked in a deep and unmixing basin. One can only guess at the adverse effect upon health that this may have had, particularly in respect of people who had moved to the area from, for example, a limestone or chalk water-catchment. Past glaciations had already depleted the soil of vital but soluble nutrients, and minerals that one would normally expect to get from one's water supply were doubly absent. (Local farmers give a wide range of mineral supplements to their stock - magnesium, selenium, copper, cobalt, for example. But humans? Perhaps if humans had a marketable value someone might ensure a *truly* balanced diet; but humans are meant to be responsible, intelligent beings with sufficient free will to take responsibility for their own diets, aren't they? Oh dear!).

    I am trying not to get too involved with aspects of diet and mental health at this stage, but plan to visit the subject in more detail where it becomes relevant to my own experience and observation, particularly in respect to my determination to take responsibility for my own health and well being. However, where the mushrooming technology of living has introduced an alien input into one of the sources of good mental health, our food, my object is to bring it into view and return in more detail at a later stage.

    Another alien intrusion into healthy life that arrived courtesy of the freely available electricity is aluminium. In its naturally occurring form in soil, aluminium is very widely present and humanity must have evolved being tolerant of this substance, or even using it metabolically in its natural evolution. Even if this is so, I have been unable to find any reference to the beneficent use of aluminium in the body's metabolism. The greater availability of electricity allowed the large-scale extraction of *metallic* aluminium from its ore, bauxite, and its widespread dispersion in the forms of cooking-ware, cans and containers. In terms of human health, I can find nothing to be said in its favour, the reverse in fact, for everything points to it being inimical to life. Much has been written about the possible contribution of aluminium to, for example, Alzheimer's disease. A more overt and practical demonstration of the adverse effects of the metal came from a friend who built yachts with hulls made of the metal. If he ever cut himself on it, the wound took an unconscionable time to heal, with the aluminium seemingly acting as an *inhibitor* of the natural life processes.

Here is a little conundrum for you to puzzle over while you nibble your after-dinner mint. Sodium and potassium are very close to each other chemically and functionally, and if one ingests too much sodium, then potassium cannot be retained in correct balance (classic heart and stroke advice). Aluminium and magnesium are also very close to each other on the Periodic Table of the Elements, and exhibit many properties in common. In the processes of human metabolism, if there is insufficient magnesium present to fulfil the body's requirements, and if there is available aluminium, does the latter mimic the former and find its way into the cellular and other activity of the body, and if so, with what consequences? Many people when the question is put say that it seems a reasonable supposition,

LISTENING TO THE SILENCES

but no one has yet been able to say whether I am correct or not. (A report that I read recently described the results of the examination of the brains of people who had died from Alzheimer's disease. Where aluminium was present in the tissues, there was an equivalent depletion in magnesium). Every modern source that I read describing various approaches and analyses of dietary needs, stresses that in Britain, mainly because of past glaciations, magnesium is poorly available, and that unless one has a good intake of organically grown leafy, green vegetables, or takes supplements, one is unlikely to have a sufficient intake for good health. Many things follow, but in terms of mental health, listed consequences of insufficient magnesium are poor memory, inertia, depression, anorexia to name but four. Obviously there is much to consider, and I am no dietary expert - a constant source book for me is *Nutritional Medicine* by Drs. Stephen Davies and Alan Stewart, which is very 'accessible' to the layperson

So if aluminium is replacing magnesium, what then? The thought often crosses my mind as I see someone slurping on a soft drinks can. Such intimate contact with the metal of a can that contains phosphoric acid - what then? Yes it does. After carbonated water and sugar, phosphoric acid is the next major ingredient in many popular soft drinks. So, does the acid leach more aluminium? I don't know, but it is well recorded that the phosphorus is needed in exquisite balance with calcium and magnesium for correct cellular function and if one gets too much of it - and if the aluminium is buggering up the magnesium... I'm just glad that it is not my problem. But at another level it is, for since some of the drinks contain caffeine in quantities that can cause hyperactivity in young children, it becomes a *social* problem for everyone as we see a developing generation of hyperactive near-cretins. And since many drinks contain caramel (E150) as a colouring agent, and since many people are sensitive to aspirin, and since E150 belongs to that group which, in aspirin sensitive people, can provoke an asthma attack, or even induce asthma...

Some of the same products are passed off as so-called 'diet' drinks i.e. having reduced or no sugar. In very many cases, the sugar substitute is Aspartame. If you have access to the Web, simply type in that name in your search facility. The Web is *full* of reports and articles from many sources, the majority listing the ninety-plus serious medical conditions that can be induced by consumption of the substance. In the context of my writing, just one will suffice, namely 'depression'.

I have carried out a further review of what I have written so far in this section and I have realised that my own enthusiasm is in danger of carrying me away from you. Reflecting that I had observed and experimented and amassed information during more than twenty years, I found

LISTENING TO THE SILENCES

that I was opening the floodgates of my knowledge and risked overwhelming you. Consequently, I have removed and sidelined several pages of discussion and, if they are still relevant, will develop the contents in appendices. I had written about the problems that can result from the presence of mercury and nickel in the mouth whether incorporated in dental amalgam or certain types of tooth crown – problems that can be of a general nervous and psychiatric nature. I had also drawn attention to the effects created by the presence of iron in our lives where it occurs in building construction and central heating radiators. Although it may not be obvious now, nevertheless I shall justify my inclusion of these topics and others that I have removed when later I include and explore them. They were all part of the thread of continuity, which was in danger of becoming tangled!

For now, I wonder whether I have succeeded in my proposition that much of modern psychiatry has stayed in a channel of thought created by the unintentional ignorance and unawareness of the early progenitors. With a mind-set having been created, how difficult it is to broaden the channel to accommodate new knowledge - just as in religion, believers in Creation refuse to accept the concept of evolution in spite of the evidence of fossils and the logic that supports the evidence. All that I have written or will write is based upon personal experiences, logic and reason and I write it to try release anyone whom I can reach through my words who is chained in the 'creation myths' of psychiatry.

While I hope that what I write will eventually be read by professionals, my principal purpose in writing is to reach you who are suffering or you who are trying to support and inspire someone whom you love and care for. Do not believe that your case is hopeless; do not, you carer, believe that you cannot help and motivate. If nothing from the field of mental health inspires you, look elsewhere. Here, try this - *Self Healing: My Life and Vision* by Meir Schneider - "The remarkable account of the author who cured himself of congenital blindness by discovering the body's own inner resources, and who taught thousands of others, some with 'incurable' diseases to heal themselves". Meir's problem was very apparent from the time of his birth in Russia. A botched operation provided no improvement, and, following emigration to Israel, he was to be registered blind and trained as such. However, he had *just* a glimmer of light in his vision, and that glimmer gave him hope, and he seized it. If the book doesn't inspire you as you read of what can be achieved by sheer dogged insight, persistence, courage, and an innate belief in the self-healing powers of the human mind and body, achieved in Meir's case in the face of active opposition from family and authority - if this doesn't inspire you to set to work on your self or the one in your care, whatever will?

LISTENING TO THE SILENCES

I know from long hard experience that it is difficult, nigh impossible, to pull yourself up by your own bootstraps, but Meir shared his struggle with other allegedly incurable comrades, and all in their own ways achieved progress. He eventually moved to California and has generated a whole new movement aimed at promoting the self-healing potential within anyone who is motivated to try the techniques that practical experience and experiment have been shown to work so effectively. Meir runs courses worldwide to train teachers, and holds workshops to help individuals, but in addition he has produced a work manual, *The Handbook of Self-Healing,* that can be used by individuals themselves or by health teachers and practitioners. If you say "This is not for me, my problem is in my mind", just remember the often quoted saying 'A healthy mind in a healthy body' and *try* it, acknowledging also that the book does not aim solely at physical defects, for there is a section on creating and maintaining a healthy *nervous system.*

In the part aimed at helping brain-injured children, the book quotes the work and practice of a renowned therapist Glenn Doman. Doman works with great success from his belief that progress and recovery must follow the original development pattern of initial arm and leg movement without body action, followed by creeping and crawling in sequence and finally walking, proceeding ostensibly through the initial embryo stages of fish, reptiles and mammals, and only achieving results if the sequential stages are followed in that order. I am personally very interested in Doman's concept, for I have developed a similar belief concerning the extent to which our evolution is still within us *in totality.*

You may never think about it, but without exception, you are mammals: if you disagree, just look at your chest and see the externals of the mammary glands there. Albeit a mammal with intellect - and that is the root of the problem. The core of your behaviour and reaction is the result of millions of years of evolution culminating in *Homo erectus, habilis, neanderthalensis* and *sapiens,* and it all continues to reside in you, that incredible journey. There is still within you all of the essence and potential reaction to circumstances that have always dictated the behaviour of the component parts of the body and their response to external stimuli and challenges. The problem for us humans is that, having intellect, we create far more situations and problems than the evolving 'us' had to contend with at any stage in our evolution, and that is at the heart of our nervous and mental problems, excluding those resulting from actual physical and chemical damage. Even some of the facial asymmetries that I shall consider later in my work may be the result of conflict between intellect and 'inheritance'. This then is the dichotomy of evolution and intellect to which I plan to return in due course as I attempt to unravel its influence upon our mental health.

LISTENING TO THE SILENCES

In the meantime, and all the while as I go about my daily chores, I wonder and speculate, as one does, whether the mammoths suffered from migraine; whether orang-utans in the wild have incurable personality problems; whether *homo neanderthalensis* was ever depressed or anxious and how he coped - perhaps he became extinct because he didn't have tranquillisers to help him come to terms with the fact that it was getting warmer and the sea level was rising, or maybe he received modified shock treatment in the form of a sharp blow to the head with a stick or club; whether any of our distant forebears were conscious of the concept of 'spirit'; whether any or all had the experience of intruding voices in the mind, and what was the response of *homo habilis* - whether he made an improved stone axe following instructions from the 'divine'. Of course, I will never know, but I do know something about 'voices' and 'divine and malign intrusions', all of which appear in the next twist of this devious maze through which I am trying to lead you.

At the outset, Paracelsus called us to view the bright new star of imagination: however, from here onwards I have to ask you to accept actual evidence, the evidence of personal experience, the experience that says that voices in the mind are *not* the product of imagination, but of a reality. This reality belongs to the people who actually have these experiences, and these are the people to whom you in turn must listen…

Roy Vincent

CHAPTER 5

If

You, yourself, have never heard

discarnate voices

in your mind,

how possibly can you tell

someone who has, that they

are

deluded?

Roy Vincent

LISTENING TO THE SILENCES

There never was a king like Solomon
Not since the world began,
Yet Solomon talked to a butterfly
As a man would talk to a man.

The Bible does not record, neither does Rudyard Kipling, who wrote the verse, whether the butterfly ever replied, and with what voice. Solomon was fortunate in that he wore a ring which, it was accepted, gave him the ability to converse with 'beasts, fowl, creeping things and fishes'; without the ring, and admitting to 'hearing voices', today's Solomon would have an inevitable fate - 'Just like Harpic, clean round the bend!'

There can be no doubt that to many people, professional and lay alike, the hearing of voices in the mind is a mental illness. In reality, it is not an illness at all. That there are people who hear voices who are also ill cannot be disputed. However, as you read on you will see that it is my contention that some voice hearers are already ill, undermined, depleted, isolated, for a variety of reasons and causes and, in that state, begin to hear voices, whilst others start to experience voices through a variety of ways that I shall illustrate, and are then made ill as a result of the treatment to which they are subjected. That a person can be made very ill by medical treatment I have already amply demonstrated, and from the fullness of personal experience - experience which increasingly, we learn, is far from uncommon.

The fact that 'hearing voices' is called an 'illness' and treated as such by those who have public authority in the field of mental health, or have the public ear through the various organs of mass-media; the fact that virtually the only times a voice-hearer features in these media is as a 'schizophrenic' - usually a '*paranoid* schizophrenic', and equally usually, by implication or directly, a '*violent* paranoid schizophrenic' - because of these facts and a variety of other related factors, there are many voice-hearers who do not reveal themselves as such, because immediately they would be labelled as 'mentally ill', categorised, made to have 'treatment', and would become stigmatised.

Is it not odd that there is no universal definition of schizophrenia? I have a recording of a BBC 'Medicine Now' broadcast of some years ago, that was devoted wholly to the topic, and in which this fact is frankly admitted by speakers – all eminent in their mental health fields - some of whom quite positively asserted that, for example, the definition differed depending on which side of the Atlantic it was made! Thus we have Harvard medical graduate and a Professor in Psychiatry at the University of California, Dr. John W. Perry, writing "Let me specify at the outset exactly which condition I am speaking of here: this is only one among many syndromes that pass under the name 'schizophrenia'..." In the preface to his scholarly, but very readable, and certainly beautifully written book, *Schizophrenia Genesis*, Dr. Irving I. Gottesman writes that "A heritage of distortions, stagnant certainty, and self-serving territoriality characterises the fields of knowledge about this dreaded disorder - aptly called 'the cancer of the mind' ", and offers his book "...to help fill the information gap between the 'ivory towers of academia', with its research 'factories' and private language, and the idiosyncratic narratives glorifying or obfuscating disorders of the mind".

"The scientists" writes Dr. Gottesman "are revealed as the fallible, egoistic, political, territorial, and *humane* beings that they are" and I can say with the certainty of one who has read his book, that Dr. Gottesman reveals *himself* to be most humane. There can be no doubt that the majority of those working in the fields of mental health and medicine strive to relieve the suffering of people, whether as individuals or in the mass, and I want nothing that I write to imply, or even to be read as implying, criticism of their intent and motives.

However, withal, many lay people are uneasy when they consider the immense social powers that are invested in these same medical scientists when they acquire the letters M.D. after their names. In matters of ethics and morals, they are expected to have God-like powers of understanding and discernment and of making decisions affecting life and death. In the field of mental health that concerns me now, there are powers of incarceration and compulsion that, in other fields of social activity, require the full apparatus of the law and courts.

An asylum, by definition, is a 'benevolent institution affording shelter and support to some class of the afflicted and unfortunate'. Would that the reality met the definition; would that the concept of asylum as an attitude, embraced not only buildings and establishments, but also the *way* in which mentally afflicted people were regarded by society. 'Benevolent', 'shelter', 'support' - lovely words, words that I found at the very heart of 'The Retreat' mental hospital in York, which I visited recently; a centre of excellence in its approach to the *care* of people, and which gives hope of an ultimate change in attitude.

Too often the reality for a voice hearer is a closed ward, drugs that have side effects that can be worse than many illnesses and which carry the risk of dependency - and even electro-convulsive therapy: treatments that it is believed will cure a condition that does not yet have a universally accepted definition, and which appears to have many bizarre causes and by-products:

> Some schizophrenics have a thicker than normal *corpus callosum*...

LISTENING TO THE SILENCES

Some schizophrenics have high levels of 'sulphite' in the urine…

Some schizophrenics exhibit high levels of copper in serum and hair analysis…

Some schizophrenics have nutrient deficiencies, especially of B vitamins, zinc, magnesium, chromium, manganese and vitamin C, while food intolerances are common in many…

   Some schizophrenics have a greater than
   normal susceptibility to arthritis…

Babies born in cities during the winter are at greater risk of developing schizophrenia in later life than those born in country areas, or in summer (possibly because of damage in the womb caused by influenza in the expectant mother)…

Some schizophrenics have a larger than normal left lateral ventricle…

Unfortunately, one could go on and on and on…

When I started to write, I did not intend to provide an analysis of *Schizophrenia Genesis,* neither shall I, except to draw one further quotation from it - Dr. Gottesman writes - "Schizophrenia is a complex disorder of human functioning. The absence so far of a solution to its origins compels me to be skeptical about received wisdom from all participants, however noble and well-intended. I am, however, optimistic about finding solutions via the energies of scientists and the canons of science within a decade."

The decade having ended with the Millennium, and no solution to the problem as perceived being even faintly in sight, I wonder whether I can be accepted as one of the 'scientists' to whom Dr.Gottesman refers? Or, perhaps, accepted as a bridge from scientists to the world of actuality, of the reality of what is? Just as in my work, I was such a bridge between scientists and the engineering functions of the practical, the possible. As I have written, by training and profession I am an electrical engineer who specialised in instrumentation and measurement. For 10 years, I was the Senior Instrument Engineer at the world's first commercial nuclear power plant, Calder Hall. The bridge that I provided was between the scientists who decided what they wanted to achieve within the inaccessible world at the core of a nuclear reactor, and my instrumentation that enabled them to try to achieve it and told them whether or not they had done so.

However, analogies can be stretched too far. If the scientists who are using the canons of science to try to find a cause and cure for schizophrenia really want the answers, they must abandon their science and become just ordinary people. The canons of science that they must apply are those of fundamental *human* science - the canons of personal experience. For unless the scientists themselves start to hear voices or acknowledge the truth of what the voice-hearers themselves say, they will never identify the true cause, which very many of us who hear voices already know with stark certainty

They will certainly never find a *cure* via science. All that will be achieved will be the creation of more mind suppressors, or variations of E.C.T, perhaps, perpetuating one of medicine's more notorious barbarisms.

Yes, I am a voice-hearer and have been for over twenty years, during which time I have never sought, nor would have accepted, the intervention of psychiatry or medicine. I know the exact moment when, and the exact mechanism by which the intrusions into my mind and body began. Yes, <u>intrusions</u>, not *delusions* nor *hallucinations.*

The scientists who would know the cause of schizophrenia must join the rest of the human race - at least that part of it which acknowledges the existence of a spiritual state of being.

Is it not odd that, worldwide, and for virtually the whole of recorded history, there are or have been popes and prelates; bishops and priests of all sorts and persuasions; rabbis; muftis and mullahs; ayatollahs and archimandrites; assorted clerics and ministers of a variety of religions; lamas, shamans and medicine men; and a whole range of other religious functionaries, all proclaiming, and at least 60% of the population of the world believing or paying lip service to the belief, that there exists a spiritual world or 'dimension'; that there is spiritual good and spiritual evil, and that the religion which each espouses is the one that will help to avoid evil, promote good and bring a happy landing in the heaven of choice? Yet, when it comes to *applying* the reality of this belief to the relief and understanding of the human condition in our 'enlightened' western culture - Oh dear me no! "Intrusive spirits, *evil* spirits? ... My *dear* chap...ha...ha... that's positively *mediaeval* and arcane!... Yes, of course I pray in my faith...To whom or what, you ask?... Yes, of course I am asking for spiritual intervention, and to be protected from evil, if you put it like that".

    My former parish priest would often deliver sermons or homilies based upon the wonderful and noble deeds of someone, now probably canonised, who had achieved so much at the behest of spiritual voices, but would invariably end by saying "Of course, if any of *us* hear voices, we should seek psychiatric help". So there you have it; look no further; the great dichotomy, the great divide! If you hear voices that encourage you to do noble deeds, or give you aid or succour at times of tribulation, well, my dear

LISTENING TO THE SILENCES

people, they must be of divine origin, coming from at least an angel or saint, or even God Himself. *But,* if you hear voices that are nasty, tormenting, obscene; voices that are threatening, or encourage you to do things that you know are unwise or wrong - well, you poor sod, you are deluded, hallucinating, you must be 'sectioned', isolated and *treated.*

When I told the same priest, as I shall tell you, exactly what happened to me, he heard me out and then said "Oh my dear chap, my heart bleeds for you, you have had a breakdown, but you're obviously all right now; get the kettle on there's a good chap". When the *religious* have lost their way in their chosen world of spirit, within which they should be guides, what hope is there for the rudderless, blown hither and thither by tormenting voices?

Once there was *certainty.* Ignatius of Loyola, founder of the Jesuit Order, in his Spiritual Exercises, defined *Rules for the Discernment of Spirits*, i.e. is the spirit that has entered your mind or presence from God, or is it malevolent? A recent writer in the same Order follows the modern trend of watering down, even abandoning, the concept of intrusive spiritual malevolence and instead writes of the 'discernment of *moods'.* He also advises his retreatants to keep a dream diary 'in case God is speaking to them in their dreams'. No doubt he, like many, was suffering from a surfeit of Jung!

From priests and religious who come under the spell of Jung, may the good Lord deliver us.
No, we must return to a third Jesuit to put the matter right and help us to retrace a step or two. In his book *Silent Music*, a study of meditation, William Johnston treats of the perils of too hasty a descent into the 'deeper realms of the mind' and quotes from Dr.Elmer Green of the Menninger Foundation, who writes:

"According to various warnings, the persistent explorer in these realms... *brings himself to the attention of indigenous beings who, under normal circumstances, pay little attention to humans...*
...Systems for inner exploration describe these indigenous beings as entities whose bodies are composed entirely of emotional, mental and etheric substance, and say that at this level of development they are psychologically no better than average man himself. They are of many natures and some are malicious, cruel and cunning, and use the emergence of the explorer out of his previously protective cocoon with its built-in barriers of mental and emotional substance as an opportunity to move, in reverse so to speak, into the personal subjective realm of the investigator. If he is not relatively free from personality dross, it is said, they can obsess him with various compulsions for their own amusement and in extreme cases can even disrupt the normally automatic functioning of the nervous system, by controlling the brain through the *chakras*. Many mental patients have made the

LISTENING TO THE SILENCES

claim of being controlled by subjective entities, *but the doctors in general regard these statements as part of the behavioural aberration, pure subconscious projections, and do not investigate further*".

Johnston continued - "I reflected that a decade ago religious people were affirming the existence of devils, while the scientist smiled with amused incredulity. But now, just as we find religious people doubting about devils, we find the scientists affirming their existence. And so the wheel turns". (The particular chapter entitled *A Perilous Journey* is worth reading in its entirety).

Dr. Kenneth McAll qualified in medicine in Edinburgh and then spent a number of years, including war internment by the Japanese, as a missionary-surgeon in China. Returning to Britain, he worked for the next ten years in general practice and from then onwards as a Consultant Psychiatrist. His experience in China led to interest in the power of 'possession', and he has devoted his life since to the curing of psychiatric illness 'through divine guidance'. In his book *Healing the Family Tree* Dr. McAll writes -

"When patients come to me, often after enduring years of unsuccessful medical and psychiatric treatment, they can be in a highly unreceptive state of mind, unwilling to co-operate and reluctant to trust another doctor…When a mutual feeling of trust has been established, the patients are usually able to unburden themselves of the 'secrets' that have been the source of their illnesses.

Many emotional problems have their roots in a purely biochemical imbalance which requires medication, and this can be remedied easily enough when once identified, although it is not always easy to discover. But many deep emotional hurts need a different sort of therapy and the supportive love of a Christian community. *We cannot ignore any means by which the full healing of an individual can be achieved.*

An increasing number of the patients sent to me admitted that they suffered from the presence of 'spirits' or the intrusion of 'voices' from another world which were apparent and audible only to themselves and which psychiatry dismissed as madness. This was reminiscent of the traditional Chinese superstitions about good and evil spirits that I had encountered so many times when I lived in the Far East. Gradually, I realised that the spirits and the voices were real and also that there was a distinction between them. Some seemed to be evil and often came as the result of occult practices, while others seemed to be neutral, harmless voices begging for help. Sometimes the patient could identify the voices as belonging to a recently dead relative, but often there was no known connection in the patient's mind.

Who were these unbidden, unquiet spirits? Why and how could they hold living people in bondage…".

LISTENING TO THE SILENCES

Perhaps we should ask a former President of the Royal College of Psychiatrists. Professor Andrew Sims of Leeds University is quoted as saying that psychiatrists should give less emphasis to a patient's sex life and more to his or her prayer life. Many people, he said, spent more time in prayer than in sexual intercourse, so "why is it therefore that prayer is given much less prominence by our profession in our enquiries of patients?" And further - "Psychiatrists have exclusively concentrated upon the mental and ignored, to the extent of denying, the possibility of another, spiritual, dimension".

I have drawn, and could draw even more, from the language and the writings of the Christian tradition to add weight to my own writing, but therein lies a danger, the danger of alienating those who have no religion or whose religion has a different interpretation. In other philosophies, some may refer to *entities* or *energies;* others will dismiss totally any suggestion of an intervening spiritual dimension. However, it is my intention to continue without trying to draw again from any particular faith or philosophy, but to write in terms with which I am most comfortable such as *spirits* and *spiritual intrusion* and to hope that my work will be read without *any* religious mind-set.

To return to the secular let me draw from the experience of a clinical psychologist:

For sixteen years, Wilson van Dusen worked in this role at Mendocino State Hospital, California. He reports that in that time in his professional work, and also out of human interest, he examined thousands of mentally ill persons. Out of his work came one extraordinary chapter in his book *The Presence of Other Worlds,* a chapter entitled 'The Presence of Spirits in Madness'. I obtained my copy of the book quite by chance in most convoluted circumstances, and began to read that particular chapter well into the night. So great was the impact upon me that I could barely restrain myself from ringing friends, even though it was well past normal bedtimes. The reason for my excitement was that what he wrote so mirrored my own experiences that it was quite uncanny.

Van Dusen is a student of the writings of Emmanuel Swedenborg - a man who claims to have had close association with spiritual beings. He writes "By an extraordinary series of circumstances I seem to have found a confirmation for one of Emanuel Swedenborg's more unusual findings: that man's life involves an interaction with a hierarchy of spirits. This interaction is normally not conscious, but perhaps in some cases of mental illness it has become conscious".

Some time later, I found the same chapter referred to in a fascinating book by psychiatrist Shakuntala Modi M.D. Dr. Modi is also a hypnotherapist, and found that under hypnosis some of her patients were able to reveal attachment, or 'possession' by spirits of differing degrees of malignancy. Using methods that she describes, Dr. Modi was able to obtain their release or detachment, to the obvious benefit, and often permanent relief, of people suffering from a wide variety of conditions, ranging from schizophrenia to obsessions, compulsions, eating and self-harm disorders. I am sure that there are those who, if they should read Dr Modi's book, would dismiss it out of hand. All I can say is that she is a reputable psychiatrist, and that case studies can always be checked independently. Additionally, she does not say "this or that is true", but rather "*this* is what I was told by this person when under hypnosis, this is the action that I took in response, and this is the apparent result, make of it what *you* will"

Would that such a frank approach was adopted by others when writing in their chosen field, particularly when they are writing in an area of uncertainty, and even more so when the greatest uncertainty in question is 'what is the truth?'. It can be guaranteed that in whatever field of uncertainty one cares to choose, there will be found zealots who will proclaim 'the truth' with a degree of *certainty*, almost in direct proportion to the lack of acknowledged truth and fact available. I have just returned to my keyboard from a mid-morning coffee break during which, much against my better judgment, I switched on my local radio station to listen to an interview with the author of a new book about King Arthur. Now, like many people, I have views about the existence or non-existence of King Arthur, and indeed make a personal analysis in which my knowledge of the Welsh language plays a part. I don't normally listen or read anymore, because I often experience a near apoplexy at some of the views expressed and 'truths' derived - thus, and for instance, when the author proclaims with great certainty that Excalibur is a Welsh word, when it isn't. But I stuck with it, and found that there were elements of what he was saying with which I agreed, but more than that, I enjoyed his enthusiasm, to the extent that I am trying to find his phone number in Kelso so that I can discuss and share some of my own ideas. But whatever we share, neither of us, nor anyone else in the field, will *ever* know the truth.

This is the unfortunate reality in many, many fields of human belief and endeavour. By post the other day came the catalogue of a publisher of Christian books - there are forty-three A4 pages filled with lists of books, videos and CDs, all deriving from a basic truth, but having such a variety of different approaches to this truth that could lead the aspirant to a feeling of being overwhelmed - even to the abandonment of a personal 'search'. But this is a Roman Catholic publisher, and undoubtedly there will be equivalent lists for Anglicans, Non-conformists, Church of Scotland - and that is just in Britain - all with as many adherents and variants of their own truth as there are individuals to proclaim them. I have no wide knowledge of Buddhism nor of Islam, but much the same seems to apply; the range of divisions and sub-divisions seems to be as large as in Christianity, and publications and personal proclamations of the 'truth' are no doubt legion – and so on, through all the major and minor religions.

Also by the same post came a catalogue of books, CDs, videos and equipment for the searchers and aspirants in 'alternative' ways - ways of healing, whether of one's self, others or the 'planet', - ways of opening the mind; of protecting it from 'psychic intrusion' - indeed, almost every field of human endeavour is covered. How about 'Awakening the Third Eye'; 'Colon Cleansing'; 'God's Secret Formula'; 'The Sirius Mystery' or 'Sacred Smoke', for starters. One can buy beautiful singing-bowls, crystals, and shamans' drums. One can enrol to be enlightened and empowered to heal within the comparatively new field of Reiki - three weekends and nearly £400 will see one emerge as a Master capable of teaching others. But what's this - 'The Lost Steps of Reiki' allegedly 'channelled' teaching from Wei Chi who lived 5,000 years ago! Back to the drawing board!

I am not writing anything aimed at deriding or undermining the beliefs of *anyone.* Indeed, I have found such a wealth of spiritually beautiful and caring people within all of the fields of belief that I have touched on, and have my own field of input into the lives of other people. Essentially, I am trying to demonstrate the varieties and range of 'truth' that exist 'out there'. Additionally, it has become so easy to get into print, and to go public, and many books, web pages, videos and cassettes are being disgorged that are not based upon adequate experience. Many people have entered alternative practices from work in communications or the media of one sort or another; people who already know the slick ways of getting something published; who know the right chat-shows on which to get publicity, and from whom books are spewed out without any depth or worth. A welter of books, that smother the market, and often overshadow the well-researched publication derived from the deep and long-experienced insights of the author, who, not having the publicity acumen of many a hack, finds his book lost without trace.

There are undoubtedly many fields of publishing endeavour where this must be the case - the one who arrives firstest with the mostest, the one who has most 'clout', the one with the most prominent backer, who gets most publicity and 'air-time', whatever the real *merit* of the work. I have only been on the fringe of academic research and publishing, but observation leads me to suspect that the urge to get into print, to get noticed, to add to an impressive list of work already published, must be a prime driving force of many. Often, it seems, volume of work published, promotion and funding appear to have a direct correlation. I recollect an occasion in my work when it was planned to merge three crafts - electrical, mechanical and instrumentation - for first-line maintenance, in order to increase speed of response, and I decided that a functional simulator would be very effective in presenting real, live, cross-discipline faults and breakdowns. I happened to mention this project to an academic whom I met at a conference, and who was sufficiently interested to want to get involved. He visited me at the Works, and had discussions with a variety of engineers, then left, but 'hit the ground running', for something got into the post that night, then shortly afterwards, and again, shortly after that. Great enthusiasm, no fault there, but no *depth*, no practicality, just a seeming, almost Pavlovian response i.e. to get into immediate print, willy-nilly.

I have read several books derived from psychiatrists engaged in research into the causes and potential cure of schizophrenia. In each case, in each book, I look in vain for something *original*, being myself someone who is desperately looking for a voice, an opinion, a *reality* with which I can identify; a *practicality* that can have relevance in the lives of people whom I know. What I find is a recycling of much that has gone before with very little added value. I can only read for a limited period, for, in truth, I find myself back in the 'Caucus Race' which Alice had defined for her by the Dodo - remember? - "…the best way to explain it is to do it, keep running in a circle until you stop, no start, no finish and everyone is a winner". Why do I say this? Well it seems that every author refers to every other researcher who has published in the field. A sort of incestuous Caucus Race. 'A' refers to 'B' and 'C' with whom he agrees; disagrees partially with

'D'; completely with 'E'; speculates about the methodology of 'F,G & H' et al, whom he cites frequently to give credence to his own views, which seem to derive from those of 'P','Z' and 'Q', with whom he is in *total* agreement, but as they have published in German there is little hope of mere mortals checking. After all, if, as I have, one has human concern for someone who is dubbed 'schizophrenic', one is desperate to know what is the relevance of *Reactions to Psychotropic Medications* by Tormatore, Sramek, Okeya and Pi (1987), or to learn more about *Cannabis and Schizophrenics: a longitudinal study of Swedish conscripts* by Andreasson, Allebech, Engstrom and Rydberg (also 1987), if only to know whether the conscripts were laid end to end to end. Or maybe Slater (1943) has a point with *The neurotic constitution: a study of two thousand neurotic soldiers.* I can just see it, can't you? Two thousand soldiers laid end to end in a longitudinal study - (with an average height of 1.75m they extend for almost two kilometres!) and then wonder why they are neurotic! Did you want to know, as I am sure you do, whether cortical pruning has any significance in the causation of schizophrenia, or whether it is caused by programmed synaptic elimination during adolescence? Why, you will find answers in the assorted publications of Feinberg, Hoffman and Dobschka.

I jest, of course, but with horribly serious intent, for, to a man, these authors each admit that, as yet, no one knows what

LISTENING TO THE SILENCES

schizophrenia is, or what is its cause or its cure. Yet, here is book 'A' - highly respected author, who, in something like 250 pages, has 494 references to published work, and cites over 500 different individuals involved in authorship; or book 'B', with a few less pages, but with 300 references, and 360 citations; and similarly with other books. In the vast reaches of Christian theology, there is, in fact, a 'Jesus Industry' that sustains endless research, analysis, discussion, conferences, synods. Likewise in the echoing corridors of psychiatry, there is a 'Schizophrenia Industry' with similar echelons, and equally immense published outpourings - there is even a *Schizophrenia Magazine!* But where, in the vast verbiage of the religious outpouring, is the ordinary person to whom Jesus was speaking? Vanished without trace. In a like manner, the 'schizophrenia theology' does not deal with *individuals.* You cannot simply take a study of 50,000 soldiers and say that you have a result that applies to *all* neurotic soldiers, unless you have 50,000 clones. So how can any study involving numbers, double blind trials etc, have any relevance to the isolated individual - not a *patient*, but a *person*? The sad fact is that in spite of all the verbiage, no one knows what is the cause of schizophrenia, nor how to cure it, yet the poor sods who exhibit (or maybe, in some cases, *don't* exhibit) what are called the 'first rank symptoms' of the so-called illness, are treated with mind bending, addictive drugs and possibly E.C.T. In other fields of human activity, I am sure that there would be great regulation and oversight, so why not here? Prisons have Boards of Visitors. Where, one might ask, are the Visitors to the prisons of the mind and to the prisoners held by the chains of these drugs – which, often, they have been taking with no remission until they are too scared to come off them, or are rendered inadequate by them? Prisons have their proportion of recidivists created by the 'system'; psychiatric recidivists are often created by *medication.*

'First Rank Symptoms' - "what are these?" I hear you ask. In the 1930s, a German psychiatrist, Kurt Schneider, devised the following list which has found wide approval:-

1   Voices speak one's thoughts aloud.
2   Two or more voices (in the mind) discuss one in the third person.
3   Voices describe one's actions as they happen.
4   Bodily sensations are imposed by an external force.
5   Thoughts stop, and one feels that they are extracted by an external force.
6   Thoughts, not "really" one's own, are inserted among one's own thoughts.
7   Thoughts are broadcast onto the outside world and heard by all.
8   Alien feelings are imposed by an external force.
9   Alien impulses are imposed by an external force.

LISTENING TO THE SILENCES

10 "Volitional" actions are imposed by an external force.
11   Perceptions are "delusional" and un-understandable.

It is only recently that I have seen such a list, but over the last *twenty years,* I have experienced all eleven reactions. I do not call them *symptoms* for I am not ill. As you read of my experiences in what follows of my narrative, you will see how this came about and you will see, written in my own words, the equivalent phenomena set in the context of some bizarre and, at times, disturbing events. You will also read of how, for a very brief period when I could not cope with my immediate circumstances, I took refuge in the local hospital, though not as a 'schizophrenic', but as someone deemed to be suffering from a bout of depression.
                It was to relate these particular events that I began to write (it seems an age ago now - you will perhaps have noticed how the view from the window beside my PC has reflected the passing seasons). I wrote with the intention that you should appreciate fully my accounts of what happened - how it was that I came to experience intrusions in the first place, and what I have learned and recorded over the intervening years. To do this I felt it necessary to tell you of all that has gone before, so that you could see the basis for my mistrust of much that passes for, and is done in the name of, psychiatry. I have no idea what will become of my manuscript when I have finished, for I am already weary of it all, and the

constant exposure of myself and my inner being, without having to contemplate the tedium of publication and possible editing and modification, for it has all come from my gut. To alter it or take much away would be to remove something of me, and I have already lost too much. And yet, I was/am prepared to give more, for I have offered to collaborate with any research programme within reasonable reach of my home, to have my brain scanned, and ultimately to leave it and any other useful bits to science. I have not made the offer widely yet, but initial response has been non-existent, as has been the professional response to my offers to share all my experiences purely for the benefit of sufferers. That is one of my chief indictments of the professional world of medicine - you appear as one of the active runners in the Caucus Race, a practitioner, or you appear as a patient, in which latter case you have no voice, no intelligent input. Or you do not appear at all, you don't exist, for, except in a few rare cases, the professionals have no interest in any contributions that you may endeavour to make.

But come, let us not be downhearted, something is about to happen…

CHAPTER 6

O, what a world of unseen visions and heard silences, this insubstantial country of the mind!

What ineffable essences, these touchless rememberings and unshowable reveries!

☐

And the privacy of it all!

Roy Vincent

LISTENING TO THE SILENCES

"This consciousness that is myself of selves, that is everything, and yet nothing at all" What is it? And where did it come from? And why?"

Julian Jaynes had not expressed these thoughts in public at the time that I had that conversation with Gilbert B... Even if he had, I doubt whether they would have exercised my mind for very long - definitely not in the context of what it was that Gilbert wanted to tell me. I certainly could never have dreamed - not even in my *wildest* dreams - where this conversation would ultimately lead me, or by what strange paths. That it induced such a major change in my life may be judged from the fact that at times I am glad that it took place, but that at others, I curse it profoundly. Yet, at the time, an interesting conversation and demonstration involving two practical and pragmatic engineers did not seem all that significant. It happened like this...

One afternoon at work, I was passing Gilbert's office when he called me in - "I've just had a rep. in from K..'s Fire Detectors, and he showed me this... (producing a pair of thin welding rods bent into the now familiar L-shape). He got me to hide things under the carpet, and he found them by holding the rods in his hands. Then, when they swung and crossed, the hidden thing was immediately below...like this", and he demonstrated.... Of course, I had a go and lo! - it worked for me also - my first encounter with practical dowsing.

At that time, (1971), dowsing did not have the exposure that it enjoys today - I had, indeed, seen only one other person use rods, and he was a professional surveyor who used properly made telescopic ones with balanced pivoting handles. Even though he was successful in locating drains, the significance of what he was doing did not register with me. In my own case, I did very little then with this newfound skill, other than finding drains and pipes for farming friends and showing them how to do it themselves.

I watched very little television at the time, thus the rapidly expanding use of rods and pendulums for archaeological dowsing, and by people seeking so-called 'earth energies' (largely and, as I keep protesting ad nauseum, wrongly called 'ley-lines' by many) in the main passed me by. It is quite probable that my interest would have waned completely had I not chanced upon a significant book, *The Practical Pendulum*, by Dr. Bruce Copen.

It was a seminal moment when, in the local library, I took out the slim book, that I could so easily have passed. As its title suggests,

LISTENING TO THE SILENCES

it was very practical, with much 'how-to-do-it' information. It also attempted, through a sort of pseudo-science, to explain the mechanism of dowsing using a short pendulum. And so it was that I made myself a pendulum as the book described, and soon found that all that was suggested in the text worked for me. The acquisition of a catalogue of new and second hand books on esoteric subjects took me one step further, for I found there a second book by the same author - *Dowsing from Maps* - which I bought, together with a professionally made Perspex pendulum. **What I didn't know was that I was about to set out on a very perilous journey on which, literally, I could have lost my mind.**

Very detailed instructions were given on how to dowse from maps, while included in the text were several charts and diagrams that one could use in a variety of analytical functions. Everything worked for me just as the book described, and the pendulum became a constant companion. What did not 'work' for me were the explanations offered for the way in which it responded. The concept of subtle energies, and even more subtle muscle responses, carried no weight, particularly when one considered that the pendulum was hovering over a piece of paper and not a piece of real-estate.

To explain why I made my next move it is necessary to describe some of my background and beliefs…

As you have read, my working life as an electronics engineer in the field of measurement and control had been cut short some three years earlier (1976) by a serious depression that had been caused, originally, by the completely unnecessary and, now professionally acknowledged, inappropriate prescription of Librium. That was now behind me, and I was beginning to revel in my total freedom in my tranquil rural home. It was a mind that was curious, but not much more, that led me on to explore and experiment with the book as a guide; a mind obviously coloured by experiences and events that stretched back into childhood.

One side of my family had been very actively involved in spiritualism. It had never drawn me, in fact the reverse, and I had not been personally involved, except to be aware of beliefs and practices. What I did have was a firm belief in *the actuality* of spiritual beings, which, when one boils it down, is the basis for all religious belief. The little experience that I had had of spiritualist practices, had been with direct voice trance mediums, nothing more. By extension, however, I knew that there was a potential for spiritual intervention in other ways. To me, it was a logical deduction, correct as it turned out, that the pendulum was being controlled directly by spiritual means.

LISTENING TO THE SILENCES

The moment one uses the word *spiritual*, one releases in one's hearers or readers all their own attitudes, beliefs and prejudices about spiritual concepts that form the basis of the religion in which they have been brought up, or which they have later espoused, or which they reject. Ideally, I would like to proceed without the preconceptions of *any* religion, but only with the understanding of the existence of a spiritual 'dimension' and the reality of individually acting spiritual beings.

As I have written, my own spiritual life and religious practice had been virtually extinguished in the void of the depression; but from whatever cause, vague stirrings were being felt. For reasons that completely escape me now, I began to think in a minor way about Buddhism, and in particular about the possibility of reincarnation. At the time, (1979), there was a resurgence of the threat of nuclear war that would inevitably create worldwide desolation. In another field, the 'experts' were predicting an imminent mini ice age. My reasoning went thus: if there is going to be nuclear desolation *or* an ice age, I did not want to reincarnate. So what did I have to do *not* to have to return? This was not *obsessive* thinking, rather was it a series of vague stirrings, and the beginning of exploration. In every respect I was buoyant and my mind was active - friends call me 'the ideas man', very much a lateral thinker and seeker of practical ways and logical solutions.

Thus, what did this pragmatic engineer do with his knowledge of a spiritual state of existence and his belief that the pendulum was being controlled by a discarnate spiritual entity, in ways that he could not determine? He did what many have subsequently insisted that he should not have done, he made an alphabet and numeral chart!

This advice should be heeded by anyone thinking about doing the same, as the experiences that follow should show.

I had never thought much about, and had certainly never experimented with, a planchette or ouija board, nor had I tried any other forms of divination. I was certainly not looking in any way whatsoever for deep insights nor for predictions. I was just *looking*, in total innocence and without expectation. The spiritualist activities of my parents and grandparents had always appeared to have assumed the presence of *benevolent* spirits. If they had any concept of, or protection against, the intrusion of spiritual malevolence, I was not aware of it. The possible existence of such never even entered my mind. (Recent conversation with my brother, who was a much more active participant than I was, has informed me that there were indeed careful and stringent precautions and practices aimed at guarding against such intrusions.)

LISTENING TO THE SILENCES

      I cannot recall in any detail the particular day in the spring of 1979 when I first sat down with the pendulum suspended from my right hand and hovering over the centre of the alphabet chart. What I do know is that immediately names started to be spelled out, names that slowly and laboriously I wrote down with my left hand; being right handed it presented something of a difficulty. I responded in my thoughts and in no other way. I would ask when and where the alleged person had lived, and how and when they had died, together with such ancillary detail as seemed appropriate - information that would, in the main, answer specifically my mentally posed questions.

      In their spiritualist activities my parents had participated in a so-called 'rescue circle'. To such a 'circle' the spirits of people who had died in trauma - accident, suicide, homicide, war - were alleged to be brought by the medium's 'guides', in order that by continued, but regulated, contact with still living people they might ultimately be reconciled to the reality of their death, and then make progress in their spiritual domain. It was in this manner that I reacted to the names and circumstances spelled out by the pendulum. Always my thoughts were of reconciliation with their circumstances and the manner of their dying, and encouragement to progress spiritually.

      As I look back nearly twenty years, I marvel at my 'innocence', lack of awareness and, I cannot emphasise too much, my *gullibility.* No, I was not controlling the pendulum in any way, nor had I any pre-conception of what would be spelled; and yes, the pendulum *was* spelling logical responses to my thoughts - and not solely to *my* thoughts. A visitor at the time used to sit beside me, and as I held the pendulum, would ask questions or make comments in her own mind, and to which I was not party. I remember quite distinctly the occasion on which the response to her was "We are not fortune tellers".

On another occasion, my friend and I had been debating aspects of abortion and euthanasia in consequence of some high profile cases proceeding at the time. When I sat that evening, the pendulum spelled out "Read Leviticus Chapters 18 to 22". I obviously knew that Leviticus was a Book in the Old Testament, but I can say, with almost 100% certainty, that I had never read it. When I did read the prescribed chapters, I found that there were elements that could be interpreted as having relevance to the debate. However, on re-reading the text to refresh my mind as I write now, it could be that I was being warned against *...those that have familiar* spirits...and *...wizards...who*, it was ordered, should be stoned to death. I shall never know! What these accounts *should* show, however, is that I was not exercising any physical or mental control over the pendulum, but that it was being controlled by a 'mind' that was separate from mine.

I was fully aware of the spiritualist concept of 'guides' - attendant spirits, whom, it is believed, have access to the mind of the medium and control the admission of other spirits. Thus, I was not surprised when a trio gradually identified 'themselves'. The identities that they claimed were, in turn:

1 *Ibn Ubar* - mid- to late nineteenth century, well placed (chief) in Masai-type people of North East Africa. Claimed that when he was old and infirm, he had deliberately set out to kill a lion knowing that he himself would probably be killed - almost in reparation for the lions that he had killed whilst protecting his cattle.

2 *Degef Gayad* claimed to have been a monk on the Tibet/Nepal border; had held a lowly position as keeper of a beacon for travellers; said that he had been killed by a bear whilst tending a remote beacon.

It is difficult to explain how a *presence* or *ambience* could be experienced whilst simply holding a pendulum, but it was actually the case in that a seriousness or portentousness accompanied the third member of the trio -

3 *U Gedafad* who, it was said, had been a Buddhist priest in Burma in the late eighteenth century. As I remember, his life and death were never discussed.

I am writing as if these were the actual spirits of real people. It is difficult to do otherwise, for while I have a different understanding now that qualifies everything that happened to me, it is something that I cannot at this stage anticipate, but must try to write of the experiences and beliefs of the time when they happened, and in the sequence in which they happened.

The Buddhist began to encourage me to study Buddhism. When I asked why, I was told, "every priest needs a pupil". I was encouraged to join the Buddhist Society, which I did, and to get hold of a book, *First Steps in Buddhism* by W.V.Trapp. Written in German, it was said, and translated into English in 1927 by Lionel Fellows, the translator being inspired by U Gedafad. When I asked the Buddhist Society Library for the loan of the book, I was told that they could not obtain a copy; I was never told that the book did not exist - whether or not it had ever existed, I shall never know.

I did not persist with the Buddhist Society for more than a few months. Many of the concepts and much of the terminology I found alien to my existing beliefs. Also, as with many Eastern religions or philosophies translated to the West, much seems to revolve around a particular guru or group of 'in' people, with which again I am unhappy. Something that I was asked to do and which I did adopt and persist with, was the setting aside of a quiet time at 11 a.m. each day, during which I practised a simple form of meditation.

As the spring merged into summer, hardly an evening passed without its time with the pendulum and chart. No longer did I need to write down each word as it was spelled, for the pendulum darted, almost just hinting at letters. 'Conversation' became very rapid - so much so that a time was reached when I really knew what was going to be said in advance of the spelling, and I was being well prepared for the events of an exceedingly significant day.

My 11 am sitting place was in an upstairs room looking north east to the nearby mountain tops - Scafell, Great Gable, Yewbarrow and others. I settled into my chair, easing my neck onto the high wingback, and rolled my head gently from side to side to smooth out any tensions, and then something happened that was so dramatic and far-reaching, and yet, paradoxically, was totally devoid of drama. A 'presence' that I could not see, moved from the space in front of me, *into* me, and immediately my mind was charged with another 'voice' or provoker of thoughts, thoughts over which, then, I had no control, and which were not initiated by me. In my head began conversation as between two separate people, one of whom was me.

I began to 'hear voices'.

That same evening, I settled with the pendulum and, as I held it over the chart, it started to whirl around rapidly and horizontally at its fullest extent, faster and faster, and continued whirling for several minutes. When it finally stopped and settled it spelled out "**we've won we've won**".

Who had won and what had been won, only time will reveal.

I have never used the pendulum from that day to this; it simply does not respond!

The fact that I was not wary or apprehensive about the events that were taking place may surprise some, but it can be explained by the reasoning that such limited contacts as I had had with spiritualism had always been of a benevolent nature, and indicated a caring practice. As an example let me quote an incident that occurred in 1950 in my home in South Wales very shortly before leaving to take up work here in Cumbria.

Quite by chance, we had a visit from the medium who presided at the meetings held at the home of one of my aunts. After chatting for a while he went into trance and I was spoken to. Comment was made concerning a proprietary medicine that I was then using to counter a sinus problem. I was advised to stop taking it and instead to use Morton's 'Nervatogen'. When we obtained some it turned out to be an herbal tincture that had the most benign and relaxing effect. My sinuses cleared, and I subsequently took the drops whenever needed for other reasons until all the bottles that my mother had bought were exhausted. After a number of years, I tried to obtain a further supply, but it was no longer available.

LISTENING TO THE SILENCES

Essentially, I believed that the named individuals had previously existed, and now, in spirit form, had access into me and my mind. Thus, when a further contact was made who was alleged to be my late father, I had no reason to doubt it.

Many of the conversations were about very practical matters. My concerns regarding the desolation that would follow nuclear war, or a returning ice age, were developed, and I was encouraged to believe that there could be survivors in such quiet places as that in which I live. It was suggested that I should learn as much as I could about basic survival techniques that would be needed if I survived, or which, if I died, I would be able to pass by inspiration to such survivors as there were and to their descendants. This seemed all the more logical as I began to appreciate that already, worldwide, there were individuals and small groups living remotely and learning and practising these skills; indeed, I came to know of one such man living not ten miles from me! Myself, I was encouraged to acquire a lurcher pup from a neighbour's litter in order to learn the skills of training a hunting dog and using it to obtain food. Many other topics were introduced for study - an activity in which I found no hardship, for I had long been active in many outdoor pursuits such as fishing and wildfowling.

As well as my physical survival, or the survival of knowledge with me, much thought was being engineered concerning my spiritual survival. My exploration of Buddhism was short lived; nevertheless, there was strong argument that I should become morally impeccable, but that I should not choose a philosophy or religious affiliation because it allowed a degree of moral latitude. It was put to me that as, at an earlier time, I had elected to be a Catholic, I should 'return to the fold', or, if not, then my rejection should be for sound reasons of belief, and not because I was looking for a path with less exacting moral standards.

I was encouraged to adopt a sincere prayer life and spent long periods in prayer each night. More and more the theme of the 'Second Coming' of Jesus was developed, and then, quite bluntly, it was put to me that He would return in a more mature person than was generally expected, and that I was a suitable candidate within whom He could manifest Himself. I cannot remember exactly how I declined such an offer that, it must be thought, no one could refuse. I do remember that I declared that I was too much of a coward to be able to accept such a high profile role.

Equally with the encouragement to be morally and spiritually 'clean', I was being urged to be most punctilious in my physical cleanliness. My underwear and socks I washed each night, and daily clean clothes became the norm, while bodily I entered another dimension. As an example I was encouraged to wash my anus each time I defecated, following, allegedly, Middle Eastern and Oriental practice. I was even schooled in how to be able to do this in a public

LISTENING TO THE SILENCES

loo. There was not an aspect of my life and thought that was free from scrutiny, for I was even counselled against a normally accepted practice that had developed in my heterosexual love life!

By a sequence of happenings that are too complex to relate, the spirit of a young (twenty-ish) woman was introduced into my 'coterie'. Her physical presence in me was most noticeable in ways which can only be experienced and not described. It was particularly apparent when any music was being played. I normally respond to dance rhythms with movement, having always enjoyed dancing. Now the 'feeling' of the movement became subtly different - feminine and sensuous.

Little by little, I was being accustomed to what some might find difficult to accept, namely the actuality of spiritual-physical contact. Thus, when I adopted my usual late-evening stance, leaning against the rail of my Rayburn cooker in the normal bum-warming posture and musing before going to bed, it seemed to come as no surprise when my head was moved by external influence: gently, from side to side, back and forth, easing tension out of my neck. Each day the interventions became more positive and, ultimately, I stood away from the cooker. 'Hands' pressed on my shoulders and I was 'eased' into a back-bend posture, where I was held for as long as I could tolerate it. When I stood up, I was eased into a forward bend as far as, and for as long as I was able to bend. Subsequently every evening I went through this routine, being bent further and held longer as time went on. My thigh and abdominal muscles became rock hard, my breathing improved, and, coupled with the dietary advice that I had been given and followed, I became as fit and healthily slim as I had been for a long time.

Again and again, I have to emphasise that all that was happening I saw as being entirely benevolent, and I was a willing participant.

The culmination of this 'body tuning' came one evening and without preliminaries. My body began to be manipulated as if by two skilled chiropractors. I was then fifty-five and my frame had acquired its share of the residue of past accidents and strains - playing rugby, being mined at sea, riding horses, plus all the rest that can be classed as fair wear and tear. Over the course of that evening and the one that followed, every one of the affected areas was worked on with consummate skill. I was stretched and manipulated as must be someone on the rack, but while it was happening, in the words of the Scottish Bard, McGonagle, "He felt no pain". Somehow my pain centre was inhibited, although there were body reactions which seemed to indicate that a natural response was taking place - towards the end of the second session I felt as if I was going to faint, while at the same time my feet were performing a little 'drumming' dance.

Yes, I felt no pain while it was happening, but as soon as it stopped my whole body screamed in agony. I literally climbed the stairs on my hands and knees, and had to take an analgesic to be able to sleep. On the morning of the third day, I was carrying a bale of hay to the stable adjoining my house when I had to put it down. It was large and was bearing against a knee that for some time had troubled me intermittently by filling with fluid. Still very much aware of the two previous evenings, I looked up and said in my mind, "You have forgotten my knee". That night I woke in bed to find the knee being worked on 'ethereally', and happily, it has never bothered me again in over twenty years.

Life carried on in the same general vein for some little time, though it could not be said that it continued 'as normal'! There was an episode of automatic writing that recorded nothing of importance, and the presence of the young woman became almost tangible, to the extent that I found myself reaching for a hand when about to cross the street.

It was an extremely wet autumn, and the work of keeping a horse stabled at night was becoming very tedious. Gradually, over this and other activities, I found myself being 'needled'. Criticisms began to invade the previously harmonious exchanges. It is, indeed, very hard, in retrospect, to recreate those particular days, and to understand how it became possible for me to be dominated by an altogether different group (or the same group acting differently). Living alone, enveloped in a foul early winter, everything outside soaking and muddy, it was fast heading for a 'bleak midwinter'. Certainly, and principally, the lack of association and the inability to put the events in perspective and discuss them with people living more varied lives completed the isolation. It was thus that I found myself being alternated in my mind between two groups - the one needling and critical, the other supportive and encouraging. (I discuss the strategies and ploys used to dominate and torment people later).

The two areas of attack were the religious practices and the horse. It is quite easy for religion to be used as a source of criticism and torment. Once one has undertaken to engage in intense practices and a highly moral life, the possibilities of being accused of backsliding and lack of devotion or compliance are endless, and need not be enlarged upon.

The way that the horse was used was interesting and quite unique. In Britain, the horse has a special place allegedly going back into early culture and worship. The linkage with the past nature/horse devotion was now being quoted at me as predating any modern religion, and which, without fail, should govern *my* treatment and care of my mare Bokhara. In reality, my care was very good, as my friends commented when later they had to take over, but because the newly introduced concepts of 'the old ways' were being cited, it was being demanded that the mare should be treated with an almost *religious* devotion, and that my management of her should be impeccable. This attitude was brought home forcibly to me in a way that, looking back, is reminiscent of attitudes and incidents from some of Grimm's Fairy Tales. If my mucking-out and remaking the bedding were of a high order, then the barrow load of dung and straw was as light as could be and was whisked along as if I had a host of helpers. If, however, I was skimpy in my work, it seemed that the barrow was filled with lead and that its progress was being actively resisted and my work impeded.

When one's family has fragmented, and there are no longer children at home around whom the celebrations of Christmas normally revolve, the ways in which it is observed away from the religious context are normally somewhat contrived. Thus, I found myself 'contriving' a merry Christmas but being pulled in several possible directions; no one else was actively contributing but all were relying upon me to 'provide'. My lack of commitment must have showed, for one by one the others found alternatives.

I am writing this over twenty years later. The sun is shining, the trees that were bare then are full of leaf and birds, the field that contained my mare is rich in grass awaiting mowing for hay and not the sea of mud and icy rime that it was then, and the mountains are hazy and cloud-shadowed not stark and snow topped. In spite of that, as I look out towards the mountains I have only to let my eyes go out of focus, and I can 'see' the reality from all those years ago, and even though I have pages of notes that I made soon afterwards, I do not need them, for every detail is as real as it was then, but now, fortunately, without the terror and torment that were building up. It may be wondered why I did not share with others at the time what I was experiencing, and ask for help. All I can say is that, exactly as I found later when I did need real help, - it is virtually *impossible* to convey or even hint at the reality of these events, just as many people, in broad daylight, cannot relate the torment and reality that were theirs at three o'clock earlier that morning.

Many times over these intervening years, I have retold my story to a variety of people in a variety of situations. What has remained with me after these various tellings has been the fact that almost no one has returned to the subject, asked supplementary questions, or followed through with any analysis, except for those in two groups. The first is the group of people who have had deep spiritual experiences of their own - they recognise and accept all that I say, and then there is nothing more *to* say, but only to empathise, with the understanding that can only come with shared personal experience. The second group is composed of one individual, one of the several Rogers amongst my friends. He used to come to stay for a few days at a time to talk and derive the healing that the house and environment provide. On one occasion, he harked back to his previous visit and what he had discerned within me, namely my anger, albeit unexpressed. In an effort to help Roger from insights derived from my own experience, I had recounted in detail all that I am writing in this and the next two sections. *His* response was to begin to analyse *me* to *myself*! He was very much 'into' Jung, and all the Jungian jargon came pouring out in the convoluted analysis of which only he amongst my friends was capable. In the 'let me be your counsellor' role in which I found myself, I could not let my anger manifest itself, but internally I was seething, and it must have showed; with his perception of it, I was able to take off the string that had been tying down the safety valve, and *express* myself.

Which really is me getting to the point of saying to you that if you are reading in a state of total disbelief or with the intention of 'doing a Roger' on me, there doesn't seem to be much point in your reading any further. What I am writing does not *allow* of any interpretation. It all *happened*, and in the manner and ways that I am describing. If you are reading with the intent of *using* what I am writing for the benefit of others, well 'welcome', be my friend; while I live I'll talk with you, enlarge, tell you all that you want to know. But now, stay with the narrative - things are getting *really* serious!

The final departure occurred three days before Christmas Day itself, a Saturday, and as I drove my last remaining visitor to the station yet more strange things began to happen. Making my way along narrow roads, I found my driving was being interfered with - at times my vision clouded spontaneously and I had to stop; on some corners I was forced to mis-steer and likewise had to stop to avoid crashing. At the station - well, you may have guessed - Saturday service; the next train was not the next train, but the one after that.

When I finally got home it was mid-evening, very dark, very cold, very damp, and there was still Bokhara to be seen to. First, I had to muck-out her loosebox, and here again I encountered the interference or help with the wheelbarrow. Looking back, I am reminded of one occasion when I was about thirteen. I had gone fishing in a small trout river several miles from my home, cycling there with my rod tied to the crossbar of the bike. When I reached the river, I had to leave the road and push the bike over some terrain resembling a links golf course. I had been joined by some lads whom I knew by sight, who lived locally and were about a year or two older. They helped me negotiate my bike over a railway line that I had to cross, and then I started to fish. I had hoped that they would go on their way, but no chance, and after a while, they got bored and started interfering with everything and behaving provocatively. Fishing was pointless and I packed up and decided to head across the mixed grass and sand to where it was possible that my parents had gone for a drive. My tormentors I had hoped to leave behind; some hope! They pushed against me, pushed against the bike, grabbed it from behind and stopped me from going forward, until, in desperation, I lashed out with my rod that I was carrying. That did it. I was set upon, harried and punched to the ground, continuing while I was lying there unable further to defend myself against the onslaught. Finally, they had their fill and left me a sobbing heap on the sand. It is amazing how the detail has come back, and how exactly it matches the interference of those harrying 'imps' of the wheelbarrow, and the reactions that they provoked in me and me in them.

Whatever, I finally got Bokhara installed and dried and fed, in the midst of what varied thoughts I cannot remember, although I have no doubt that I was being forced to concentrate upon aspects of my moral life, and my fitness for a life of improving spirituality. Let me again emphasise, there was nothing in my moral life, past or present, with which I could reproach myself to any significant extent, but somehow, everything was trawled, examined, and even the most minor peccadillo could, in my then state of mind, be made to seem to be an enormous 'sin'. Gradually, the whole thrust of the 'catechism' and analysis wound around the 'Christmas story', and subtly, and by allusion, around all past relationships with my parents. Any misunderstandings, any 'wish lists', were extracted within the 'Holy Family' context, as if my parents were near at hand and conscious of all that was transpiring. Yet again, the wheel turned and there was being stoked a feeling that I should go to the local church on Christmas Eve, but only to stand outside, not being fit to proceed to join the 'good' people inside. It all sounds so ludicrous as I write it down, and I do so solely to show how ones sense of proportion could be made to be so distorted as to accept such dominance as reality.

What next I remember, is going into the storeroom side of the stable to get some hay to fill the manger. Before I could start to cut the strings of the bale, I found myself forced down onto it on my knees, and made to stare downwards, but it was not to look at the assorted feed bags and twine that I would have expected to see. No, I looked into a void, but not a void. Picture the most *drear, cold* landscape of your imagination. I was in a narrow steep-sided valley, and it was *grey,* and *cold*. A white, snow covered landscape has some charm, but not this that I saw. The wind blown, snow blown terrain and scree was so grey and lifeless; not a plant grew, not a creature moved, not a bird flew, and it was soundless. And on my back was a great weight of ice, as if the whole of a glacier lay there, bearing me down. I was so *utterly* cold and alone, and I knew inside me that this could go on and on and on for ever. But in spite of that, I could muster the shadow of a wry smile, for I knew that this could in fact be a state that deliberately I had chosen, for, in essence, I was being shown what Hell could be. What I was seeing and feeling would be the equivalent of having once known and experienced the warmth of Divine love, and then of having deliberately rejected it, given it a derisive gesture, in full knowledge of what I was doing, and the remembrance of what I had lost by my rejection would be with me for eternity with no chance of recall.

I have no knowledge of how long my 'vision' lasted, though lasted it did sufficiently to have stayed with me unabated for over twenty years. Nevertheless, gradually the warmth returned and I was eased to my feet as my benumbed knees regained their function, and so, standing comfortably again, I turned and looked out over the half stable door. The clouds had cleared, and the sky was full of stars. So full of stars. And the reality of Christmas, and the *unqualified* unique love that it had brought with it into the world, swept over me.

It is impossible, and I will not even try to convey to you all of the sensations and reactions and emotions that engulfed me during this and the next day. Even now, when considering some of them, I only take a sideways look with half an eye, and I marvel that I could have become and been so embroiled in a situation that emotionally took me from feelings of deep and abiding love and commitment, to those of absolute despair and terror. I know and understand more now having lived with and thought much about the consequences, but *then,* then much was so incomprehensible, and yet it was all interwoven with the everyday functions of making meals, making the bed, doing what had to be done.

And so I did what had to be done during the following morning, a Sunday, and two days before Christmas Day. Whatever I did, it was completed by noon, and experiencing a total urge to escape from everything, I went to bed. But escape I did not. What a fertile ground is the mind; what a source of memory; memory that can be stirred and trawled by skilled spiritual inquisitors. The strange thing is, on reflection, that I did not question the *right* of this particular inquisitor who dominated the 'examination', for that is indeed, what had developed. And how strange it is, and awesome, to realise that *everything* is already known - everything that I had ever thought, had done was accessible - or was skilfully extracted. What a catechism followed! And all set by reflection within the Easter 'story'. For three hours I stayed, wide awake - held enthralled and being forced to confront *everything*.

It was only by conscious reflection sometime afterwards that I realised that I was being purged, stripped of any 'handholds' in my mind by means of which my composure or credibility could be undermined - just as a Greek wrestler of Classical times would oil his body and remove all hair to deprive any opponent of an anchorage for his grip. I am sorry that I cannot share with you what was being awakened within me - not awakened then for I was exhausted; the core of my being lay like a skinned animal and I was *sore* inside. The awakening came with time - the realisation of the *actuality* of the fundamental message and essence of the Christian faith, and the *reality* and individuality of the Holy Family. It is not that I do not *want* to share what I came to experience and know - I just find it impossible. To return to an earlier analogy - experiencing the summit of Mount Everest. One could go there with all of the sophisticated video and sound recording gear and give a detailed commentary, but never ever bring back one's own inner spellbinding thrill of experience, and of knowledge gained.

Always it is only by analogy that it is possible to convey the wonderment and awesomeness of an experience, and analysis is often banal. Yet, on another plane of understanding, it can induce further appreciation. Take the actual Everest. We know that what is now the summit was once at the bottom of the sea, and that the huge forces of tectonic plate movement have thrust it up to its incredible height. Likewise, by analogy, it might be said that Jesus has appeared as a pinnacle thrust upwards by the turmoil and pressure of human spiritual developmental forces, to become a focus and goal that the aspirant soul seeks. Opposing the height of the mountain is a deep core descending far below the Tibetan plateau which, in my analogy, reflects the core of evil influence and aspiration that the perceptive will know actually exists, and is allowed to flourish.

But Everest is composed of a type of rock that can be found in many places all over the planet, and likewise Jesus was/is human and, equally, can be found anywhere that he is sought. This was a reality that I found with the passing months, as I did with the other members of the Holy Family, each in their own role. The reality and its effect upon me will emerge as my narrative progresses - as has my experience and understanding of the opposing deep root core of evil which, had I but known, I was to experience in full measure, and soon.

Vulnerable and open to any influence, I undertook the chores of horse and stable management with all of the intrusive domination at its most intense. Detail is pointless, sufficient to say that I was threatened, and accepted and believed the threats of what would transpire if I attempted any of the escape routes open to me. If I was to take the car, I would be so influenced in my driving as to swerve and cause an accident killing someone. If I set out on foot, I would find myself run down by someone else who had been forced to swerve. If, nevertheless, I did set out in the car to either of two possible refuges and arrived without accident, in each there were young girls and I was threatened that I would be found committing some sort of sexual assault. *And so much more.*

In spite of it all, I completed my stable work and went indoors, very bemused and not knowing how or where to seek help. How, or to whom, is it possible to convey the reality of what, after all, was unseen, and in my mind and body? Yet, for me, the physical presences that invaded me were oh so very real and potent. By a process and sequence that I cannot now recall, I was nevertheless encouraged to clean myself thoroughly and get into completely clean clothes - I can see myself now, white shirt, navy seaman's jersey, strong riding breeches and stockings, and slippers. The kitchen has undergone some significant changes since that night. The decor is vastly different, and the Rayburn cooker has gone, replaced by some gas hobs of my own design. The changes have been made for essentially practical and aesthetic reasons, but, withal, they have achieved a sort of exorcism of that evening. Then, the Rayburn was a place of refuge, an anchor.

I think that, possibly unconsciously, people choose this type of cooker for the ever-present comfort that it can bring - not just its warmth, but the focus and stability. But my stability was not to last for long. Back to the brothers Grimm, and the teasing tormenting imps, hobgoblins. Little puffs of air started to be blown on my face and head from all directions. Tugs and pushes from all around caused me to let go of my 'anchor', and I headed for the phone. I cannot remember who I was going to ring, but as I attempted to do so the dial achieved a life of its own and whirred randomly and tormenting. I stood, temporarily defeated, one hand on the phone shelf, the other on a high backed chair, and then found my head nodding up and down. You will perhaps have seen a braying donkey doing just that between brays. Well I became that donkey - *inside* the donkey, looking out through its eyes in a world of heavy loads and thoughtless beatings. Now, I knew that it was *me* within the donkey, but I had absolutely no way of letting anyone know, nor of getting out - and this could be another form of hell, I realised.

Then I was back in the kitchen. At one stage, I remember winding my wristwatch and seeing the hands, as I tried to set them, whirling round and round at their own volition, as had the phone dial. Next, totally trapped, I paced up and down, back and forth - you will also perhaps have seen polar bears in the zoo mindlessly to-ing and fro-ing on the terraces of their enclosure. This time *I* was the polar bear. I was inside the bear looking out through its eyes. I could look down the terraces at the deep pool and the wall and the people beyond, and, as with the donkey, I knew all, and again realised that this also could be a view of hell.

I cannot now put a time scale on any of this, and I know that my writing is shortening the span. If I were writing a 'lost week-end' type of novel, I would enlarge and draw out every nuance of horror, for horror there was aplenty. In actual fact, it is all that I can do to recall objectively, and I only do so in order to inform, so that everything in its context leads to a logical understanding - that is if you are prepared to believe the actuality of what I am writing. If you are not, why, I thought that we had parted company long ago.

Somehow, and I cannot remember how or when in the sequence, I rang my GP friend Sandy. He, as I found out later, had been alerted by another friend who had suspected that all was not well, and, although I could hear the sound of a

LISTENING TO THE SILENCES

pre-Christmas party in the background, he promised to come at once. And so he did.

I let him in, but cannot recall what, if anything, I was able to tell him of my recent torment. The next that I remember is being seated in an armchair, while Sandy stood beside a small table to my left. He had longish side-burns and wore glasses that had fine gold frames; his bag was reminiscent of a Gladstone bag - and all of this conspired to make him look like a doctor from many years ago. He stood there filling a syringe, and I am sure that I was trying to talk to him, but I was aware of no response - and I could see myself, held in a time-warp, for ever trying to communicate with Sandy while he just stood, and could not hear my anguished calls. And this was another potential hell. It was odd, all these 'visions' of possible hells, for I have never ever thought about hell as a concept, nor as a possible reality - whenever I had had cause to think analytically about any spiritual belief or practice, I had always looked for the positive, the buoyant, never the downside. So this was new territory for me - and yet more was to come.

Suddenly, yet again I wasn't there; instead there were disturbing, tormenting voices - "Let's get him! What does he fear most? Hanging - yes, let's hang him" - and there I was, standing on a gallows, ready for the drop, staring down into eager, gloating faces, terror in my every fibre. "What is bliss?" -"Yes, Pentathol, that's it", and I was floating. "What does he fear more than hanging? Yes, beheading" -and the scene changed to the headsman - then back again to bliss. Once again back to terror and the prospect of being impaled, and then back to bliss. Finally, the prospect was of being frozen to death in some dark, alien landscape... Then I opened my eyes, only to look down at my arm and saw blood down the forearm. "Oh shit", I thought," I've tried to commit suicide". In reality, Sandy had had difficulty in locating a suitable vein and there had been a dribble of blood. Finally, tranquillity arrived and I sat chatting with him, the terrors subsiding. He wanted me to go in to the nearby cottage hospital, and I willingly agreed, and so, next, we were involved in practicalities. What did the horse need? Where were clean nightclothes? How do you turn the Rayburn off? How do I contact your brother, daughter? Who do you think will help look after the horse? Then the ambulance arrived and soon I was ferried off to the cosiness and security of a small room that I shared with a ninety-year-old rabbit catcher from a small hamlet near my own.

Living as I do in a fairly unsophisticated area well off the mainstream, it is not surprising that one's activities embrace a range of people who keep popping up in other guises. Thus, here was the nurse whom I previously had met in a violently mauve leotard, moulded to her every ample curve, in a yoga class. Then there was Dorothy, Bob's daughter-in-law, who lives not far from my home. Thus word got to Bob, and here he was visiting me and having good crack with the rabbit catcher, whom

LISTENING TO THE SILENCES

he had known for many a year. This was Christmas Eve, and a day mostly in bed, a bath and company having restored some equanimity. My daughter came with some presents, and life was becoming rounded again. Christmas Day, and well-decorated Dorothy and her colleague were in the room with a song and a dance and breakfast on a tray, with presents that they had acquired and wrapped for us. And thus there began for me a process of enlightenment, a process that has continued without cease to this very day.

During my stay in the little hospital, attached as it is to a retirement home, and during the events that followed over the Christmas and New Year period, I met at first hand the people who *care*. They don't figure in the pop-charts; their obituaries never make the national media; most don't figure in the New Year's Honours lists - in fact they get very little recognition at all, and most would probably get a little embarrassed if you went out of your way to praise or thank them. How about the Salvation Army musicians who brought carols and joy; the volunteers who had time and something for the older people in the next door home, many in temporary residence over Christmas, as their families had respite and a chance to visit elsewhere; the clergy of the different denominations; the man with the accordion who played while we danced? And many more.

Thus I danced my way to an appearance of normality, and as the beds were allocated by medical practices for their own emergencies, Sandy wanted his for the sorts of emergency that the time of the year frequently generate. And so it was, eventually, that arrangements were made for my departure and transport home on, as I remember, the day after Boxing Day, the 27th of December. I had not, in fact, been thinking very clearly, and had not forewarned my daughter, who had my house key, of what was happening. Thus it was that I found myself set down by the ambulance in my slippers at the minor road junction adjacent to my house – set down into a light powdering of snow. "Woe, woe, thrice woe" he cried! Cursing myself for a fool, I went around to the back of the house, broke a window in a small conservatory, and managed to get into the house.

I will not labour you with the tedium of restoring warmth, rooting out food, and of getting myself organised, all with a mind that was again under attack. One event, however, deserves mention. I still had my practice of praying by my bed, and the next night I was thus engaged. I often held a bible as a focus and possibly to read a little, and I had not been on my knees for very long when the book itself was being 'attacked'. I found myself wrestling to hold on to it, while at the same time my head was being plagued by a horde of physical knocks and tugs - for how long, I am not sure. While this was happening, or just afterwards, it was put into my mind that this was 28th December, the Feast of the Holy Innocents, the day dedicated to the remembrance of the infants who had been murdered by Herod in his attempts to slay the infant Christ. Far from being honoured by the fact that their lives had ended so that, effectively, Christ could survive, frankly, they were not best pleased. Thus, on this day dedicated to their memory and honour, so I was told, they went world-wide creating as much havoc as they could, joined, one suspects, by the spirits of *all* the infants and young who are slaughtered or aborted for the sake of 'expediency'. Whatever the truth of this, I know for sure that I had not been in the least aware that this was, in fact, Holy Innocents day.

And so it came to pass that on the next day I spoke again to Sandy, and managed to put something into words to Peter and Tricci saying, as I remember, "I have more problems than I can cope with". Again, the wheels of caring started turning, and arrangements were made. During this time and that which followed, Klaus and Brenda had taken over the care of the horse and cats, and eased my mind of many problems, though, throughout, I was never able to convey even an inkling of what was besetting my mind, nor give adequate thanks for all the help that I received. Eventually, seeking refuge, I was taken by a volunteer driver, and delivered to the familiar scene of the psychiatric ward of the main local hospital, on Saturday evening, the Saturday between Christmas and New Years Eve, 29th December 1979, when the ward would probably have been expecting a variety of admissions, many the product of the festivities and the season.

On arrival, I was interviewed by the duty Consultant Psychiatrist. I cannot remember what I said to him, and I certainly did not know how he had been primed by Sandy. I know that I tried to describe some of what had happened to me - with what success I have no way of knowing, but, on a busy Saturday evening, with the bustle of the season and other new admissions, it was of necessity not a long interview.

I was allocated a fairly stark room - probably one used for all emergency admissions, some of whom would be the worse for drink or drugs. I was free to mix generally, but in that room when I went to bed, the sense of isolation and of being spied upon was intense. In the wall opposite my bed, was what remained of a chrome bell push, and in my state of mind, I feared that this was a viewing channel through which my behaviour could be studied. My feelings of isolation and persecution became almost unbearable.

Fortunately, after two nights, I was placed in an open ward with about seven beds, and my composure gradually began to return - very slowly at first as I started to realise that I was not being spied on, and then more positively as I began to observe and talk to my fellow inmates. I also had a second interview with the psychiatrist that I found difficult to respond to, the principal reason being that he was accompanied by a male nurse. Had he been alone, I am sure that my story would have flowed, but, for whatever reason, I simply could not talk about voice hearing and the recent terrors, and went along with the suggestion that I was suffering from a recurrence of my previous depression. And so, for the rest of the week I found myself being 'infused' with an anti-depressant via an intravenous drip. As I was not suffering from depression, it had no apparent effect, except to stabilise my bowels, which had become disturbed. Notwithstanding that, I appreciated greatly the care and concern with which I was being treated.

The care and concern extended outside the hospital to my friends, and soon I was being visited and supplied with items that I had not even begun to think about in my sudden departure from home. One friend in particular, Val, who had been my secretary at work, and who, because of a long-standing problem, was a frequent inhabitant of hospital respiratory wards, provided the practicalities of 10p pieces for the phone, writing materials and tissues. The feeling of 'normalness' induced by these everyday necessities, her thoughtfulness and concern and the similar responses of other friends, contributed greatly to the rebuilding of my self confidence and assurance, which was doubly strengthened by the arrival from London of my brother. His practical application was inspirational. Remembering that this was early January, he had driven well over 300 miles to arrive at a home that was bitterly cold and not as salubrious as it might have been. My brother cleaned the kitchen, cooked a good meal, discussed my affairs at the hospital and extricated me for the first weekend.

Although my financial affairs were essentially in good order, obsessive thoughts about such things as tax matters were being forced into my mind, and a whole ambience of anxiety was being engendered around me. Fortunately, again, my brother took everything in hand and, in a comparatively short time, had the imagined problems examined and proved them to be non-existent.

Back in hospital for a second week, I was able to see more clearly and assess the thoughts that had begun to emerge during the first week, and to understand why I found myself to be so alien within my surroundings. I found that I was able mentally to detach myself from these surroundings and the reason why I was within them, and to look objectively at some of the others with whom I was sharing them. In time, I saw a pattern of individuals who just could not cope with the season 'of good will' and to whom it had, in fact, become a burden. There was, for example, the middle-aged bachelor, still living with his parents who had become alienated and depressed by other people's apparent enjoyment; the younger man, whose brother I knew, who immediately previously had been seeking spiritual 'enlightenment' at several isolated monasteries, and who had somehow 'lost it' in his own spiritual isolation at Christmas; the Evangelical preacher with a drink problem who found Christmas overwhelming, who, nevertheless, was able to

LISTENING TO THE SILENCES

make his mark with gentle 'preaching' to the young isolated man. It turned out that I was learning, as I had been in the cottage hospital, something of the nature of this particular time of the year, this particular season of celebration. I was learning of different peoples' inability to cope, and also was seeing the wealth of 'caring potential' that exists. From all of which, and over the intervening years, there has come my own determination to try to understand, and to be part of that same 'caring potential'.

All of my 'insight and understanding' lay yet in the future. In the sequence of events, I had encountered the Consultant Psychiatrist (MC) of my previous 'incarceration' and who agreed to let me transfer to his care. I was able to tell him that my difficulties were psychic rather than psychiatric, upon which he stopped the intravenous medication and just left me to take stock. The next weekend saw me being driven home by some good friends and starting to cope again, returning to the hospital solely to sign myself off. When I say 'cope', the word seems inadequate in the context of an entirely new ambience that began to be created around me, and seemingly within me. At all stages in writing this account, I am meeting many problems of communication; not with the mechanics of communication, but in finding suitable words with which to convey the reality of experiences that are not part of the everyday life of the majority of those who will read my work. Thus, and for example, how can I describe to you the exact nature and function of a wordless communication through which I was encouraged to achieve, and shown the means of achieving, goals for which my previous life had not prepared me?

It was not to be plain sailing. Once the door to the body and mind has been opened, it is most difficult, if not impossible, to close it again. One can learn or devise techniques to control access, but one is dealing with immense subtlety and cunning. There is, however, the great consolation that the same routes, the same channels are available to, and can be used by, sources of spiritual help and 'goodness'. How to recognise each for what it is, minimise the potential harm, accept, and enhance what is good and profitable, is the subject of the chapters that follow.

Before I move on, I reflect on what I have written, and particularly on the three original 'characters' that were first on the scene. Of these, 'Ibn Ubar' is the one who has left the greatest impression. Following an interest that has nothing to do with the foregoing but more to my study of exploration and ancient routes, I found my thoughts and reading being focused upon the lost city of Ubar (or Iram, as it is referred to in the Koran). Long sought by explorers such as the legendary T.E.Lawrence (of Arabia, fame), it had eluded discovery until an American, Nicholas Clapp, had the brilliant idea of having taken from space-shuttle and satellite, visual and ground-penetrating radar photographs of the area of Oman where legend had it that Ubar was located.

LISTENING TO THE SILENCES

The city had allegedly been the centre for distribution of the frankincense that is produced in the area, and was fabled far and wide for its beauty and lavish water supply, and for its verdant surroundings. Until one day it, or a large part of it, collapsed into the ground, and the area was reclaimed by the desert.

The satellite photographs showed faint outlines of the arrow-straight caravan routes from times long gone, routes that converged on a place that an expedition later revealed as, indeed, the lost city of Ubar, called by some the Atlantis of the Sands. Built over a huge limestone cavern, the source of its abundant water supply, the city had fallen into the hole created when the cavern roof collapsed. Thus it was destroyed, and not by an angry God, as subsequent legend would have it. Just across the room as I write is a copy of Clapp's book *The Road to Ubar*, which makes fascinating reading. Now there are those who would make a big thing of the coincidence of the two 'Ubars'. As for me, well....

Roy Vincent

CHAPTER 7

If you have

a

thousand reasons

for

living,,,

Roy Vincent

LISTENING TO THE SILENCES

If you have a thousand reasons for living,
if you never feel alone,
if you wake up wanting to sing,
if everything speaks to you
from the stone in the road to the star in the sky,
from the loitering lizard, to the fish, lord of the sea,
if you understand the winds, and listen to the silence,
rejoice, for love walks with you,
love is your comrade, your brother, your sister!

Dom Helder Camera

Someone who always had my interest at heart once expressed the wish that a magic wand could be waved and somehow everything could be restored to a state of serenity. It was a lovely thought and wish, and at the time I am sure that I fully agreed. Now, having lived for over twenty more years, I am not so sure. Somehow, I think that it would be rather like being lifted to the top of Mount Everest by helicopter - *great* view, but sense of achievement? Not really. For successful climbers, I am sure that the actual climb will figure more in their thoughts than the view from the top. For myself, at the time - the early days of 1980 - I hadn't yet come to terms with my new knowledge and experience, let alone realised that there might be a goal. I had yet to meet anyone who showed in their face that they had seen the 'twin peaks of Mount Meru', and so, basically, I went about the business of regaining my confidence and coping with the reality of living.

      Even if I had had my 'visionary's' goal, I doubt whether I would have proclaimed a pilgrimage. Always I have kept my emotions and inner desires and ambitions private except to a limited and close 'few'. Public and ostentatious displays of sentiment, or spiritually inspired emotion, have always embarrassed me, and so I sought not my palm from the Holy Land, nor my *coquille* badge from Santiago. My pilgrimage, if one there has been, has been into myself, exploring myself and my actions with a new vision, and becoming aware of the possibilities and potential that reside in practically everyone. I have always been a Christian - was I not baptised in the chapel-of-ease of the abbey church? Did I not attend regularly at the Sunday School and services of the close-by Calvinistic Methodist church, when we moved to our new home; and did I not become a communicant there and, later, in Glasgow? And did I not then become a Roman Catholic, with full conviction, at the time of my marriage? And then did I not put much into the local church life and belong to the St. Vincent de Paul Society that is charitably working for young

LISTENING TO THE SILENCES

people? Having absorbed the tenets and practices of a Christian life with my childhood breath, I had only deviated from them in minor ways, and yet looking back from the stance of maturity, I wonder and speculate whether I was confusing form with substance. There was obviously not a deep and abiding spirituality, however that may manifest itself, for where had been my resources when I so desperately needed that extra 'something' in hospital in the 'sixties and afterwards?

There were, anyway, new and imperative factors in my life that I would find difficult if not impossible to ignore. Could I put aside, turn away from the new knowledge that I had acquired, and the experiences that had been mine during the previous nine months? Had I wanted to do so, I would have found it impossible; entry had been gained into my mind and into my person, and now the question was to try to maintain control of as much of my thought and function as was humanly possible.

Yet again I have to ask your indulgence over this problem of communication; partly the choice of words with which to describe the indescribable; partly in how to assert my own personal certainty without in any way conveying a sense of 'spiritual superiority', or any form of exclusiveness. There are those who, having gained what they see as enlightenment in one or other of the world's esoteric philosophies, crushingly put down the neophyte with "If you have to ask *that* question, you obviously won't understand the answer!" No, there is nothing of that in me, nor in what I am trying to convey. I, myself, have never been a seeker after hidden truths - if anything, I went along in a sort of humdrum acceptance. I didn't see much future in the sort of analytically religious debates that sometimes went on in one particular naval mess in which I lived - the books of C.S.Lewis were making their appearance at the time and provoked new ideas - and yet, many years later, my friend David said that he had then admired my certainty. Who knows? Maybe I did have a solid belief that I applied in my life. My religion, if I thought about it at all, centred around the way in which I lived it and applied it, as a matter of *practice* rather than endlessly debating it, particularly if that debate was at the expense of another and different denomination or creed.

Possibly that is one of the keys to my way of thinking, to the ways in which I instinctively act, for the practical always seems to prevail - again a component of the intake of my infant breath, for the 'if you want it but can't afford it, you make it yourself' philosophy was around me from the beginning. Thus, in my early years, I wore clothes some of which my mother had made on her machine, or which she had knitted; ate food every bit of which, apart from bread, she had cooked; sat on chairs, or used other furniture, some of which my father had made; listened to a radio that he had constructed - I can still see the coils being wound, smell the solder and flux, see the outdoor aerial being strung between the chimney and a tall mast that he erected. I can still remember the tedium of taking accumulators into him at work where, as an electrician, he put them on charge. (Though there were benefits, for if I went to the works at a convenient time, I could stand above the coke ovens and watch the red hot coke being pushed out, and be smothered in the clouds of steam as the heat was quenched, and long to be the one who had control over this great big jet of water. Or I could go, preferably at night when it was all so much more dramatic, and watch the blast furnaces being tapped, and see the flow of slag into the huge ladles, and the molten, glowing iron run into its pig moulds.)

This was the father who, outside work, slaved away as the local union branch secretary: who didn't smoke or drink, but instead was able to buy a small car long before they became a common possession; the mother who, with her north-country canny thrift, ensured that we were buying our own house, and also had money to finance an annual holiday, well before holidays with pay became the norm. Within the family from which my father came, there were the beginnings of a parallel innate 'compulsion', for want of a better word; a compulsion to be involved in activities for the benefit of others. Thus my grandfather, who had served and been wounded in the Boer War, had come back from service under Baden Powell and, inspired by him, had founded the first local Boy Scout branch. It was he, who, with my grandmother, had created the first local spiritualist church. They both worked according to their convictions and desire to help others in the early developing new approaches to 'healing' - as also, as I was later to find out, did my Uncle Gwyn. If I wanted to, I could go and watch Gwyn at the local copper works, where he skilfully turned the vibrating sheets of copper as they passed between the rapidly spinning rollers. Or I could watch him and my Aunt Grace in their other life as market gardeners, where the hands that healed had a way with plants also.

It was a family from which I came that, as far as I was aware or can recall, never sought 'preferment', never pulled strings. This has been the way of my life, of self-enrichment in the intellectual sense, of avoiding absolutely any self-seeking, self-advancing 'brotherhood' or whatever, and rejoicing in developing my life as much as I am able by means of my own efforts. How could it be any other way? One hears more and more of 'foetal programming', well, I haven't had much time yet to think about that and its consequences, but certainly there was 'childhood and adolescent programming' in its broadest sense, and for that I am most grateful.

I could not have been kept in closer touch with reality and the practical, than when ultimately I left home, and became a number, C/MX 656045, in the Royal Navy (where I did learn the *negative* preferment of a Welsh accent!). The greatest 'hands on' reality was in my work as a Radar Mechanic, which I have already touched on. The equipment for which I was responsible *had* to work and be kept working by my efforts, and it *had* to be accurate, whether it was 'ranged' electronically, or pragmatically from the harbour at Haifa to the distant Crusader fort at Acre. Without its function, it was useless hunting terrorist infiltrators at night along the Palestinian coast, while it also contributed greatly to the safety of the ship as it 'went about its business in great waters', as the daily Naval prayer has it. I had experienced the reality of German bombs and V2 rockets; had looked *down* from my training establishment, HMS Ganges, onto 'buzz-bombs', as they sped up the estuary of the Stour in Suffolk. I had faced the reality of Irgun or Stern Gang terrorists in their attempts to put limpet mines on the ship as we lay at anchor in Haifa Bay. I had seen the reality of the destruction of cities and the impact upon their inhabitants, whether in Britain, Valetta, or Naples.

I began to experience a new reality when, following graduation, I began my career at the Windscale Works at Sellafield, for what could be more real than the nuclear weapons, that were the original purpose of the plant? I had no problem with that, for such was the thinking at the time, and nuclear bombs had been seen to bring to a horrible end, an incredibly horrible war. Nevertheless, I was more at ease within my involvement with the peaceful application of nuclear energy at the Calder power plant, even though I had an exceptional reality in my responsibility for its measuring and safety devices. Perhaps the *ultimate* responsibility and reality came on the day on which the Queen opened it, and the world was watching. Because of this very public gaze, it would obviously have been a great embarrassment if the reactor should shut itself down automatically, as the result of failure of any of the safety devices themselves. As many of the devices were new and innovative, it was a possibility that had to be faced. *So*, a piece of wire was put in place to bypass all of the automatic shut-down circuitry, and, during the Queen's tour and the official opening, I stood ready to snatch off that wire if there had happened to be a genuine operating reason which demanded that the plant should be shut down quickly.

If it is not obvious, what I am trying to demonstrate is that I am not some head-in-the-clouds, ethereal, self-deluding being who is totally out of touch with reality. The converse is by far and away the truth. At a basic level, consider the room in which I am now, and every aspect of its function, in which I can see something from my own hands and mind. It is upstairs and runs at two different levels, north to south through the house. The computer is a bit of an oddity in this setting, but I have grown used to it. At the moment, a bright November sun is streaming in at the far end through a large picture window of my own design. The opening was enlarged by Oliver, whose house I can see nearly half a mile away, now that the trees are bare. Oliver is brilliant at working with the cobble construction of these thick walls. The window was made, installed and glazed by my joiner friend Alec, who has supplied me with much good wood and also contributed his handiwork over recent years, as time has become more valuable to me and I pay to have things done that hitherto I would have done myself. Beside me as I sit, and with a view to the west, is another window, hole courtesy of Oliver, window from Alec, and the distant Irish sea, viewed between three century-old pines, is where I often lift my gaze when short of inspiration. In the same west wall, towards the far end of the room, is another window, this one courtesy of my long dead friend Bob, also a genius with a cobble wall, while immediately on my right is a north facing window that I renewed myself. My gaze through the latter takes me to Lakeland's highest mountain, already with its first winter snow touching the summit. It is a room that is so full of light, and which is so nice just to be in, just to sit and look out to sea, or south, through some more mature pines to the 'earth-mother' rounded contours of Black Combe.

However, going back to the early days of 1980, which is where my narrative had taken me, the room had more of the feel of a furniture showroom, so uninspired and cluttered it was. That was also the general perception of the house, for at that time, in truth, I still had no specific direction, no particular goal. Overcoming the hollowness left by the events that had caused me to retire from work, and still somewhat disturbed by the culmination of the happenings of the previous nine months, I see myself, in retrospect, rather like Mole in *Wind in the Willows*, as he emerges from his deep winter sleep, blinking at the sun, wary of predators and getting his bearings afresh. Just as Moley had Ratty to 'put some wind in his sails', to buoy him up and show him that there was a huge, undiscovered world, albeit fraught with unimagined dangers, but with exciting new experiences and such *interesting* new friends - just as Moley had all of that, I had - what? I had a new world, the existence of which, in reality, I had never truly sat down and considered as actuality; neither had I thought of the consequences of acknowledging its very existence. I had the parallel, interweaving world of the 'spirit' (Capital 'S' or lower case, you choose yourself, for you *have* to choose yourself, I can only tell you of my own experiences and derived beliefs and practices).

      I can only write in the language and context of the contact that I was experiencing, namely the Christian one, but fortunately not the one of entrenched 'theology'. No, it was to be very 'hands on', in more ways than one. How, though, can one enter into something, ask for light if one doesn't know that one *is* blind - blind to so much that is possible once one's 'eyes' of intellect, knowledge and experience are opened? Thus, not knowing that I was blind, I had not stood by the roadside like Bartimeus of old and shouted out loudly "Son of David, help me, have mercy on me". Nor was I struck blind like Saul on the road to Damascus, only to see truly when his vision was restored.

LISTENING TO THE SILENCES

Now, I had actually been on that self same road to Damascus - it seems a lifetime ago - in 1946. With the advent of peace, the Navy was able to resume many of its traditional peacetime practices, and one of these was to lay on transport and visits to whatever was worth seeing, wherever the ship visited. Thus it was that I had been driven along the Grande Corniche road in the South of France, visited the perfume distilleries at Grasse, and Monte Carlo with its palace and casino. When the Fleet was at Naples, I had been to Pompeii; when at Nauplia in Greece, I had seen many antiquities; when in Cyprus for the ship's boilers to be cleaned, I had 'holidayed' under canvas near Famagusta and in the Troodos mountains, and had fished all night in his boat with a local fisherman; later I had swum in the crystal waters off beautiful Skiathos. So what was I doing on the road to Damascus? Well this time we had tied up in Beirut, principally for oil, but there was also time ashore. Time to see such a jewel of a city; untouched by war, and certainly not aware then of its ultimate devastation during the internecine wars fought around it and along its sweeping boulevards. And so it was that I (who "didn't smoke, drink or go out with dirty women", much to the disgust and total incomprehension of Scouse 'Spud' Murphy, whom I had encountered in a minesweeper on the Clyde) opted for the 'culture' and exploration, and found myself with several mates of similar persuasion in the back of an open truck as we creaked our way inland towards the Beka Valley and ancient Baalbek (or

Heliopolis if you prefer the Greek). The road over the Shu'uff mountains was very hairpin-bendy, and very hair-raising in a truck with bald tyres and a body that indisputably had a detached life of its own, as the tailboard hung over a precipitous drop, while we edged and reversed, edged and reversed around any one of the many hair-pins. Up through the clouds, past gangs of men and women breaking stones and restoring parts of the road itself; then over the summit of the pass and the sight below of a road that seemed to vanish as a thread into the floor of the valley beneath. Unforgettable, as with so many other sights along the way - moving walls of straw that turned out to have camels inside them; people harvesting and threshing in ways that were timeless and so much more. But then, there it was, totally insignificant and unexpected, but awesome in its recollection, a simple signpost with the one word *Damascus*>... and in a moment we had passed. The day has many recollections, of Baalbek itself, but especially of friends who were killed at Corfu shortly afterwards - but no, I didn't experience blindness and revelation.

I didn't experience them in 1946, nor yet as 1979 changed to 1980, where I am in my story. Yes, my story. Sometimes when I stop and read what I have written in total, I spend a lot of time reflecting on *why* I am writing, for whom, and wondering whether I am achieving what I set out to do. Remember, I set out to inform and help and *encourage* individuals who are suffering in their minds; who cannot cope with intruding voices and

LISTENING TO THE SILENCES

presences; who cannot get anyone, lay or professional, to comprehend or believe what it is they are trying to convey; who suffer the indignity - yes, shout it loud, *the indignity* of constant disbelief; of being treated as a 'syndrome'; of having to submit without choice or understanding to mind altering drugs and 'therapies'. Partially isolated in my tranquil setting, it can be so easy to lose sight of you, or you who are trying to cope and give support to someone who is so difficult to understand and live with, someone whom you loved, still love so dearly, but who is not the same person you once knew. Sometimes as I write, I wonder whether my own reminiscences get in the way of my intention. Part of the reason, an almost instinctive ploy, is that reminiscing helps me to cope with the release of so much that is/was personally painful. If I can show to myself that so much of my life so far, the greatest part indeed, has been happy, formative and positive; that my personal distress and disasters had a cause and eventually a solution; if I can show this to you, then maybe you will derive comfort from the thought that there is a way through your own particular morass, if you can find the right guide or means of support. Acknowledging, however, that you may have to find the courage to go it alone. For sometimes it is necessary to reclaim an identity from the amorphous categorisations and identity obliterating processes in which you find yourself.

      More, and more, and more, life and technology are conspiring to obliterate the individual. It is the information age, we are told. Before long I am sure, people will be desperately seeking the age of the 'person', a living, breathing, walking human, not a web page, totally anonymous, without an identifiable author, devoid of human emotion and contact (except perhaps something 'interactive' and self-degrading). Returning to a point that I was trying to make in an earlier section - I was trying to illustrate how the world of academic, and particularly psychiatric, research is far removed from the individual. No test yet devised can equate the mental distress and problems of one person with those of another individual; nothing can harmonise symptoms and reactions sufficiently to use averaged results for the treatment of all, no matter how strongly it is believed to be so.

Yet here is the statistical 'you'. Another tea break, and switch on 'Westminster' on TV, and what have we got? Mental health questions. Health Minister - "One in four people in the country will develop a mental health problem". What a prospect - and here is the point that I have tried to make in sketch outline, and to which I shall return in detail after I have completed the narration of my own story, - here is the point: I can guarantee that many of the so called mental health problems will have resulted from people being undermined and submerged by all the consequences of modern living - all the man-made and natural influences that I have touched upon, plus stupid diet and lifestyle; the very panic of trying to keep pace with all the 'must have', 'must do' compulsions that skilful marketing ploys thrust at one. Just take, for instance, computing - bigger, better, faster, more memory, this and that software, outmoded today, faster tomorrow. Must have it, must have it; and the kids have to keep up for school (if they aren't already mind-blown, overweight and asthmatic from the intensity of computer games and a computer in the bedroom), and *they* want the latest so they can have street-cred, school-cred. How my heart bleeds for you. If you haven't already fallen victim to the system, you had better take hold of your life or you will become the one in four who does end up as a mental health statistic!

    But what chance does the poor, overworked G.P. have to help you as an individual? (He, possibly, is already a mental health statistic *himself!*). He has six or so minutes to analyse and probably prescribe - are you anxious, depressed, how's your sex-life -good indicator (or maybe the media have led you to believe that you must have bells and whistles, multi-orgasms and earth movement every time you perform, and maybe you feel inadequate)? Get your head around all that and try to describe it lucidly, then listen to what he tells you about the side effects of the drugs that you are going to take - *six minutes* - it would take six bloody minutes alone to read out and explain all the side effects of some of today's 'designer' drugs!

    But you are at the far end of the chain that began with the original research - harking back to my 'second opinion' interview with

Big Wheel, I sometimes wonder whether the reason that he didn't sit during the time that I was with him was that he would not have been able to see me because of the stacks of books ranged around his desk. If the length of time allocated to me is a guide, one wonders how much of the endless research that he has published is based upon direct human contact. I have a very good friend who has a son who is a professor in earth sciences, with many responsibilities world wide for projects initiated or funded by government or international bodies. Bolivia, Bangladesh, Mexico or Marakesh - the postcards arrive - from projects being advised, post-graduate students being supervised. Then there is this advisory body or that conference to attend - (while his mother frets about the effects upon his health that she can observe). He is, in fact, an expert in his field, and is doing a first-rate and very worthwhile job. Yet as he clocks up enormous numbers of air-miles, I am left to wonder in what manner, and from how many levels removed, does he have an impact upon my cretinous dwarf in Bangladesh, who only needed a bit of iodine in his diet. Or on the life of the riverside fisherman, whose fishery and livelihood are being destroyed so that some international conglomerate can build a dam to make electricity for the purpose of smelting aluminium, neither of which will benefit the fisherman (nor will the profit, that belongs to the shareholders). The aluminium will, of course, go to make soft-drink cans to create more health problems in the 'civilised' world! (My friend's son

LISTENING TO THE SILENCES

is, in fact, involved with many fundamental and valuable projects, and I don't want the hyperbole of my argument to detract from that.)

Nevertheless, my point is still this: you are, or the one you care for is, the individual at the end of the chain. A *unique* individual. How can anyone study, advise, prescribe unless that individuality is seen and acknowledged at every stage? But who can allocate time in the hectic world of national health, and the often under funded, under-resourced world of mental health, to cater for the needs of the individual? Obviously I am in no position to prescribe for you - wouldn't dare, anyway - but I can continue to do what I have been doing up to now and tell you what happened to me, and how I coped and developed a completely new life, and maybe I can help you to create your own coping strategy.

Possibly the greatest help that I was given came from a family. Not my immediate family; my brother had his own work and family to attend to, while my daughter was developing a career of her own at UMIST in Manchester. So what family? Whether you have a religion or not, it is profitable to look at the brilliant concepts involved in the origins of the Christian one. A family - the Holy Family - so called. A family with which anyone, no matter what their own circumstances, could identify. In this rural area where people stand out as individuals, the concept and working of a family unity can be seen all the time - craftsman father being followed by son or daughter; mother closely involved with the 'family firm', contributing, supporting - and the same in farming. An old-fashioned way of life maybe, but an effective one, and seemingly devoid of mental problems, if my observations are correct. A family that, in this case, my case, came and absorbed me. I, as I keep on saying, had not been looking for *any* sort of outcome or development. However, as I came to absorb and understand a little of what I was experiencing, and what was opening up to me, the realisation and understanding of some of my personal 'revelations' within the tormenting time around Christmas, began to open my eyes. I am writing with the benefit of more than twenty years' subsequent experience, and the 'smoothing out' of my lack of immediate acceptance and collaboration - itself the product of a wariness that had been derived from those same Christmas experiences. I laugh sometimes at recollections of my own rejections of what I saw as intrusions, interference; but as the further realisation dawned at the time, and I *accepted* what was on offer, life took on a new meaning as I found help and support within a family that I never knew that I had. Just, as I shall relate in a little while, I found in Scotland a human family that I hadn't known existed, and which was to absorb me and make me part of itself.

I have some friends who, some years ago, were expounding their own attitudes to religion, and who came out with a memorable statement, that "Christianity would be all right if it wasn't for *Jesus!*". Jesus was perceived as some sort of wimpish adjunct that could be dispensed with, leaving the rest - a way of life. In some ways, you cannot blame them, for that is often the way religious art has portrayed Him and His family, and the whole of the apostle band. Dramatised with no doubt the best of intentions, but, more often than not, a set of ethereal wimps. I have had no personal visions or revelations on the matter, but recollect this - they were the working people of their day, and I see shepherds and craftsmen virtually every day that I live here. I also remember a fisherman.

    I have mentioned already the time when my ship came to be tied up in the little harbour of Famagusta in Cyprus for the regular boiler clean, and watch and watch we had a week's leave. The first part was spent in tents beside a lagoon where the local fishing boats beached. A friend and I had a keen interest in fishing, and indeed had some tackle that we had bought in Malta to fish from the ship's side. But this was the *real* stuff, and we went to see what the form was. We watched and chatted as the long-lines were prepared for that night's fishing, and soon we were invited to go along. Thus it was that in the early evening we went down to the shore with our little packs of NAAFI sandwiches, and were soon afloat. The boat was typically Mediterranean, double ended and rowed facing forward. In the stern deck was a round hole, and in it sat our fisherman friend - yes, his name was Peter, believe it or not - baiting the myriad hooks that hung over the edges of a number of round baskets, each basket containing about half a mile of line. But this wasn't the fisherman who was so memorable; it was the one who rowed. His bare feet on the deck of the open cockpit were spread from years of thrusting at the oars - would ever shoes fit them? - and they were the roots of a veritable tree that sprang from them, a tree that spread as it rose through huge leg muscles to a torso that would have a sculptor reaching for clay or stone, and upwards to shoulders so broad and to arms that made the stout branches; and all so effortlessly swaying as the oars swung and the boat thrust through the reef and out into the sea. Hardly a wimp.

And shepherds - what wimp would spend his days, made easier admittedly since the advent of the 'quad' bike, going up and down the fell-side tending hundreds of sheep - not now and then, but constantly, day in and day out? Atrocious weather, snow drifts, sheep that seem to be prone to a multitude of ailments - scrapie, louping ill, gid, sturdy, foot rot and maggots, to name but one or two -and predators such as foxes or vagrant dogs. I see them, the sheep that is, being gathered and brought down from the fell-top to be dosed or shorn or tupped or to lamb, returning to the fell between-times. I have, myself, helped at times, at gathering and shearing, and sorting the lambs, male and female, each to a different future, and corralled the tups in my fields as they waited for the autumn 'off' - and been rewarded with huge meals in the family kitchen -

LISTENING TO THE SILENCES

"Reach up" is the welcome command. Wimps? No, *real* people. I could go on, drawing examples from my carpenter and metalworking friends, but I hope that I have already made my point.

It has only come to me over the years, this brilliant concept of a family - the Holy Family, so called, - a family with which, and with whom anyone, whatever their rôle or status in life, could identify. Mother, sister, female friend or confidante; brother, exemplar and rôle model - hero, even; and then the father figure, the universal worker, craftsman, home-maker.

So many individuals over the centuries have tried to convey their inner reactions and feelings as they have responded to the realisation of the core message of Christianity. The ecstatics such as Teresa of Avila, John of the Cross, Julian of Norwich, Hildegard of Bingen, have used language of the deepest love as they have tried to express the inexpressible - the language of the heart and viscera. Heroic was the language of a hero, Edmund Campion, as he uttered his famous 'Brag' from the scaffold at Tyburn as he was imminently, and literally, about to lose his heart and viscera to the executioners' knives. How can one compete if one wants to express one's own inner state? And yet, there is the desire both to shout from the housetops and at the same time to hug one's joy to oneself.

Can you recollect the first time that you were in love? *Really* in love; when you walked on air, unable to believe that this was really *you* that this was happening to? The sheer disbelief that this divine creature could actually love you in return? Recall that desire to go to the steeple top, ring the bells and tell the world "She (he) loves me" - yet at the same time, recall the great desire to hold on to this wonderful secret and, as with a jewel in your hand, contemplate the thought and the revelation just for one's private self, for *surely,* no one had ever been in love quite like you before in the history of time.

Recollect the words of Julian Jaynes that I quoted earlier:

O, What a world of unseen visions and heard silences, this
insubstantial country of the mind! What ineffable essences,
these touchless rememberings and unshowable reveries!
And the privacy of it all!

Yes, the privacy of it all. For what is visible of the mental processes and inner core feelings as one goes about the daily doing, of living, of performing the humdrum?

And yes, the humdrum. For revelation does not produce instant everything, like winning a lottery. Life still has to be lived in all its never-ending detail; yet it was through this humdrum side of living that the 'magic' started to appear. There can be little doubt if you have kept in touch with my day to day living through all that I have written, that my home lacked a certain order and deep-down cleanliness. Unlikely though it may seem, this is where I first became aware of what was 'on offer'... If you had been in this room with me now, you would have seen me gaze unseeing for some little time, almost oblivious of the brilliance of the orange of the sunset to my left, and very nearly 'unmanned' as I recollect that time.

In spite of the fact that I had very good friends on whom I could draw whenever I had need; in spite of the fact that I had been shown the wonderful actuality of what having a brother *really meant*; in spite of all that, I was at core so very alone, so deeply lonely, isolated by my experiences and a new knowledge that I was finding difficult to understand myself, let alone to share. And it was a recollection of that loneliness that swept over me now as I drew from my memory - but more than that, for there also came a recollection of a total *spiritual* ambience that began to be generated around me, and the warmth as from a deep and all-pervading friendship - memories that time certainly cannot erase and which are as potent now as they were immediate then.

I think that if one could see at the outset, or in any way catch an inkling of the potential, the reality, the knowledge and available power, one would be so overwhelmed as to be rendered overawed and impotent. And so it was that, little by little, virtually by infusion, the practical results of a new collaboration began to appear within or through me, at a pace and level with which I could cope. It might be assumed that with such strong spiritual association developing, all power would have been drained from the adverse spiritual intruders and that *they* would have been rendered impotent. Had this been so, I would have become totally reliant upon the cocooning and protection and would have learned nothing. I certainly would never have been able to write this account.

No: what I was being given were the *means* by which things could be accomplished, goals could be reached. When, on joining the Navy, I had begun to learn the skills of seamanship and all that that entails, I found that suddenly I was able to tie the most complicated of knots, knots that I had seen in diagram often before, but which had defied all my efforts of interpretation. Indeed, it is hard to forget the first time that I had a complete and neat Turk's-head at the end of my practice piece of rope; give me a rope now and well over fifty years later I will tie you one with no effort - because I was well taught. Stage by simple stage the knot had developed under the tuition of someone skilled and patient, himself the product of a long tradition of skilled and patient instruction and practice, for the result, the product of the teaching, had to be someone upon whom others could put their trust, and upon whom others might have to rely for their very lives. Even if it was done by rote or by simple mnemonics, or by repeated practice or 'evolutions', it was done, and skilled individuals, part of a greater whole, gradually developed and integrated into a single acting body with a common purpose - the crew, the ship's company. It is unlikely that I shall again have to protect a rope from being chafed, but I know still how to do it, and that I "worm and parcel with the lay, and serve the rope the other way", or that when meeting another ship at sea at night, if it's "green to green or red to red, then perfect safety, go ahead".

Subtly and without fuss my new 'instructors' got to work. It is difficult now to recall that I, then aged fifty-five, should have *needed* instruction in life skills, but when I also recall how undermined and demoralised I was, then my appreciation, even now, is boundless. Although some of this may sound so banal or trite, it wasn't a game that was being played. My mind was very, very vulnerable, as I was, and I was then facing real and exceedingly potent and cunning adversaries.

Take a simple activity such as shopping, involving a round trip of twenty miles to my nearest 'metropolis'. My mind had to be collected positively, and lists and memory pads became the order of the day. In the car, before setting out, I was worked through a 'drill' that was aimed at focussing myself and my faculties. In the town, I had two or three 'stability' points where I knew that I could collect my wits before the next sortie- the library; a friend's men's' outfitters, and so on. Thus, slowly and imperceptibly, my confidence and my horizon both enlarged.

Or returning to the mundane, the domestic, the *cleaning*. Consider the small conservatory attached to the back of the house. The floor had become a depository for all sorts of bits and pieces, items in transit, in or out, with only a narrow 'trod' enabling me to pass through to the back door. It was a clutter and scrow that I didn't see any more; I simply walked through it. Then, one morning, the 'day dawned', the sun shone, and imperceptibly I was guided. The junk from *this* side all over to *that* side. Scrub the exposed floor. Everything from *that* side over to *this* side, taking the opportunity to 'skop' (lovely northern word, full of meaning) anything that was dispensable. Scrub exposed tiles. Re-examine all items, and continue the 'skopping' process - I learned the importance and joy of a *large* waste bin (essential for skopping). Result: one clean and *usable* conservatory. By extension, the process began to become part of my personal repertory, and the orderliness of domestic work and an understanding and acceptance of its inevitability conspired to remove much of the attendant tedium, making what followed so much easier and even pleasurable. For the reality of the concept of a 'Holy Family' whom one desired to take up residence and for whom the house, and by extension, one's personal life and thought, must be immaculate, was particularly potent.

It is difficult, virtually impossible without resorting to what could be construed as hyperbole, to describe this developing reality: so please accept that for me this is what was happening. However, just as in most normal families individuals don't live in each other's pockets, but are 'there' for each other, so it became the case then, with the core knowledge that love and support were unquestionably available, and prayer became as normal and acceptable as everyday conversation.

And so it came about that, after about twelve years absence, I began to go to church again. I had thought about it generally at Ash Wednesday; much more actively at Easter; then finally, on a bright Sunday in the spring of 1980, I was there, to a liturgy that had become even more open than the one that I had left, to the voices raised in 'Morning has broken' and, at the (to me) newly instituted exchange of a 'sign of peace', the firm handshake and welcoming look of the man standing next to me. A new communion and a sense of homecoming. Yet, it was not the presence and participation in the Mass that was so important as what was released, what flowed from it all, and what I became involved with as a result. Thence, life began to flow with an increasing force and into several widening channels, although, just as a rope is the sum of its strands, each interdependent, so it was that the total flow of my life became the sum of the seemingly independent channels.

Inevitably, the house became the centre and focus of much of my activity, although it would be tedious for you to have to read through an inventory of everything that was attempted and achieved. I shall confine myself to the developments and achievements that are germane in the rest of my tale, or in the ways that they relate to the flow in the other channels. Essentially, my first moves were triggered by the consideration of the plight of a friend of my daughter, and one of my regular visitors. She had been crippled whilst in a psychiatric hospital. Confined in a first-floor ward, disturbed by the sudden change in her drug regime and wanting 'out', she had chosen the first available route, namely a window that was in process of being repaired. A broken spine, severely damaged feet and legs, left her wheelchair bound, and with limited social outlets. Conscious of the lack of holiday accommodation specifically adapted for disabled people, I began the process of creating on my ground floor, facilities suitable for the ambulant disabled.

Anyone who has become seriously involved in DIY will recognise what I have discovered over the years, namely that it moves on from being a chore, a necessity, and becomes more of a hobby. I need no excuse to buy a new tool or piece of equipment, particularly when I soon realised how life could be eased, and jobs speeded up and completed more professionally, by using the specialist devices, and whereas in the past a lady might buy herself a new hat to give her spirits a lift, I buy a new tool. I frequently ponder upon the *honesty* of tools. They are inanimate but not soulless. Each is the result of years, centuries even, of pragmatic evolution, and provides a link within one's hand to countless generations of craftsmen long gone. I recently made on my lathe a couple of carvers' mallets,

LISTENING TO THE SILENCES

each of subtly different design, but in all respects replicas of a design that was old when the Romans ruled. No one has ever bettered it. How could they, for the mallets sit in one's hand in perfect balance; left or right hand it doesn't matter, and always presenting a correctly angled face to the butt of the chisel or gouge. A masterpiece of simplicity and suitability.

      The earliest records relating to my house that I have seen date back to 1715 - annual letting agreements as a small holding - and there can be no doubt that it existed for an unquantifiable time before that. It is of random 'cobble' construction - an outer and inner wall linked by 'throughs' and resulting in walls at least two feet thick. A construction that requires the skill of a 'native' to modify. Fortunately I have had the ready help of two such craftsmen, Bob and Oliver, without whom, over the years, I could not have made progress. Times I have viewed with trepidation the enlarging hole, as cobble after cobble was removed and the remainder subtly propped, then gradually breathed again as the lintel was worked into place, window sides rebuilt and sill constructed - and a wonderful view was opened up and light allowed to stream in.

      Internal development has been made even more 'interesting' by virtue of the fact that there never seemed to be a true vertical or horizontal, nor a corner that met at ninety degrees. But I learned, and as my skill and confidence grew, enjoyed the learning and doing. Carpentry, plumbing, central heating, additional wiring, tiling have all come together into a home that affords me much delight, and in which I take immense pride. Purists and fundamentalists will tell you that pride is a sin. Poppycock! Pride in achievement is natural, justifiable and healthy, and not just in one's own successes, for I am equally proud of the accomplishments and association of all who have contributed over the span of twenty years. I have mentioned already Bob and Oliver, whose skills ranged well beyond the manipulation of stone (Oliver is as fine an amateur plantsman as you could wish to meet). Then Klaus, and sons Patrick and Jason, can be seen in different metals, from the beautiful copper hood over my fireplace, to specialist brackets spread through the premises. Alec and son James figure in wood everywhere, in pieces that they have made, or in the raw materials for my own handiwork. The Two Geordies come to life in many places - porch, garage, sunroom, stable, which all rest on the foundations created by the 'heavy gang' - Graham, Andrew, Joe and Ian, who also reside in memory in the paths in the garden and in the structure of ponds. Myles, Jack, Peter, Bill and his grandson, Des, all have a real presence throughout the house and workshop in a variety of artefacts and constructions.

And the ladies; who could ignore or forget the ladies? The results of their skill with needle, paintbrush and trowel are everywhere in house and garden. I hope that I remember to include them all. The two Jeans, the several Margarets, Annes and Marys; Stephanie, Brenda,

LISTENING TO THE SILENCES

Diane, Edna. Not to mention washing and ironing and mending and cleaning, and lots of lovely, lovely grub!

Help also came from anonymous sources, via the mind. Does that sound strange? I write at great length about the adverse spiritual intrusions, but what about the positive? Yes, *what about the positive?* I have written about this new territory of craftsmanship in which I found myself, tackling projects in which I had no previous skill, and working into a construction of heavy granite boulders and thick, iron-hard plaster, or plaster that would not take a fastening. I could have been way out of my depth, and there was a limit to the frequency with which I could call upon Bob. But then it started to come, virtually by direct transference, subliminally, as it were, the *total concept* of a process or mode of construction transferred without 'words', but rather by complete inspiration. But not only the knowledge, the know-how, but the *resolve* and active support to help me to go forward, for many times I was daunted and demoralised. Let me illustrate. I was needing a link unit between two elements in my kitchen, and had constructed something almost in desperation, then went to bed not truly satisfied, aware that I had virtually 'cobbled' something together that would just about do.

I woke early next morning to a feeling that, over time, I began to recognise - the feeling that the right day has dawned, that the tide is flowing, the wind is in the correct quarter, and that nothing will hinder progress. Thus I was encouraged and buoyed up, as I completely dismantled the efforts of the previous night and reappraised the design. Although much more intricate work was involved, I, nevertheless, achieved a much more satisfactory result, aesthetically and functionally, having been given directly into my mind, insight into a mode of construction of which I was not previously aware, and about which I had no other source of information

Advancing with my physical and practical activities were the internal and spiritual, and yes, the *reality* of interactive spiritual beings - you can deny their existence, wish the concept away, but I'm afraid that you are on a loser. Have no doubt about it, such do exist. Take for instance the little shelf above the cooker in my kitchen. I was building in a large electric oven into a previous cupboard space and needed a shelf to link the upper and lower sections. It could not be regular, and would involve a different curve at each end. I drew these out on my chosen piece of wood one evening and took the wood to my bandsaw the next morning. Unfortunately, the tide was not flowing, nor was the wind in the right direction, and I made a bit of a cock-up of the curve at one end. Disheartened I went and had my breakfast and considered the situation. My craftwork prayer focus was St Joseph - he the craftsman and worker, and the ear to which I raised my invocation. I finished my breakfast and washed up, then took my shelf back to the

LISTENING TO THE SILENCES

bandsaw and presented the other curve to the blade. Immediately I, myself, was 'locked on', and the wood went through the saw in such a way that even if I had wanted to, I would never have been able to deviate from the curve. So remarkable was the feeling that even if I had been levitated and propelled out of the house I would not have been surprised, so great was the sensation of being held in a strength and focus that I am afraid defies description. This second curve only required a touch of sandpaper; the other needed a rescue operation with rasps. But there the shelf is, a constant reminder of what is possible.

Not everything was portentous and awe-inspiring, for there were light-hearted events and humour aplenty - take this for instance, as when I had cause to replace the hot water cylinder in my bathroom. When installed, no provision had been made to allow the cylinder to be drained, and there was quite a residue of water that prevented me from completing an awkward lift. So I connected up a pipe that reached to the loo, and then blew into the top of the cylinder in order to displace some water. It was quite a blow, and I paced myself so as not to do myself a mischief. After one such blow, I sat back gasping, when a voice in my head said, "We would love to help you, but we've all run out of puff". Not the most hilarious of jokes, but in the location and circumstances I found myself rolling on the floor in laughter.

On another occasion, I had been following on the radio a serialisation of Fielding's

Tom Jones. It was broadcast at nine on Sunday evenings, and this particular Sunday was to be the last episode. It was a beautiful evening and I had had a number of friends for meals during the day. I was finishing off, washing up and musing as one does after a very enjoyable occasion, and was completely lost to the world, when suddenly there was *blasted* into my mind the rumbustious 'voice' of Squire Western, - "Zounds Tom - a pox on it!". I managed to keep hold of the dish that I was drying, and came to my senses realising that it was exactly nine o'clock and time for the finale of this radio romp.

      I can put no worthwhile time scale on the progress of the work and developments, but I am almost at the ultimate point of completion. For some time I have had a ground floor that is very accessible to anyone in a wheelchair - bedroom with en suite shower (which could be fitted to take a loo), cooking hobs at knee-height for a wheelchair, two accessible loos and a sun room with easy access and paths with gentle slopes. Though, strangely, it has not been the *physically* disabled who have come to take advantage of the facilities, as time will reveal.

      After a few weeks of regular church going, I found a sort of pattern developing, although attending either of two available churches required a round trip of twenty miles. On shopping days, if I arranged my timing correctly, I could hear Mass and receive communion on occasional weekday mornings, while at the weekends I decided to return to the church that I had formerly attended. Such is the way in which the liturgy works that the 'vigil', i.e. the evening before a particular day, has the validity of the day itself, and thus attending Mass on a *Saturday* evening was the equivalent of Sunday attendance, which is required of Catholics. This became a regular feature of my weekends and allowed me, having descended from my 'mountain fastness', to follow on with some social visiting, and at the same time leaving me free to be at home on Sundays when friends were most likely to call.

The sense of 'homecoming' and belonging added greatly to my inner composure and developing strength, and my 'world awareness' began to re-emerge as I took my part in an organisation that reaches to the remotest regions. One could not fail to have been aware of the African tragedy, as famine killed millions. Not having a lot to be able to give to charity, I wanted what I gave to make its mark without loss to any administrative costs, and so I chose to join an organisation called *The Little Way Association,* which guarantees that every penny will make its way to the needy through a network of missionary priests and nuns. I also participated at home in the regular prayer activity aimed at supporting these front-line people and their works. This was fine up to a point, but the far-flung individuals remained as shadowy figures working in the remote desert or bush. I needed a face, a focus. Such a face came via a photograph in the *Catholic Herald*, which I had started to take again.

The face was that of a nun, a 'Missionary Sister of Our Lady of Africa', a so-called White Sister - they and the White Fathers used formerly to wear a white Arab-style burnous to identify themselves with the local populace in Algeria and North Africa where they first operated - and thus they got their name. Joy was then an assistant chaplain at Liverpool University, and I wrote to tell her of her new role as my 'focus'. She replied, and sent me details of some prayer events and retreats that were scheduled at 'St. Beuno's', the Jesuit College in North Wales, one time home of priest and poet Gerald Manley Hopkins. In particular, she had circled and recommended a weekend in February (1981), and thence I went. This was an entirely new venture for me, as was the setting; and new was the contact with a young Jesuit priest, recently returned from a part of his training in Japan, at the Jesuit University there.

He brought to us concepts of stillness, breathing, sitting, meditation, derived from Eastern, and particularly Zen Buddhist, traditions, for part of the remit of this University is the promotion of dialogue and understanding with Zen Buddhism. I also, for the first time, became aware of the spiritual ambience of a place, a group of people, for the place had focused many years of prayer, while in the group there were a number of nuns of teaching orders taking their half-term break, and nuns are not strangers to prayer. Practically, I brought away the design of a simple meditation stool, a virtual bridge across the ankles that enables one to kneel/sit effortlessly and comfortably for long periods.

Much flowed from that encounter with Joy. She, additionally, had a job as an 'outreach' worker at a school in Liverpool's deprived Toxteth district, and, amongst other things, she asked me to pray for these needy children. Prayer, for me, is a call to action, and so I asked what I, personally, could do. Reply there came: the children needed holidays. And so it was that the house began to find its purpose, and the combined forces of the Seascale churches kicked into action. A group of ladies, the Co-workers of Mother Teresa, were the first to answer the call, and a posse descended on the house with besoms, mops and polish. Jack came with wife Edna and helped me to lay some new carpet on the stairs, that I hadn't yet got round to. Fresh curtains appeared; bunk beds were donated by a local hotel; towels and sheets, crockery and a *large* cooking pot arrived courtesy of a local Spastic Society school that was closing, as did some extra kitchen chairs. And the *large* cooking pot would definitely be needed, for, whereas the first contingent was going to be West Indian lady, Jenny and her five children, it was now also going to include her friend Carol plus her son. Good old Val, who twisted arms at a local bedding manufacturer and obtained additional duvets and sheets. And so we were ready, and with extra transport as the train rolled in, and out poured a seeming host of black faces as Peter, Alicia, Nicola, Darren, Sonia and Wayne descended to the inevitable Cumbrian rain - it was spring bank-holiday week.

A book would be necessary to relate the mixed activities and emotions of that first encounter, and all that followed in the subsequent summer holiday as Little Ground became fully booked for the season. Evenings in that first week provided a memorable picture as the area around the fireplace filled with a variety of sitting, lying, wrestling bodies, while to one side hair was being teased into tight, tiny plaits. I soon found myself whittling knitting needles and huge crochet hooks from dowel to occupy idle hands, and looking around, I saw my mini harem, but without the sultan's privileges! We alternated the catering, and the large cooking pot did full service, although its walls were fully proof tested by the force of cayenne pepper and chillies, as chicken or sea-fresh fish were absorbed into its interior, emerging as highly charged but superb meals.

The summer holiday filled a much greater need for these and other children, for it was in the intervening months that the infamous Toxteth riots occurred, and while the visitors weren't actually traumatised, they were all glad to be removed from that violent atmosphere for a while. Jenny and her gang returned for a fortnight, when they found a much wider range of activities as the sea became warmer and the shore beckoned, and beckoning also were the ponies of my neighbours' daughters. Next to arrive were Elizabeth and her mother, who immediately found a place in my life, where Mum stayed until her unfortunate early death, and where Liz now remains, a science teacher, married with three young children. They also came twice, once by design and the second time to fill a gap created by the early departure of a family - mother (plus her sister) and six youngsters all under eight. They were overwhelmed by the open space and silence, and having come on a Saturday, vanished on the Monday. The immediate gap was filled by two delightful girls, their mother and an unpleasant, and basically unwelcome partner, whom I hadn't bargained for. The girls were left mainly to my charge as mother and mate went around pursuing his activity of trying to wheedle antiques out of unsuspecting country folk. I later had police enquiries about him and his local escapades, and also heard about his imprisonment for GBH. Interesting times!

Once one opens one's door to life and its huge diversity, it seems impossible to stem the flood of so much that is new and exciting, and, well, *interesting.* I recall one particular day on which I heard a Radio 4 broadcast that effected a major change in my life - as if there hadn't been enough already. But, as the Bard correctly says, "There is a tide in the affairs of men which, if taken at the flood...". My tide was certainly flooding, but was it I who was allowing the flow to increase by continually opening the sluice gates myself? The broadcast centred on a man who was to have a significant role in my subsequent life, and continues to have even after his untimely death. I refer to Bruce Macmanaway. A former Major in the army, he had, as a subaltern during the Dunkirk retreat, been inspired to 'lay his hands' on wounded men, resulting in bleeding being arrested and pain eased. He went on, both during his career in the army and subsequently, to become a renowned practical and very effective Healer and teacher, who influenced *many* people, as I was to find out in the years immediately following,

I still have a tape of that broadcast, and revisit it and the two key elements that stood out to me at first hearing. The first was that Bruce described quite openly the use of a pendulum, and his own use of one in diagnosis. It made me quite concerned, because I was so very fresh from my own pendulum adventures, and concerned because he included no reference to the unwise uses of pendulums, or the possibility of unwelcome intrusions. The second element, which jolted me and my life, was his description and use of 'hands on' healing. No great hype; just matter of fact acceptance and practice. Now it so happened that a number of individuals had responded to the touch of my hands in a way that had been puzzling me. I had learned and freely gave gentle massage to anyone who would 'submit' as I improved my skills. People reacted to my touch in ways that suggested that there was more coming out of my hands than I was consciously putting in.

So I wrote concerning these two matters, and received a reply that said that after forty years practice he was truly aware of the first, and that also included details of courses that he was about to run, courses which, he assured me, would give me some answers to the second. The courses that year were to be at two centres, the one at his home (and teaching and healing centre) at Strathmiglo in Fife, and the other at an hotel in Mickleton in Warwickshire. I opted for the latter, for a plan was forming in my mind. The first part of the plan was to travel via a place in Carmarthenshire where I could buy some first-class leather to feed my burgeoning hobby of leatherwork, and then to stay a few days in my hometown of Port Talbot, where I planned to visit my remaining relatives who had formerly been involved in healing work. Remember, I had shied away from any contact with this aspect of the family's activities, being embarrassed by the whole involvement and concept. Now I was curious.

I had arranged to stay at the home of 'the girl next door' and her husband, who still lived in the family home, my last visit having been when my father lay dying in a nearby cottage hospital. I soon went to call upon Aunt Grace and Uncle Gwyn. Only Gwyn was at home together with my cousin Eleanor. We chatted a while and it emerged that he had withdrawn from his mediumship and healing work because his breathing was becoming limited following years of exposure to all the fumes of copper and other working. But, surprisingly, he was soon showing signs of 'actvity', and then lapsed into a trance. Gwyn had two of what are generally called 'guides', and who, almost inevitably, seem to be North American Indians and Chinese. Thus the two, Great Heart and Xiang, began to speak through him. There were initially domestic comments about the health and general well being of Gwyn and Eleanor, and some remarks to me and what I was embarking on. Then, as I was waiting to see or hear what next would transpire, my cousin gave a gasp and an exclamation - "It's Uncle Tom!" Now Tom had been my father, and as Gwyn stood up his whole demeanour, stance, and walk as he came over towards me were indeed those of my father. I stood and met him, and the hugs and emotion were immense. Then he took my hands, which were so hot that they were almost steaming, and held them towards Eleanor saying, "Look at the power, look at the power".

I cannot remember how we parted, and though the next day produced another domestic 'séance' with Grace being present, nothing as dramatic and so personal emerged. However, I felt that I had received the family accolade, and travelled east two or three days later, to my destiny!

The Macmanaway course assembled in an hotel run by a group of people united in a form of religious association, and which was in a delightful setting. Bruce and his wife Patricia led us, and talked to us on a variety of topics. Principally, we were shown Bruce's techniques of using a pendulum to dowse for trapped nerves within the spine, and for other structural abnormalities, and then we learned basic manipulation methods for their release. We started the day with yoga, which was skilfully led by Patricia, ate superb food, and mixed with each other in a close association of like minded and spiritually committed people. So close was the bonding that one evening when Bruce, in the middle of a manipulation, made a throw-away remark, slightly inappropriately, we were all conscious of a cold 'stab' that went through each of us in a remarkable way, sufficiently for a number of us to exchange comments afterwards. There were undoubtedly areas of disagreement and dispute, such as Bruce's propagation of the 'mystical' ley-line concepts, but for the rest, the whole week was inspirational.

Undoubtedly I learned many things, one of which was that in a skilled led meditation it was possible for one's own mind to enter a trance-like state. I only allowed this to happen once, and kept my own awareness thereafter, for I was determined, following my own experiences of the previous eighteen months, not to relinquish control again. I had a long conversation with Bruce about these past happenings, and one also with Patricia, out of which came some good advice, and an agreement that I could go and stay and *learn* and gain experience at Strathmiglo in the near future. A rewarding and genuinely mind opening week, and the beginning of so much more.

Returning towards home, I detoured via Liverpool, staying for a few nights at the White Sisters' house there, and to where Jenny and her brood and a number of their cronies came to give me a party, ending in a West Indian knees-up, or 'merry neet', as in Cumbria. Also to this house there came two nuns, sisters from the Mother Teresa missionary organisation. They had got wind of my presence, and came to ask whether a day visit to my church in Seascale could be arranged for a number of their down and outs. They could provide the coaches, could we, i.e. the church, arrange the rest? And so I came back with a project to put to our small congregation. Instant consternation, then realisation, as ideas came forth and a combined churches task force swung into action. It had to be on a Wednesday when the many alcoholics would be all spent up, and there would be no truants to the nearest pub. Food was planned, extra cooking organised, the hall booked, sightseeing planned and entertainment by the 'Evergreens' laid on. Apart from a major delay because the coaches took the longest route to travel, everything went as planned, and another organisational milestone was passed as the sisters and postulants marshalled their charges, did a head count and vanished into the night.

What a year for new faces, and how easy they can be recalled - Joy, Jenny, Carol and all the kids; the Macmanaways and many on the course; Sisters Jose-Ann from India and Aurore from France; and many faces in the two church congregations and in the prayer group to which I now belonged. As time went on, I saw more of Jack and Edna and a strong friendship developed, and their roadside home became a frequent and convenient stopping and 'watering' place. It was in their lounge that another face came into focus. Judith. In a photograph. Their elder daughter, she had died of leukaemia a few years earlier, leaving a husband and two young children, and in the picture she was in profile, looking into the cot at her baby as only a mother can. Every time that I passed the photograph, as I did on entering and leaving the room, I felt a pang at the poignancy of it, and yet felt the warmth of this lovely view of motherhood.

      Gradually, over a period, I began to sense Judith's presence in an indescribable way. Not as a wraith, ghost or physical presence, yet certainly full of obstreperous 'life'. I do not like messages from 'beyond the grave'. I do not seek them, and resist any that are apparently there, until I have tested and re-tested. But increasingly it kept coming into my mind that Judith was happy, and that I must tell her mother it was so. For some time, several weeks possibly, I resisted, for how do you broach such a subject? Then one Saturday evening, I called on my way to church, to give Edna a lift to join Jack who was umpiring a cricket match. As I was passing the photograph on my way out of the house to go to the car, I felt such a thump in the middle of my back between the shoulder blades, and 'heard' the command that was intensely strong in my mind - "Tell her now. *Tell her <u>now</u>*". During the short journey that followed, somehow I managed to find the words, and was so relieved when I had done so, for

Edna's joy was boundless. She had fretted inside since Judith's death, conscious of her (Judith's) loss and potential for unhappiness, and to learn now that she was indeed happy so gladdened Edna that, she told me later, she walked on air for days afterwards. She also confirmed that Judith had been so full of life, but also was so definitely *obstreperous!*

It was about this time that the 'Africa connection' began to develop and expand. "Could you" wrote Joy, "manage to send copies of the *Catholic Herald* and *Observer* to a friend in Uganda?" How could one refuse, and weekly I rolled newspapers to send to Marie, and began a very long and enthralling correspondence and association. There were four White Sisters staffing and running a dispensary in the bush some distance to the southwest of Kampala, a dispensary that had been a hospital until Idi Amin had wreaked destruction on his own land. It was functioning again, fulfilling a vast local need and stretching meagre resources beyond limit. Regular probing produced for me an appalling picture of shortages and lack of funds, and of a national economy so completely devastated by Amin's depredations. So affected was I, and disappointed at my own inability to do much financially, that I used to look begrudgingly even at the tin of cat food that I dispensed daily to my two moggies. Fortunately, one could be returned to its former home where the family generated enough waste food to feed it, while sadly the other fell

LISTENING TO THE SILENCES

victim to one of the occasional car rallies that like to use the narrow winding roads of my neighbourhood.

As soon as I was able, I covenanted the cost of my one daily, medium sized tin of cat food for the benefit of Marie's dispensary where, and it still amazes me to recall, it paid the wages of *two local nurses and a midwife*! Even now, after twenty years, I cringe at the sight of the stacked super-market shelves of pet food.

Much developed from this contact with Marie, some of which will emerge as my narrative continues, but I must move on as the flow in the other channels gathers force. However, before I leave Africa temporarily I must tell you about George. Once the doors of awareness of need and suffering are opened, it is impossible to close them again, and one would indeed be hard hearted even to try. George brought into my ken a swarm of blind children who needed people to write to them. He was actually in Kenya. A Scot, he had lived in East Africa since the end of World War 2, and now, after a number of traumatic events resulting from the Amin regime, resided in a school for blind children for whom he wrote letters, sought contacts and read replies. So it was that I began to write to Mary, Ruth and Respe. I had been fortunate in acquiring a decent type-writer, courtesy of Edna, which had revolutionised my then letter writing almost as much as my PC has done in recent times, otherwise I could not have managed this burgeoning correspondence.

Roy Vincent

I still have the letters written in George's tiny hand, and some of the copies of my replies, which I retained to be able to keep track of the three individuals and George himself. Character and life story began to emerge, and how one wished one could do more. Mary was completely sightless from river blindness; Ruth still had vestigial sight and went on to the high school at Thika (of *Flame Trees* fame). And Respe, who could not weep for Respe? Let anyone try to tell me that *real evil* does not exist! Respe at twelve, a strong healthy girl, was raped, and so that she could not recognise him, her assailant gouged out her eyes.

After some time had passed, the letters via George ceased. On enquiring, I found that the staffing policy of this Salvation Army run school had changed to employ solely local people, and that George, who had also succumbed to malaria, had left for England. Surprisingly, and after much phoning and detective work, I tracked him down to a hospital not twenty miles from my home; and so we met. Gradually, as he recovered from the stroke that had put him into hospital, his story emerged - far too intricate to relate, even in synopsis. However, it was an inspiring story that fired many to emulate his dedication to the needy of Africa, and each time I visited him, beside his bed would be at least one nurse or therapist listening, and being inspired to take up voluntary service overseas.

LISTENING TO THE SILENCES

George went later to a Salvation Army retirement home in Bath, where he eventually died. But he left me a sort of legacy. Divorced, George had married a Ugandan lady with whom he lived in Kampala until the uprisings and civil war, during which his wife had been killed and, beaten and injured himself, he had moved to Malawi, losing touch with his daughter Doris and stepdaughter Kate. I had written for him to Kate, now tracked down at University in Kenya, but heard nothing. The letter must have had a long gestation period, for nearly ten years later I received a letter from Doris. She was in London, to where she had come earlier as a refugee. Kate had remembered my original letter, and so I found myself involved in yet two more lives, as I wrote to an uncaring bureaucracy to support Doris' attempts to get a British passport on the strength of her parentage. Kate, meanwhile, has worked for a Master's degree in Kenya, but, like many single African girls, is facing a life of chosen celibacy because of the prevalence of AIDS in a country of male promiscuity.

However, I have gone ahead of myself, so let us return to the spring of 1982 and my journey north to the Kingdom of Fife, where.........

Roy Vincent

CHAPTER 8

Enough, if something from our hands have power to live, and act, and serve the future hour.

Wordsworth

Roy Vincent

LISTENING TO THE SILENCES

Horatio : ..but this is wondrous strange.

Hamlet : There are more things in heaven
and earth, Horatio, than are dreamt of in your philosophy.

It was John who always quoted these words of Hamlet to me as his life and the lives of others began to mesh with mine. But not just yet: they were all in the future, and nothing that followed would have happened if I had not taken the road over the Scottish Border in that sunny late May in 1982, to determine whether there was in reality '...something in my hands which would have the power to live and act and serve the future'.

The auguries had been consulted and it was indeed deemed auspicious that I should begin my apprenticeship with Bruce Macmanaway at his centre at Strathmiglo, and there I arrived near midday one Sunday to a kind welcome. I was placed in a flat in the village that I shared for a short while with a young student, Nicky, who, it turned out, originated from a place not fifteen miles from my own South Welsh home. We did not share for very long for she departed, ostensibly to stay with a sick friend.

Roy Vincent

      I spent the Sunday evening taking stock of my surroundings and musing upon what might happen, though I was not in any way certain exactly what I would be doing, for I wasn't to get my 'induction' until the following morning. In a sense, though, I had company, for since my visit to my Uncle Gwyn it had been put into my mind that I was to have transferred to me his two 'guides' - 'Great Heart and Xiang'. I cannot remember how I reacted to this intimation, and had not speculated much upon what, if anything, it might mean, nor what might follow. I was still very wary of *any* form of intrusion or overt spiritual association, as I am right up to this present day, for I have never been without them, good and bad, as I shall write in detail later. In addition to the alleged African, Ibn Ubar, who, I assumed was still active and party to the developments, I had my new duo, and thus equipped, but not thinking specifically about any of 'them', I slept well and rose early to meet the day.

      It was such a beautiful sunny morning, as indeed it was all week, and I walked the short distance to 'Westbank' - a sturdy former farm house with its buildings converted to a variety of other uses, though there were still horses. At the entrance and vying with the sun was a rosebush in full bloom, a rose that I have grown myself ever since. It is the first of any to show in spring, and although its flowers are single and just a couple of inches across, the whole bush presents such a joyous picture, truly living up to its name of *Canary Bird*.

LISTENING TO THE SILENCES

How very much I regret that I can do no more than give you the merest inkling of the impact that this week, and particularly this first day, were to have on my life and development thereafter. At one level, there is a whole crowd of superlatives jostling to be used: at another, and so very potent, are the images that so easily return to my mind's eye. In every one of these images there was the sunshine that was all pervasive, especially in the part of the treatment area in which I was to work closely with Bruce. The sunlight poured in through a large area of glass, which itself gave onto a beautiful and imaginative garden, the product of Patricia's mind and hands. It illuminated a long room divided by curtains into several consulting and treating areas, and shone onto Bruce and two young women, friends, who had arrived together, each needing help.

Both were professional violinists and, as with many of their calling, had upper back problems. Bruce used to declare that he could muster at least one full orchestra from among his clients! Permission for my being there having been sought and willingly given, I sat to one side, watched, and listened. A decision having been made as to which would go first, Bruce sat and chatted to her, pendulum in hand. I already knew what he would be seeking in his mind, but it soon became apparent that he could work simultaneously on two levels. A pendulum is used in these circumstances simply to indicate a definite "Yes" or "No", giving answers to the mental questions - "Can I help this person?" "Are there any problems in the spine?" And so on, following a sequence that had been established over years of practice, and through which an easy conversation could still proceed.

It was determined that this young woman's problems lay in the muscles controlling the shoulder blades, and these in turn were subjected to some subtle and skilful manipulation. She was next sat upon a high stool, I stood behind and responded to my instruction to "Put your hands there, Roy" - 'there' being parallel with her spine and between her shoulder blades. So simple, but such a seminal moment, especially as the response was almost immediate. "Phoooaaah!" was the ecstatic sound, followed by attempts to put the inner sensations produced into context, the nearest analogy being, I think, that they were the equivalent of being in a microwave oven. It was the response that I needed, for I had had no inkling of what to expect, as through my hands I felt nothing, no tingling, no excessive heat, nothing exceptional. And there I stayed, applying 'hot hands', as my mentors used to phrase it, while the second violinist received the equivalent from Bruce. I know that this was commonplace to the workers at Westbank, but to me that ecstatic sound had told me all that I needed to know, just as I knew that my life would never be quite the same again.

If I needed further demonstration and confirmation, it came with the next client of the morning, a Russian Orthodox priest who had arrived with his interpreter. A diminutive man, bent and hobbling with a stick, he looked very un-Russian, and more like an ancient Chinese intellectual. He was riddled with arthritis in knees, hips and shoulders, and kneeling for prayer or his beloved gardening was impossible. The conversation, travelling as it did via the woman interpreter, who also had an input, was fascinating, but all the while the pendulum was reacting. Following a series of manipulations, Bruce sat with his hands in place on hip and knee, while I was placed to stand so that I could have my hands at the back and front of a shoulder. The animated conversation continued, while I felt the crabbed little rounded shoulder between my hands. But what was this? My hands were slowly coming together, and between them it felt as if the intervening shoulder was melting. From time to time a hand came up and stroked the one of mine that was at the front, and again, occasionally, the head turned and bright bird-like eyes shone up at me from above a beatific smile, which itself emerged from a wispy oriental beard. I have no real idea how long we stayed thus, but magic moments always end too soon, and there he was, being escorted out by Bruce, while his interpreter sat holding herself with laughter. What amused her so was that the little priest no longer hobbled and had gone off without his stick, totally oblivious to the extent of his now upright stature, while it was being slowly explained to him that Bruce never took payment from the ministers of any religion.

Roy Vincent

It would be inappropriate for me to give, and I am sure that you would not want, a recital of all the problems brought by such a wide variety of people, who had variously come from Northern Ireland, the Outer Hebrides, parts of Scotland, as well as from the local village. My week was so full, so very, very full, and full still is my mind of many memories. Right up until the last session, when the contrast could not have been greater, between an ox-like Jock from the Black Watch who had done his back a mischief as he had helped to retrieve a gun from a ditch, and a petite and elegant former ballerina, one, it turned out, with whom I, like many, had fallen in love a number of years before when she had entranced us all, as she had danced and acted through her films. What a finale to an incredible week.

But that wasn't all, for additional things happened during some of the other activities at the Centre; events which in themselves were equally memorable. Each Monday evening a number of people gathered at Westbank for a general group meditation. Formed into a horseshoe we sat, positioned relative to each other by Bruce. He conducted the spoken meditation theme in a way that I had experienced at the earlier course. By my own determination, I did not let myself drift, but there were obviously a number of this group of about twelve or fifteen who were 'away with the fairies'. When the meditation had ended and everyone had returned to the planet, Bruce asked each in turn what, if anything, he or she had experienced. The replies were obviously quite diverse, but my ears pricked up when one lady said that she had been involved with black people in some sort of lion hunt. My ears positively waggled when another lady said that she had been presented in her mind's eye with the head of a North American Indian in full feathered head-dress.

Bruce left me until last in this catechism, when I had to confess that, whereas I had no personal experiences to report, I believed that I was responsible for the lion hunt, for reasons which I explained, and that also the Indian was one of 'mine'. But where, I said, was the representative from China whom by now, I thought, must also be present? "Well," said the lady who had seen the Indian "part way through the meditation the head changed into that of a Chinaman, but I rationalised that this could not be possible, whereupon it had returned to its previous Indian form".

Wednesday noon produced a gathering with a different purpose. Every one of the Centre's many clients, and all the people for whom requests had been sent, were to be made the focus of a combined direction of absent healing. Into the assembled names I had put that of Sandy, my GP friend who was slowly dying from a strange wasting illness (motor neurone disease, as it turned out). Neither I, nor anyone else, expect miracles, but one has to try. Again, there was a led meditation and prayer for each of the named individuals, at which point, for Sandy, I felt intense internal emotion, but no, sadly, no miracle. At times one feels let down when something dramatic does not occur, but I was very much a beginner in this ancient 'craft' of healing, and it was only later, when I became closely involved with the so-called 'gentle approach' to cancer, that I was to learn that there are many different ways in which individuals can be 'healed'.

As on the Monday, at the end, Bruce asked each to relate any experiences. Mine had been obvious to all, and others had been internally involved with thoughts of the many unnecessary deaths resulting from the sinking the previous day of the Argentinean cruiser *Belgrano*. Nothing of particular note came forward, and I might easily have forgotten the laughing comments of one young woman, who said that she had been presented in her mind with what looked like a peculiar cage of filigree gold, shaped, as best she could describe, like a pumpkin with a handle on the top; though I had to wait until I subsequently arrived home to realise the significance to me of her 'vision'.

After lunch on my final day, I was sped on my way, still in the bright sunshine that had blessed the whole week, by a collection of such memorable people, and with a mind brim full of a vast range of experiences and phenomena. It was not all that far to the Kinross service station, but I pulled into it simply to let myself descend slowly and a little closer to the planet. I don't know what my thoughts would have been had I known then that Westbank would figure even more significantly later in my new and burgeoning life, or that, in spite of the apparent total benevolence of all that I had experienced, there was a trap laid by the 'Auld Enemy' (that's his name in Scotland), in which Nicky innocently figured, and which would not be sprung for another eight years. The context and happening are not truly relevant to my ongoing tale, and so I'll have to leave you speculating on that one (though don't go too wild in your ideas), but the events subsequent to the trap being sprung served to show me, in my naïveté, just how two-faced even the nicest people can be at times. No, entirely unaware of a whole variety of impending developments, I took to the road again, somewhat more focussed than I had been on the first part of my journey. At Carlisle, I staged myself at the home of a cousin and her companion and shared some of my experiences, and then on again, wanting to get home and yet not wanting to. My final diversion was to visit the farmstead of Peter and Tricci, which was very close to my route, and as I walked across the yard, Tricci came out to greet me saying, "Where have you *been*? You're positively *shining!*"

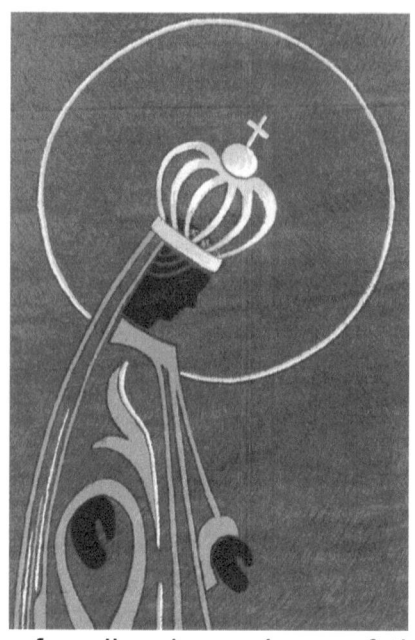

The final event that closed this particular sequence materialised when I had collected and sorted my mail. Enclosed with a letter from Marie or Joy, I forget which, was a prayer card issued by the Missionary Sisters of Our Lady of Africa, and on it was a picture of the statue to Our Lady of Africa, which stands in Algiers, the founding home base of the missionary order of White Fathers and Sisters. Surmounting the head of the statue was a crown – a filigree gold construction, which did, in fact, resemble 'a cage shaped like a pumpkin' while the cross at the top did, actually look like a handle. (On the wall opposite me now as I write is a larger version, painted in blue and gold on brown bark cloth by one of the White Sisters in Africa, and the gold crown with its surmounted cross totally fits that description).

What a range of memories and consequences there are to recall and put in some sort of order and sequence, as each of the strands of my life unwound and wove again one with the other. One of the principal ones, undoubtedly, was that concerned with an understanding of many of the factors involved in my own health and that of other people, which had been made all the more relevant with my direct opening into the field of 'healing'. As my body and mind had cleared themselves of all the residues of my unfortunate sixteen years of being polluted by the drugs that I had taken, I found that, in many ways, I had been going through a process of rebirth and of rediscovery. What was coming back to life, and what I was rediscovering, were normal body functions and reactions that had been suppressed by all the invasive medications, whose prime function had been, after all, to suppress or alter the body's natural functions and reactions via their effect upon the central nervous system. Even now, nearly forty years after my initial encounter with Librium, I am still trying to re-educate my centre of reaction that I would call the solar plexus, which went into a sort of rebound after so many years of being suppressed, and has never truly regained a stable and natural function.

After having been subjected to a sort of medical 'rape' of my mind and body, my one overriding approach to anything to do with my health was that which also governed my burgeoning activities in the home - Do-It-Yourself. My encounter with Richard Mackarness' book, *Not All in the Mind*, and Sandy's realistic attitude to medical intervention, prompted me to start learning in earnest, and from all sources, and at every juncture. As I encountered anything to do with health, I read and read and asked questions. One learning leap occurred following my hearing of a broadcast of the radio programme 'You and Yours'. The name 'myalgic encephalomyelitis' has thankfully been shortened to M.E. At the time, i.e. 1981, and when also known as the 'Royal Free disease', it was not commonly recognised nor talked about. As the broadcast progressed, I found myself recognising in myself so much of what was being described, sufficiently for me to write to an address given for further information. With the information package came a very detailed and wide-ranging questionnaire, which I duly completed fully and honestly. The answers were assessed by a group of doctors who had volunteered their services, but, inevitably, it was a procedure that took some time. The reply, when it came, said that there was a distinct probability that I could be suffering from M.E., and offered several suggestions about how next to proceed. In the time between sending my questionnaire and receiving the reply, I had decided that whatever the outcome I had no intention of being saddled with *any* illness, and had moved on, with a determination that I should take as much responsibility for my own well-being as I possibly could.

In spite of this decision of mine to disassociate myself from any personal connection with an illness, it is worth looking briefly at those of my own reactions that I had felt matched the ones that had been used to define M.E. The reason

LISTENING TO THE SILENCES

why I do so is that they appear severally or alone in a setting that will emerge shortly. The effects that I thought that I recognised, or with which I identified, were: intermittent difficulty in sleeping; unexplained and unpredictable mood swings, particularly to 'lows' that went as inexplicably as they had arrived; periodic difficulty in achieving coherent thought; physical sensations that were hard to identify or specify, as they incorporated aspects of tingling, twitching, numbness and aches, which were worse in bed and cumulative through the night, and so on.

One positive and fruitful area of study derived from my increasing use of herbs, and was stimulated by a delightful and remarkably informative book *Grandmother's Secrets* by Jean Palaiseul. Over the years, I have acquired other herbals, but this is always my reference book of first choice. From it, and allied with the information disseminated by the Henry Doubleday Association, I learned of the properties of one herb that, in particular, has become both efficacious and influential in my life. Comfrey, or knit bone, or any of the many other country names by which it is known, has a prolific life in my garden, where it provides the core of my composting activities. But it is the remarkable healing properties that it possesses that have kept it to the fore ever since I learned of them, and it was these that were to have a major influence in my continuing contact with Marie and her dispensary.

Sometime in 1982-3, she had written describing the even worse economic situation that was enveloping Uganda. In particular, they were desperately short of medicines; could I help? I did the first two things that came to my mind, and through which I believed that I could achieve *something*. I contacted the Medical Department of my former employers, who most willingly and generously provided a quantity of materials and drugs, which I sent. Secondly, I sent a copy of *Grandmother's Secrets*; a book by Lawrence Hills called simply *Comfrey*, and all my available supply of comfrey ointment. This may appear to some as naïve, but many of the ailments being treated in the bush were on the surface of the body, where I believed that the direct healing promoted by comfrey would be effective. Anyway, I did what I could, and invited other agencies to help as well. The ointment duly arrived, on a Friday, and was immediately applied to an ulcer that was on the leg of an old man who had walked for three days to reach the dispensary. Marie wrote that such an ulcer would normally take a fortnight to heal using the standard treatments available to them. However, by the following Monday new pink skin started to appear, and within a very few days the healing was complete. The old man departed joyfully, calling down blessings on Our Lady, while everyone else who was there at the time was most impressed!

After such an auspicious start there had to be a follow up, and that came through the assistance of a remarkable man, Lawrence Hills of the Henry Doubleday Organisation. He could not have been more helpful, for he obtained seeds of comfrey for me to send, and also supplied me with several kilograms of ointment, having himself sent an equivalent amount directly. My contribution went to Uganda courtesy of Marie's sister, who was about to depart for a holiday there and who carried it with her. The ointment was so valued and applied so freely to all manner of skin complaints that it disappeared like the proverbial snow off a dyke, so that when Marie returned to work following her own break, there was not much left. This remainder was applied to a varicose ulcer that had defied all other remedies, and yes, that soon healed as well.

      The seeds grew into plants, and when they reached maturity and their form could be seen, the nuns found that there was comfrey growing in their own garden already! But having the plants available led on to other things, for one of the sisters took note of a photograph in the book *Comfrey*. This pictured a woman who used to buy at her local cattle market, calves that no one else wanted because they were scouring i.e. had diarrhoea. She took them home and fed them milk in which was chopped comfrey, and the property which the herb has of being an internal vulnary, helped heal the calves' guts, and they went on to thrive. You may be aware that one of the prime causes of infant death in tropical regions is dehydration following prolonged diarrhoea, and by feeding the infants in a similar way to that of the calves, many of them recovered and likewise began to thrive. Marie moved on to a different location soon afterwards, and so, eventually, I lost touch with this fascinating development.

However, this was not to be the end of the train of events set in motion by the comfrey saga, far from it. I had asked Marie's sister, Wilma, to take some photographs during her visit, so that I could appreciate more fully the work of the dispensary, and its location. Following her return, Wilma and husband Tony, together with their three daughters, came for a week-end visit, bringing with them a large collection of slides, which were all-encompassing in the way they in which brought the Ugandan bush to life. I, in turn, was invited to visit them in Dundee, which I elected to do in the coming September. I broke my journey with a friend at Livingston, and set off northward again early-ish one morning. I planned my journey so that I could call at Westbank, principally to renew acquaintances. I had hardly crossed the Forth Bridge than I found myself subjected to heavy intrusions and obsessive thoughts as to whether I would have enough petrol to cover the motorway part of my journey. Having learned that the safest course during such disturbances is to stop and take stock, I left the motorway at the first opportunity, bought petrol, and sat awhile to compose myself before continuing north, feeling rather more secure and focussed.

When I arrived at Westbank, I found that the reception arrangements had changed since my previous visit, and that the people whom I had expected to see were no longer there. So I stood composing in my mind what I was going to say to introduce myself to the new secretary. She, meanwhile, was attending to a woman who had just emerged from treatment. Also waiting patiently nearby was a clergyman. The lady having departed, the secretary turned to my neighbour and addressed him "And now, Mr Grieve"… I stepped back and looked at him, and thirty-seven years fell away, to the sea off Corfu, and my friend David standing at the foot of the accommodation ladder of the aircraft carrier, HMS *Ocean*, down which he had helped me and into the pinnace that was to transport me to the nearby hospital ship. "David, Shepherd, Alan Grieve?" I said, and I treasure to this day his look of mixed surprise and consternation, while I hastened to identify myself. I will not even begin to try to describe the encounter; words just would not do it justice. Patricia, alerted, came out to take in the spectacle, and, when all was reasonably composed again, I went in to assist with David's treatment, which seemed fair, as the last time we had met he had been tending me.

My visit to Dundee was most enjoyable as Tony and Wilma went out of their way to make me welcome. Theirs was a lovely warm and *caring* household, caring manifested in virtually every one of their many activities and work. My visit was broken in the middle to respond to an urgent invitation to travel to David's home a short distance to the north, where I was to meet his wife Marjorie, and their youngest daughter, Margaret, the only one of their four children still at home. Additionally, I was to renew another friendship, and how delightful that was. During our training, and when we had been comparatively close to London, David and I had hitched to the north of the city and to Brookmans Park, where there was a Free Polish Radio, and where, helping to man it, was David's new brother-in-law, Bruno, who had married his elder sister Rae. The epic of Bruno's escape from Poland when it was overrun is well worth the hearing, but here he was and Rae also, so welcoming, and such warmth. And here it was, the other family that I wrote about earlier, which I hadn't know that I had, but which absorbed me as if I had always been a part of it, as did David and Marjorie's other children, Allison, Michael and John and their partners, when I was to meet them subsequently. But I have to warn you: Bruno's Polish generosity with a tumbler and whisky bottle exceeds even that of a generous Scot - and you get one nationality *added* to the other, and you need a strong head!

It is interesting to pause and reflect for a moment that if I had not responded to the intense intrusions in the way that I had, and left the motorway to compose myself, my arrival at Westbank would not have coincided with that of David. This pause for reflection really acknowledges the fact that the spiritual intrusions, good and bad, were a feature of my every waking moment. That I had coped thus far, and continued

LISTENING TO THE SILENCES

to cope satisfactorily, says a lot for the strategies that I was developing, which in turn owed everything to the fact that I was fully aware of how the voice hearing and physical intrusions first began. I write in analytical detail later describing exactly the variety of forms that the intrusions can take, and how they can exert their influence, but for the moment please accept that *anyone* can be imitated, or any situation conjured up within one's imaginative mind, and the skill with which this is done is considerable. A 'voice' resembling that of Inspector Clousseau, or the subtle effects of a sensual female presence, can be generated so easily - and all the while I was trying to cope within and through this barrage, and wondering whether, indeed, there *were* these three individual 'guides', as had been represented. Fortunately the issue was to be resolved, and soon.

Still reeling from all the amazement and excitement generated at Westbank by my encounter with David, I had, nevertheless, remembered to ask Patricia whether I could come with my friends to the absent healing meeting during the coming week. She had agreed and so we duly arrived. All the gatherings took place in a spacious and light upstairs lounge, and while I haven't consciously tried to copy it in the arrangement of my own room, there is, nevertheless, a similarity of ambience and outlook, which makes it easy for me to recall this particular day, and sequence of events.

We were a small gathering, for, apart from myself, Tony and Wilma, there was just

Patricia and a woman who normally assisted with her healing work. Patricia began a gentle led meditation, and, virtually as she started, and always conscious of my intention never to lose control of my own thoughts, I was strongly aware of the presence of my supposed quartet of 'guides' - four, because my father was sometimes represented as being present. It is difficult to describe one's awareness of 'manifestations', but, by whatever means, I was conscious of four 'individuals' close to me, and almost as soon as this fact registered, they moved rapidly to my rear. Suddenly, I became aware of a huge body of available resource, support and power. It was as if I had become the spear point of a huge phalanx of infinite size; my back was ramrodded, and with that came the knowledge that there would be unlimited support and assistance available in all my endeavours, but - and this is the most crucial element of the whole event - everything would be delivered *anonymously*. Simultaneously my view out of the window opposite ceased to be that of the garden, and instead I was presented with the concept of my far distant goal from which I was separated by a varied and difficult terrain. I knew that if I was to arrive there, it would only be through my own efforts in walking every step of the way, but, provided that this goal was the *right* one, the available support would be immense.

Through it all, I had not lost the thread of Patricia's narrative. Symbolically, she was taking us to the ultimate centre of healing and the ultimate 'healer', as we journeyed steadily up the abstract mountain to the divine temple at the top. "But", she said, "you may not feel it necessary to go fully to the top, you may decide to pause". That, I thought, is for me, and immediately there was fed into my mind a view looking down on the small plateau on which my house sits, and I was indeed looking *down* onto my own house. Patricia continued upward to arrive at the temple at the top of the mountain in which would be the person, source of all healing, but essentially unseen, the 'ineffable'. "Hold on" I thought, "this is not my understanding" - all my recent experiences following on from recovery from the initial spiritual trauma, had been of a growing *openness* in what I was trying to do, and in respect of relationship with the 'Holy Family' of my prayer and response. So where did that leave me? Stuck on a mountain with nowhere to go? No, for again I was looking down at my house, only this time the 'lid' was off, and I was looking down into my kitchen and there at the table, the arrangement of which was still in the planning stage, sat my 'ultimate healer', talking animatedly with some children.

I could not have had plainer answers to my inner questions and to questions that I had yet to ask. I would know that in future *every* voice would be suspect, and that, as I further found out, everything that came from a desirable source would be entirely by deep 'subliminal transfer', and without being represented as coming from *any* nominated 'person' - the origin should be obvious and clear. That, unfortunately, did not mean that henceforth there would be absolute certainty about the source of anything that came into my head. I wish that this could be so, but it is not to be, and constantly one must be on one's guard: constantly. There were many gifts that came via the Holy Spirit at Pentecost, and one of these, perhaps the most important, is Discernment. It has become customary in certain political circles to say everything in triplicate, so I must do the same. Discernment. Discernment. Discernment. There is no other option; constant alertness and never drop one's guard. Intelligent people become familiar with the ploys of the advertising industry, from the full frontal assault, to the subtle, low-key, almost subliminal insinuation. The supermarket does not have to advertise its bread; it lets the smell of freshly baked loaves diffuse through the air-conditioning. Coffee shops used to let the smell of roasting coffee beans drift down the High Street. Who can resist? (Just mention a bacon butty, or the smell of frying onions, and I am sure that in some mouths the saliva will start to run).

In a similar manner, thoughts, concepts, perceptions of taste or smell even, can be subtly drifted into the mind in such a way that one does not realise that they have come from anywhere but one's own intellect. It is hard to write of these situations without going into an immense amount of detail, and obviously, the perception and reaction will differ from person to person. If possible, I shall try to describe typical scenarios later in my writing as I enlarge other concepts, although I cannot guarantee that I shall succeed. But I must try, for in addition to the direct voice hearing experience, there can be created in susceptible individuals obsessions, cravings and addictions, self-image fixations and eating disorders.

For my immediate purpose, the additional statements and answers that emerged during the course of the meditation could not have been more plain, either. There would be no ethereal, unreachable 'temple of healing' in my predictable future other than here in my own home. Neither need I look further than these four walls for my rôle model; he would be here, both inside me as I attempt to emulate him and at my side or in my hands when I ask for help for others. I am sorry that I cannot comment further, but my spiritual life and thoughts are very private to me, as are the dedications of my self and my domestic resources to the needs and care of others here or where they are reachable.

When I had returned from my first visit to Westbank, I found myself essentially on the edge of a void. Full of thoughts of my new found talents, having no point of reference, no one with like experiences to consult or with whom to explore ideas, I felt as a painter must when faced with a blank canvas. But whereas the painter has been there before, has had tuition and had tutorial experience, and has a whole tradition of painting deriving from early times from which to draw inspiration, I was looking at my own canvas, but finding that there was no living tradition of healing there to guide me, nor practitioners to consult. It might have been said that I had my rôle model, and that his healing exploits have been fully written about in the New Testament. Quite so, but at times this association with Biblical healings turned out to be a major disadvantage in addressing the expectations that many individuals have. Some people preface the word 'healing' with 'spiritual' or 'faith', and from those two words many things flow. Firstly, the word 'spiritual' has, for some, a connotation of 'spiritualism' that they find unacceptable; for others it betokens an interaction with spiritual beings, which they are not prepared to experience. Yet again, there can be the unspoken expectation of a 'Jesus'-type miracle, a concept that an individual could find overwhelming. Secondly, 'faith' also releases a whole gamut of reactions; is it the faith of the practitioner or the faith of the patient that is implied? If it is the faith of the patient, does that mean that he or she has to take on board any *religious* beliefs or practices, and if there is no cure or improvement, does that mean that the person did not have enough faith, or that past 'sin' was an impediment?

I found all these reactions, either expressed openly or implied, as I started to offer to individuals what I thought would be of benefit to them. Gradually, as these responses started to become apparent, and as my own predilections came to the fore, my approach, technique and strategy started to develop.

It may be asked why I did not follow exactly the methods and techniques that I had witnessed and assisted with during my time at Westbank. That would be a fair point. There are two reasons why I did not do so: the first is that, as you may recall, I no longer used a pendulum: the second is that I never felt myself to be sufficiently competent to perform any physical manipulations upon a person. In the event, and as will emerge, I adopted, and gradually developed, a practice based upon and more suited to the analytical engineering method that governs my approach to most situations. You may remember that in my work with measuring devices in the nuclear plants, if any piece of equipment failed it was not sufficient simply to repair it, but the *reason* for its failure had to be known and eliminated before a repair could be considered complete. Similarly, with any illness there must be a cause or causes, which if found could be addressed and hopefully eliminated, although I did not reach a sufficient degree of competence to follow this investigative path for some time. Initially, and continuing while my understanding and experience increased, I simply applied my hands where and for how long seemed appropriate.

The simple and the practical - that sums up both my original and continuing approaches. As I have written several times before, I am embarrassed by the showy, the exaggerated, and I did not want to inflict anything of that nature upon the people whom I was trying to help. Thus, there were no elaborate manual 'passes', no 'aura stroking', no adjuncts such as crystals or essences, no overt 'religious' or mystical ceremony. Just the simplicity of my hands and intellect - and who? Without going into detail, I had committed myself completely to my own *intent* when trying to help someone, and had committed myself unequivocally to the spiritual association in which I totally believed. Having made that commitment privately there was no need to produce it on show; I simply carried it with me into every healing encounter, in the absolute and certain belief that, as and when needed, help would be forthcoming from an ethereal source. So far, I have never been disappointed.

In mentioning or discussing such interventions I am always conscious of the danger of presenting myself as one of the 'chosen', or of appearing to be a sanctimonious prig: neither, I hope, is the case. In mentioning or describing any overt spiritual or ethereal participation, I do so simply to affirm that such *does* happen. I also do so to balance what may appear to be the solely *terrestrial* and pragmatic approach that was developing as my response to the individual ailments that were being presented to me. The fact that, as I continue writing, I shall give much more space to this latter approach, reflects the nature of the process of exploration with which I found myself involved. In addition, I find it necessary to readdress the issue of continuing adverse spiritual intervention and intrusion. Like you, I would have supposed that with such powerful and benevolent spiritual allies, all aggressive opposition would be swept away. Not so. In real life, no matter how powerful the civil law enforcement and protection agencies, there are thieves, muggers, delinquents of all kinds, and violent and 'road-raging' individuals. Equally, within a life of developing spiritual openness, and throughout one's attempts to put the results of one's spiritual awareness into practice, increasingly one meets the equivalent from the adverse spiritual world. Direct mental aggression, traps and trip-wires are all there for the unwary, as are the 'con-artist' and deviant.

As events moved on, I began to recognise more and more of the ways in which one can be taken over, demoralised, undermined and tricked, and sometimes dominated. Different 'ploys' began to emerge, as did an awareness of the times, circumstances or occasions when certain attacks were made and were effective. Increasingly, I began to observe and recognise these for what they were, and to record the various ones as they happened. Some will emerge as I write, but in the main, I will describe and analyse the modes of attack all together in a later section.

Somewhat fancifully, and without being specific, I imagined the great and the good being carried on their palliases to my home to be made whole. Such imaginings, which I do not think that I took very seriously, were soon dispersed as I found my 'great and good' amongst the farmer, the coal man and the housewife. Again, a catalogue of people and their ailments would be inappropriate and frankly boring. There are, however, a few encounters within which pointers can be seen, indicating the way in which my thought and practice were developing, and that are worth describing. In some, I perceived strong evidence of 'ethereal' involvement; and there were others within which I was permitted to see the inner resource and heroism of individuals, as they confronted a potentially fatal illness.

I happily adopted the word 'ethereal' from Patricia Macmanaway. I had discussed with her the situation that was created by the fact that I did not dowse nor manipulate people's bodies in the ways that were practiced at Westbank. She told me of others who did neither, yet were able to achieve results, as their clients could be manipulated 'ethereally'. I saw no problem with this approach since my body had been physically 'restructured' by such means during the earlier events of my spiritual encounters, and in this manner I proceeded, initially simply placing my hands where seemed appropriate. I did not dispute or question the fact that I believed what I had had demonstrated to me, namely that there was immense resource available, and that I was participating in a 'combined operation'. I did not find it necessary to keep voicing a disclaimer to the effect that "I am but a channel", but proceeded as simply as I could, and explained to people as well as I could what it was I was trying to do.

On some occasions, I felt that my rôle was to act as an 'anaesthetist' while others went about the *real* work. For example, I was once asked to help a woman who had mental trauma following a difficult breech birth and episiotomy. Beginning with my hands covering her upper back and shoulder, which itself is very tranquillising, I ended with a hand each on her lower back and abdomen. It was then that I became 'aware' (again the difficulty of describing awareness in these circumstances) of two 'individuals' close by, and of her 'ethereal' legs being placed in the birth posture, while that which was required was done. On many other occasions, I recognised my personal inadequacy in the face of very serious illness, and appealed directly to 'higher authority'. I did so for Esther. She had an inoperable brain tumour at the base of her skull, and had had much exploratory surgical intervention. Now she was about to have radiation therapy along her spine. One evening as she lay reclining, I placed my hands adjacent to her head and asked fervently for help for her. Soon we were enveloped within a cocoon of love so strong that I felt that I could reach out and touch it. All Esther's treatments and therapies produced favourable results and she lived actively for another year, when unfortunately she succumbed to meningitis. She was one of many individuals from whom I learned of the determination and inner resources that can reside within a person when faced with the fatal potential of their condition. But this was only a part of the learning process through which I was going at the time, because within Esther's flat I came to realise the insidiousness of geopathic stress, for where she slept was awful. This was also the situation that I found when I visited John's house, for where he had slept, I could not. But I jump ahead of myself, for I have not yet arrived at the time when I became a supporter of the so-called 'gentle approach' to cancer, and I have so much to observe and to learn about many things.

Returning to events in their sequential order, I must describe the outcome of *another* broadcast from the B.B.C. Radio 4, 'You and Yours' programme. This particular one was about SAD - the so-called 'seasonal affect disorder' - and described experiments that were in train at the Maudsley Hospital, which were trying to confirm the hoped-for beneficial effect upon sufferers of exposure to high intensity light during the winter months. As with the previous M.E. broadcast that I had heard, I thought that I recognised in myself a broad swathe of the symptoms and reactions that were described. I can almost hear you thinking, "We've got a right one here, a paranoid hypochondriac, no less". My attendance at my local surgery should give the lie to that, for apart from annual flu injections and a visit to become acquainted with a G.P. on whose list I chose to go, in well over five years I have only consulted about a minor fungal infection and

LISTENING TO THE SILENCES

nothing more. No, there are specific reasons for my apparent over-sensitivity that began to emerge, and which have prompted me to engage in a study that has been continuous since about 1981.

Certain aspects of my home and its location have emerged as my narrative has developed, but nothing has been written directly about its tranquillity and freedom from pollution. There is no source of industrial pollution within twenty-five miles; traffic along my adjacent (very) minor roads is so minimal that each passing vehicle is almost an event to be remarked. Apart from occasional gunfire from a nearby M.O.D. gun-range, noise, other than from tractors working nearby fields and the bleating of sheep, is non-existent. The only electrical pollution comes from the two low voltage wires bringing the supply to the house, while the effects of microwave transmissions are diminished by mountains to the south and east, and the sea two miles to the west. Added to all of this, I have my own private water supply, originally from streams running off the nearby fell-side and, since 1996, from a 50 metre bore hole in one of my fields, so the only additions to the water are solely what nature puts in - no chlorine, no fluoride. Thus, compared with most urban living, industrial working individuals, I can and do live with several layers of protective 'shell' removed, and that is why my urban visits are curtailed, and my last visit to London was in about 1989. It also means that I, as with many individuals in similar locations, have developed an awareness of extremely subtle variations in my ambient environment and of my responses to them. Thus, I have a very suitable 'laboratory' in which to observe myself and what are, it transpired, very sensitive reactions to subtle, and mainly electrical, phenomena. I am not alone in this sensitivity, for about forty percent of individuals are similarly sensitive, but their reactions are often masked by the gross effects of the polluted environment in which many have to live.

None of these many facets were visible to me when, following the programme broadcast, I wrote asking whether it was possible to obtain for domestic use the type of light that the experimenters described. The response when it came was a surprise, for it materialised as a phone call from a doctor actually at the Maudsley Hospital. He was one of the research team and quizzed me for some considerable time. He judged that I was of the type that was being studied, and invited me to the hospital for a fuller discussion and examination. We spent the greater part of a morning together, taking my history and analysing my reactions in particular circumstances. Although I could have stayed nearby with my brother while participating in tests through a winter, I new that my reactions would be distorted by the urban environment, and even though the researcher concluded from his observations that indeed I could be considered as suffering from SAD, we opted, in the circumstances, for a different strategy. We agreed that I would study my reactions through the coming winter, keep a diary and ultimately report.

Thus began my close observation, and the study expanded as I started to identify reactions, but also, and increasingly, began to identify *causes*. However, before I launch into a description of what and how I studied, let me make what I consider to be a significant observation. I had responded thoroughly and honestly to all the questions from the M.E. team, who had concluded that in all probability I had M.E., and now a researcher from the Maudsley Hospital, to whom, again, I had responded completely and truthfully, had concluded that I was one of those who succumbed to SAD. In both cases, what had prompted me to contact the radio programme had been a set of virtually identical symptoms or reactions.

Slowly, as I began to observe and record, but definitely, I became aware, as I never had before, of the natural world, the world in which we evolved and continue to have our being, and became aware, also, of some of our reactions to its variables. As time went by, I realised that SAD-type reactions could occur at any time of the year, but, as they might not coincide with the dark, drear days of winter, and because they were transient, they passed almost unnoticed, having possibly affected me for a day or two. My acquisition of the book, *The Ion Effect* by Soyka and Edmunds, provided me with an understanding of the electrical nature of our surrounding world and atmosphere, and gave me insights into some of the causes of my reactions. And so began an observation of weather *systems* - not 'hot or cold', 'wet or dry', 'windy or still' - but an attempt by me, through seeing the entire system, to be able to judge from *where* the current ambient air had come, and thus to form some conclusion about its electrical qualities.

One by one, other variables came to light, and were included amongst the subjects for study. One such became apparent from the unlikely event of having a new pair of glasses. I had chosen the then comparatively new variable-focus lenses. Because they need to be positioned precisely, and because I was very active out of doors, I had decided upon close fitting frames with curled, springy loops over the ears. It took a little while to get used to the accurate positioning of the head that viewing required, (Little Noddy is the appropriate name as the head is moved slightly up or down to achieve focus), but when I had done so, I enjoyed the freedom that the lenses gave me. However, from time to time I found myself getting irritated with my new acquisition, for the frames became tight on my head, and they needed frequent adjustment to restore them to the proper viewing position. The irritation lasted for three or four days at a time, and then things returned to normal. It took approximately six months for the penny to drop. The periods of irritation coincided with the new and full moons.

LISTENING TO THE SILENCES

"...but this is wondrous strange!", quoth Horatio. Not so, when one considers that our body has within itself such a high percentage of fluid. I can still hear the voice of my then GP as she shot me down - "*With respect!!!* Roy..." - never having allowed herself a moment for reflection. Consider this: if you take a bowl of water to the equator and pull the plug, the water goes straight down, without a swirl: take it one bowl-width either way, north or south, pull the plug and the water swirls, anti-clockwise in the north and the reverse in the south. Fluids are *remarkably sensitive* to the forces acting upon them, and 'the moon, mistress of the floods' exerts a significant pull. So, I had another factor to observe and insert in my human reaction equation, and a greater awareness of the moon and its movements developed. And not only the moon, for, over time, the involvement of the whole planetary menagerie emerged. *But* - before you have time even to form the thought - there is nothing of *astrology* in this. What emerged, and what I will write about fully in an appropriate place later, is that the moon, alone or in conjunction with other planets, or these planets together in significant groups, can have an actual *physical* effect upon people, their well-being and interactions. The effects are engineered through subtle gravitational changes and variations in the natural electrical/magnetic environment, which, in turn, have an impact upon the solar wind and its components.

If I had any doubts about the electrical functioning of our bodies, they were dispelled when I got to know someone who practices the electrical form of acupuncture. In traditional Chinese acupuncture, imbalances within the body and between the various meridians are detected by feeling for variations in subtle pulses at the wrists. The electrical version uses a measuring instrument to detect similar imbalances - measurements being made at the meridian ends on feet or hands. Naturally, I wanted to know more, and went to experience this particular therapy. Correction of imbalances is effected either by using a traditional needle as in normal acupuncture, or by feeding into an appropriate acupuncture point a small electric current through a moist conducting pad. The input to the pad can be varied, and is usually under the control of the clients in order that they can decide upon their own discomfort level. My friend was frequently surprised that I reached my discomfort threshold at such a low level of input, a fact that reinforced my developing knowledge of the vastly different electrical sensitivities of various individuals.

Any further encouragement that I needed to explore these phenomena came from the growing realisation that part of my own personal contribution to the healing process came from what I began to see as a subtle body electricity. This realisation, in its turn, proved to be a deciding factor in the way in which my approach to healing developed then and subsequently. Marrying the concept of body electricity with the understanding of the electrical nature of the acupuncture points and meridians, led me to experiment by directing my healing 'energy' through appropriate points, simply by touching them with my fingertips for a suitable length of time. Over a period of time, I acquired a number of texts and atlases of acupuncture, covering both the traditional Chinese methods and the newer electrical methods, in which Dr Julian Kenyon has been a prolific author, sources of reference that are never far from my side. My choice of this approach was further strengthened by the realisation that I could practice on myself, which I do either for my own benefit or for experiment.

A series of programmes on television initiated my next quantum leap. The so-called 'Bristol Approach to Cancer' was featured in six weekly stages in which the nature of the approach was described, and in which the progress of a number of individuals with cancer was observed and monitored. So strongly did I admire the pluck and resource of these people that I determined to add my own support if the opportunity arose. I did not have long to wait, for a friend told me that one of the original 'Bristol' founders had started another base within reach of my home. I made contact and after several months found myself spending one day a month trying to help. I drove for about an hour and a half to a school that, on this day each month, was transformed - transformed into what? The concentration of supporters and helpers providing organisation, superb food and therapies galore, was intense. If a therapy was available and was thought to be of value, it was added to the galaxy - reflexology, music and movement, art, nutrition, healing, counselling - *anything* that it was felt would enhance the prospects and quality of life of the individuals who came seeking help.

But there was another sort of 'concentration' which was quite indefinable, and which was voiced by a lady who came to my 'pitch'. She was near to tears. "I can't take it" she said, "I can't take it. For years I have cared totally for my parents to the exclusion of myself, and now, coming here, I find so many people wanting to do the same for me...so much *love*...". When our period together was ending, she looked beyond me and said, "Who is that man? How I wish I could find just what it is that he has got". I looked behind me to see John standing and patiently waiting, for we had overrun our scheduled time. "That's John", I said. "He has leukaemia". But he didn't just 'stand', for he walked and stood inside a smile.

John and Vanessa. It is impossible even now, several years after John's death, to separate them in my thoughts; and speaking on the phone to Vanessa, as I do from time to time, it is still as easy to talk *about* him as it was *to* him when he was alive. Together they exemplified the whole concept of the 'Bristol' approach that encourages partners to work as one against the cancerous intrusion. ("*We* have cancer", Arnold used to say when speaking of his wife Muriel). But more than that, John and Vanessa studied and followed-up every conceivable remedy or therapy that might help to improve John's condition. They were very rigorous followers of the 'macrobiotic' diet, a practice that benefited me considerably whenever they came to stay, for they brought all the wide ranging and delicious ingredients with them, and while I gave John his healing 'fix' in a quiet part of the house, Vanessa was busy preparing the most appetising and visually delightful food. "Love on a plate" I used to think, as I gorged on exquisitely prepared and cooked vegetables, with perhaps a 'Swiss-roll' of grains rolled in seaweed. ("Sea *vegetables!*" I was constantly reminded).

It was in their home that I began to take seriously the actuality of geopathic stress. On my first visit, I was put in a double bed in a room that John had used in a previous marriage, but had almost no sleep because I was constantly beset by aches, twitches, tinglings and numbnesses the whole night through. On a second visit, I asked if I could turn the bed at right angles in case it was the orientation that was causing these effects, but experienced little improvement. On my *next* visit, I was put in a different room and slept very well. Several of us had gone to stay with Vanessa and John to take part in a series of workshops that were particularly aimed at exploring the so-called 'muscle testing' method of identifying a person's allergies, opening yet another avenue, to which I will return later. Participating with us, and returning later to join in the evening meal, was a man who took his dowsing talents wherever he went. A great enthusiast, it was natural that he should make a full survey of the house, where he detected two earth currents. One current occupied a narrow strip about 30cm wide that went the length of the house, while another, equally narrow, crossed it diagonally towards one end. The first ran down what had been John's side of the bed, the side where I had been unable to sleep; the other crossed the first, exactly under the location of his relaxation chair.

The whole visit was highly educational, and not only with respect to the information that it revealed to me, but also because it helped me to see aspects of human nature and behaviour that I had never experienced before. One interesting consequence came later from the man who did the dowsing. He carried out a survey of the gypsies who regularly attended the Appleby horse fair, quizzing them about their lifestyle, diet, domicile, smoking and other habits. He found that the genuine *travelling* gypsies had an extremely low incidence of cancers and heart conditions, irrespective of diet and other factors, compared with those who had stopped travelling and had settled into permanent housing. His deduction was that the traditional sites used by the travellers had been assessed for their safety through the fundamental, unsuppressed instincts of these 'natural' people, and, furthermore, by never spending long at any one place, their exposure to anything adverse was greatly diminished.

I do not think that I had returned home for more than a day when I had a phone call from the friend who practiced electrical acupuncture. She had been to a very interesting talk and demonstration on the subject of muscle testing for allergies! Floored by the proverbial feather, I picked myself up and asked for more. It transpired that the practitioner was well known to me. Graham had first come into my orbit as a young graduate electrical engineer whom I was instrumental in engaging during my stint in charge of Training at Sellafield. Now, about sixteen later, our paths were converging again. Much has resulted from this convergence, some of which will emerge as I continue, but in the immediate time it was such a relief to have another electrical engineering mind with which to share ideas, experience and information, and one that also thinks highly of Nikola Tesla! Graham was himself completely committed to exploring the concepts of geopathic stress and the consequences of the electrical phenomena that I had been discovering and studying. He was impelled by a very strong motive, for his wife has multiple sclerosis, and he was convinced that her sensitivity to electrical interference was a major contributory factor. In a similar manner to John and Vanessa, and the way in which they had set about studying leukaemia in all its aspects, Graham and his wife were equally zealous in doing the same with regard to M.S. Some of their investigations and what they have found will emerge fully later.

If I needed any *further* convincing about the existence and effect of geopathic stress, I received ample confirmation in two separate locations. Esther had lived with her partner in a particular flat, which I visited. Standing at the bed head, I experienced a feeling of acute nausea, which subsided as I moved down the length of the bed towards the foot. One of the pair used to experience heavy, disturbing, teeth-grinding nightmares, and morning depression, while the other regularly awoke feeling the equivalent of a heavy weight on the chest, following very disturbed sleep. Houseplants, of which they had many, would deteriorate rapidly if placed on the bedside tables, but regained full health when moved to other locations. Esther had returned to her parents' home, but her partner, alerted to the unhealthy sitting of the bed, moved it within the room and experienced normal sleep.

The second location was inside the home of my cousin in Carlisle. Calling there as I returned from Westbank, I had been concerned to see how she was deteriorating from a condition that was developing in her spine, which, it turned out, was the consequence of treatment that she was receiving for severe muscular rheumatism. She was on a 'diet' of steroids, and her spine was disintegrating slowly. Ivy had been a nurse, a late entrant to the profession, having nursed a crippled mother until

LISTENING TO THE SILENCES

the latter's death. She had been a gold medal winner at Edinburgh Royal Infirmary, and her compassion and caring shaped her every activity. However, her training had also given her a misplaced acceptance of the authority, nay, *majesty*, of Consultants, and even though she knew the dangers of continued ingestion of steroids, nevertheless would not override the advice of someone so revered. And so she continued taking the tablets, until, bent nearly double and unable to breathe, she died in her sleep.

Ivy had moved into this particular house a few years earlier, joining forces with a nursing friend who also had never married. Visiting them one day, and sitting in a particular seat, I was concerned to find an intolerable ache developing in my back. I rearranged cushions, but the ache persisted and got worse. Then suddenly it dawned - geopathic stress. I excused myself, ostensibly to the loo, and on returning took a different seat. Instant relief. I came home and pondered, and then raised the question with the two. Ivy's condition had only developed since moving to the house - she normally sat in this horrible area, and slept immediately above it. Her friend, sleeping in a second bedroom that was in an area of lesser stress, had, nevertheless, developed the most atrocious teeth grinding, of which she was unaware. Importantly, however, the friend's dog would not remain within that particular downstairs room, solely entering it if called, but immediately retreating. I tried to give

Ivy a device called a 'Raditech', that I shall describe in detail later, which, using the natural resonance of its inbuilt electrical coils, can significantly diminish the effects of the earth currents. Unable to be convinced, and worried about incurring any expense, which I assured her was non-existent, she carried on as prescribed, and sadly died.

Teeth grinding, nightmares, night-time depression, unexplained aches, cancers, psychological problems, incessant crying of infants, are all listed in two books that I own, as consequences of remaining in stressed areas. I have mentioned earlier the book by Gustav von Pohl; the other is called *Are You Sleeping in a Safe Place?* Written by Rolf Gordon, it provides clear information about the sources of geopathic stress, and its effects upon people. There are clear instructions on how to dowse for earth currents, and also descriptions of the sensitivity to them of plants and animals. The responses of the dog belonging to my cousin's friend, and of Esther's plants, should help to convince sceptics that the *human* reactions are neither subjective nor psychosomatic. Rolf had a son who died of a cancer that he is convinced owed much in its origin to geopathic stress. He has since become a zealot in the promotion of knowledge about the phenomenon, and about devices such as the 'Raditech', which he sells, the beneficial effects of which have often been demonstrated. Anyone who is interested in keeping up to date with current knowledge and experience will find a considerable amount of information on the Internet, as they will about most of the other topics that I introduce.

My own reasons for including so much about a diverse range of phenomena are two fold. First, there is the appreciation of the way in which my knowledge and awareness were expanding, and, in doing so, were affecting the direction in which my life was moving. Second, many of the phenomena affect sensitive and vulnerable individuals in ways that make them even more susceptible to adverse spiritual intrusion. The circumstances in which this can happen, and the methods used, will be revealed later when I write the appropriate section.

Many people refer to the 'Swinging Sixties' as having been so very influential upon the subsequent development of their lives. If asked, I would cite the 'Enlightening Eighties' as the years during which many aspects of my life came together as a coherent whole. I do not know if you sense it, but I am having something of a struggle in riding the verbal flow. I feel somewhat as if I am rafting down a fast flowing, boisterous river that is being joined at unpredictable intervals by equally turbulent confluences, as all the new sources of information and experience pour their contribution into the main flow, and to which I have to adjust in order to continue to stay in control without losing a sense of direction. One of the counsels given to mariners in charge of vessels at sea when things appear to be getting out of control is "Ease her, stop her, go astern". Well, I certainly cannot slow the river, nor go astern, so let us steer into an eddy and pause to take stock.

Reflect, I would not have been in this particular flow, nor in this actual channel, except for the events of 1979-80, and the spiritual traumas and awakening that occurred then. Coincidentally with that time, I had been discovering unexplored talents in artistic craftwork, and in particular in the field of leather carving, which I hoped and planned to take it to an advanced level. The lady who introduced me to this craft, someone who herself has much skill and artistry in many directions, subsequently has become a very good friend. It was she who effected my introduction to the retired art professor, carver and sculptor who gave me many insights, and who effectively taught me how to *look*, that essential prerequisite of any artistic or skilled craftwork. Many times since then, and currently, even, I have regretted that I did not commit myself entirely to *that* particular channel, for I recognise that I could have been competent in several fields, and would have gained much satisfaction from my achievements.

But with my spiritual awakening and the discovery of my healing talents, my eyes of compassion had been opened and I could not shut them again, no matter how hard I tried. My compulsion grew and grew as I realised what could be achieved. I have never been so egotistic as to believe that, alone, I could effect significant change, but nevertheless have persisted in learning, learning, and experimenting, in order to achieve the maximum of which I, myself, was capable, and to maintain myself as an effective partner in this human/spiritual exchange. One outcome of my study was that I learned or developed combinations of acupuncture points through which much could be caused to happen. This was especially so in the relief of pain. What a joy it was to be able to give even just temporary ease. George certainly stands out in my memory. He came and sat on my stool at the cancer centre, looking entirely robust, as robust as his attitude was to the death that he said was inevitable from the asbestos induced cancer that was destroying his pleura. Using chosen acupuncture points, I had developed a strategy that I could use to good effect in the all too short time that one had with each person. My first move was to use points called 'Spleen 21', which are at the side of the rib cage. I put my hands there on George, and was startled to find close to the surface the cut ends of ribs, the result of his most recent operation. But what surprised me more when it came, was his gasp and exclamation as, almost with a whip crack, the constant and intense pain went. The down side was, of course, that the pain would come back, for one could not achieve much that was permanent in half an hour, once a month, and George had come from a distance, as I had, and we could not meet.

What did persist within me and for some time was the combined effect of everybody's contributions made throughout the day. Undoubtedly there was much input from spiritual sources, and one tried to play one's own part. On my windowsill, there is an object that constantly reminds me of these particular days, and the many people who came to the school. It is a small, conical glass bowl, into the surface of which is engraved the image of a pair of hands that are seemingly holding the empty bowl. The hands were fashioned for me by a Scottish lady, who has exquisite artistry in the art of glass engraving. The bowl and the hands represent what I saw as my rôle in some circumstances - effectively to hold a person in tranquillity while their inner 'bowl' was filled. How I wished that the allotted times were longer, for some were so *transported*, were so obviously 'elsewhere', that it often required a touch and the sound of their name to bring them back to awareness. How memorable and moving were the deep hugs and kisses of unspoken shared experience that sometimes accompanied these returns.

What was perhaps remarkable was that of five of us who offered this type of healing, three had been 'inducted' by Bruce Macmanaway! What an input that man had into this field, for within a small number of years, I had encountered yet three more, all within fifty miles of my home, as I shall relate. Yet, in spite of the high endeavours and dedicated motivation of most of whom I met, there were, nevertheless, individuals who seemed to have their own personal agenda directing what they did. I seem to be particularly naïve in not recognising soon enough the female of this species. No purpose is served by revisiting such occasions of disillusion, but, with one such, when there seemed to be a friendship, I fell in with a suggestion that I should go and talk to a woman, who lived some distance away, and who gave so-called 'readings' or 'channelled'. Green as grass I went, always expecting the best from a situation. Certainly the person in question could not have been more attractive or 'wholesome', to use an old fashioned word. Within the family home we sat, while she talked for some considerable time, with a break for a snack. Her intentions were of the highest, and she believed implicitly in what she was doing and in the veracity of whatever it was that she was saying, while her demeanour was purity itself as she blessed each 'spirit' that she could apparently 'see' in her ambit. However, after I had listened for some time, I began to think, "This is a pointless load of twaddle" - and much more pungent thoughts. What surprised me was that these 'irreverent' thoughts were not intercepted by the, one assumed, spiritual source of her 'channelling', but that she went on talking in similar vein.

I did not, as had been suggested, record her delivery, and on reflection, I am glad that I did not, for, of what I remembered, enough remained to have a long-term effect. There is a problem with being the object of such attempts at prescience, of 'divination' or supposed spiritual analysis, for no matter how much one is saying to oneself, "This is a load of cobblers", inevitably some of what is said sticks in one's mind and memory, always to be on hand in an appropriate situation. For example when, having been told "I give you X and Y", these being names of people, but without any actual context, inevitably, no matter how hard one tries not to, when one meets an X or a Y, one thinks "Is this the one who was meant?" - and one starts endless speculation in spite of oneself. Or, "You will write a book in collaboration with someone who already has a reputation in your field" (not naming the field). Thinking that it was most likely that what I would want to write would be of a medical nature deriving from my work in healing, I said something about 'a doctor'. "I didn't say 'doctor', but meant a professional person". So again, in spite of oneself, the speculation starts rolling whenever an apparently 'suitable' individual crosses one's path, and even more confusing, as there were other topics on which I knew that I could go into print. I did not speak subsequently of this encounter to the person who had suggested that I should go, and kept my thoughts to myself. Whether this aggravated her, or what, I do not know; what I do know is that she began a vindictive undermining campaign against me among certain people at the cancer centre, which was most unpleasant to experience, particularly in what it revealed about the way in which *others* so easily allowed themselves to be influenced. However,

LISTENING TO THE SILENCES

fortunately, she was detected in her malice, and was hoist by her own petard. (I've always wanted to write that!)

Unpleasant though it is to recall, I have done so in order to introduce the topic as a means of exploring the dangers of implicit belief in one's self as a 'channeller' of 'wisdom' or advice from an apparently etheric source. And also to explore the equally great danger of accepting from others the product of their activities, whether as channellers, clairvoyants, Tarot card readers, astrologers or practitioners of other forms of divination. It is important to consider this topic and all that is implied within it in great detail, for concealed in such seemingly innocent attempts at divination are other 'channels', channels through which malevolent intrusions can enter people's lives and minds. This may appear to be a melodramatic concept, but I hope to demonstrate the truth of what I write when I discuss the topic in detail at a later stage.

The turbulent and rapid passage of the river of the nineteen-eighties has whirled me past a number of topics so quickly that I have been able only to give them a brief mention - diet, acupuncture, geopathic interference, ion imbalance, electromagnetic fields - and some that I have been too 'breathless' even to mention in passing, such as hypnotherapy and Alexander technique. To all these I shall return, and explore, and, hopefully, explain why I believe them to be important within all that I am trying to convey to those whose problem is within the mind, or with the spirit. Yes, inevitably, one cannot separate them - body, mind and spirit - and acceptance of that inevitability would be of immense benefit to anyone trying to regain control of a disturbed mind.

In case you think that I have left behind my own struggle with spiritual intrusions, let me reiterate, as I do from time to time, they are always there in some shape or form. The actuality of these intrusions will emerge when later I present my records and analysis of these times. However, before I leave the comparative tranquillity of this eddy where we have been regrouping, and before I thrust out into the last brief turbulent flow of the decade, let me leave you to ponder one particular incident that was perfectly unique in the midst of the whole collection of the experiences of those ten years…

I have written earlier of how I read and came under the spell of *The Old Straight Track* by Alfred Watkins. In his book, and briefly, he describes how he became aware of the concept that, long before the days of roads, wheeled traffic, large towns and enclosures as we know them, in fact, considerably before even Roman times, people communicated and travelled along straight-line routes. When one considers that all traffic would be on foot or by pony, with goods carried by porters or slaves, this would have been the most logical way to journey. However, the routes were not haphazard, but were predetermined by surveying, and, from my own analysis of routes in this area where I live, the surveying was remarkably precise. Watkins found that the routes passed through many places with 'ley' in their name e.g. Hartley, Bentley, and from this observation, he named the alignments 'ley lines'.

Identifying and walking some of these alignments in my own area soon became a key hobby, as I could, in fine weather, explore routes that I had identified from my maps in the long dark evenings of winter. It was for such an exploration that I went one evening in summer to take some compass bearings along a particular route that I wanted to explore later in some detail. It was a brilliant, sunny evening, and I clambered up an old peat track to reach a broad plateau, disturbing a feeding roebuck that quickly clattered away over rocks. The plateau is most interesting in itself, as it contains the site of an ancient Bronze-age settlement, although this was not my goal. It was an evening for just sitting and looking. Anyone familiar with the watercolours of W. Heaton Cooper will recognise the type of light that flooded the whole land - so lucid and transparent. I was totally alone and intent on observing the scene. A fox trotted leisurely across my view about 100 yards distant, only to turn away suddenly at right angles and run off at high speed, tail and ears low, escape imperative. Such breeze as there was drifted from me to the fox and, picking up my scent, it lost no time in putting as much distance between us as it could.

Roy Vincent

However, I had come to take some bearings, and took out my compass. I had bought the best that I could afford, and took pleasure in it, a modern version of the much respected military prismatic marching and surveying instrument. I identified my distant point and put the compass to my eye, getting the sights truly on my objective, and then, totally to my amazement, the compass card, of its own volition, moved slowly and deliberately through ten or twelve degrees, and stayed there for a while, before slowly returning to the required bearing. You will recollect that in my profession I was an instrument engineer, and familiar with most aspects of measurement and measuring devices. I had already made sure that my spectacle frames were non-magnetic, even to the extent of having some minute screws replaced. I did a recheck on my jacket to ensure that there were no zips or metal buttons that could interfere, and that I had nothing in my pockets of a magnetic nature. I looked around to confirm that there were no wire fences nearby which could exert any influences. Satisfied with my checks, I put the compass to my eye again and settled on the distant peak. Once again the card moved, this time through fifteen degrees, and stayed there steadily for a significant time before returning slowly to the bearing of my desired objective.

I pondered long as I packed up and came home, and have often done so since. I have used the compass many times in subsequent years with no repetition, and no, I do not drink, nor ingest any drugs or hallucinogenic substances. Having had the experiences of spiritual intrusion and body manipulation that I have described, I have no illusions about the 'physical' power and actual presence of a spiritual domain paralleling and interacting with our own, and personally have no doubt that I was being given another demonstration of this ever-presence.

So, there it is. As I ease the raft into the last turbulent flow that carries us into the broad river of the nineties, I'll just leave you with your own thoughts to ponder, and while you do so, perhaps you would like to read some verse that David's son-in-law Barry Applin wrote following a visit during which we wandered the hills, and I explained to him just what it was that I was seeking…

Roy Vincent

A PATIENT EYE

Tracing paths
on the hillsides,
lingering shadows,
straight as arrows,
crisscrossing the land.

Visible only to a patient eye,
their meaning determined
by what we want the world to be.
Some wrap them in their dreams
of a new renaissance
of the ancient gods.
Other eyes,
less misty,
see age-old trails
of trade and tribal messages
picked out by the autumn sun.

Who knows? Who cares?
Few are prepared
to venture
from their pre-planned courses.
Locked behind the screens
of shiny new machines,
the detail of the land
blurred,
the lines of God or Man
lost,
to all but a patient eye.

Barry Applin

CHAPTER 9

The Wings Of the Morning

Roy Vincent

LISTENING TO THE SILENCES

And Lo! If I take the Wings of the Morning,
And dwell on the furthermost part
Of the Sea...

Even though more than half a century has passed, those words still come to my thoughts as I view in my minds eye the scene that used to greet me as I came up on deck each morning. Our ship was ploughing its slow and straight furrow parallel with, and a few miles off, the very shore upon which the psalmist author may have trod so many years ago. It was quite early, 5 a.m., for we were working 'tropical routine', and for a day-man (or 'idler' as the Naval parlance has it), the day began at that hour. The iron main deck and the entire superstructure were awash and dripping with dew from the cool of the night, while the shore was a line of opalescent shadow to the east, back-lit by the near-to-rising sun.

      Many writers, both ancient and modern, have tried to describe the colour and placidity of those eastern Mediterranean seas with greater or less success, as I used to try in my letters to my girl friend at home. Nothing disturbed the surface, other than the long line of our wake connecting us astern to the far horizon. And then there they were - the 'Wings of the Morning' - the caiques and coasting schooners, sails full set but hanging still, with no breath to fill them, but somehow 'ghosting' along and waiting for the morning breeze.

In the moments as I watched, the sun broke free of the land and even at that hour it burned. The dew vanished at a touch and the sails took on a brilliance as the light enveloped them - and the day's work began. How long it seemed, confined in the small radar cabins as I did my maintenance checks, until blessed noon when work ceased for all but the duty watch and the hands were piped to swim. The ship slowed, the whaler was lowered, and we dived so eagerly from the ship's side and into the cool depths.

What contrasts life throws at us, for within six months I was in an aircraft carrier battling its way around Britain in January storms of probably the worst winter of the twentieth century. The mountains of the Isle of Arran were snow-laden as we sought shelter within its lee and behind Holy Island, and icy were the winds as we then made our way past Cape Wrath and John o' Groats and finally to the Forth. But in spite of, or because of their contrasts, I have never lost my fascination with the seas nor my desire to be close to or on them. As I stand on my near-by shore as I often do, the expanse of the sand and the vastness of the dunes trigger memories of seemingly never ending sunny days on a similar shore where I grew up in South Wales - of fires of

LISTENING TO THE SILENCES

driftwood and smoky tea, and the long weary trudge home at night. And the high tides and gales of the autumn equinox bring back clear memories of my mother and her love of the driving spray on the rocks on probably our last outing of the year.

I wrote earlier of this attraction that water has for me and of the feast for the imagination with which I have been provided for virtually all of my life. There must be many individuals who, like me, can just gaze out to the horizon for seemingly endless time - and what do *you* see? In reality or in your own mind's eye or your own imagination? Do you look for, or even see, Tir Nan Og? Do you believe in the past existence of Atlantis, and do you give credence to the tales deriving from the alleged reincarnates from that mythical/real land? And do you gaze horizon-ward in the hope that some day Atlantis will re-emerge from the depths where 'of its bones are corals made'?

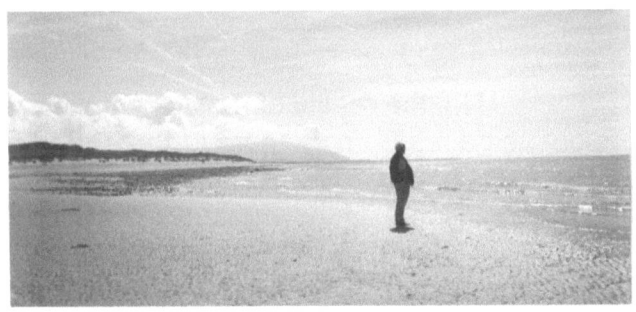

Can I ask you to put aside what you see, or imagine or hope for, and instead to join me on the self-same edge of the ocean, there to contemplate the real magic, the magic of the reality of our origins? Through the medium of television, and taking advantage of the courage and resource of undersea explorers in their minute bathyspheres, we can descend in mid-ocean to the bottom several kilometres below, and there see the origins of the tectonic plates of the continents and some of the substances of life itself. In particular, I want you to look at a 'black smoker'. ("Oh dear" said Alice to herself, nearly scared out of her wits at the thought of a Black Smoker. The only Smoker she could think of was Grimes the gardener, and he frightened her sometimes as he puffed continuously at a huge pipe stuffed with coarse twist, pouring out clouds of smoke which merged with that from the bonfire he was tending. "Now he always looks very *dark*" she said to herself, "but no, he grows such nice flowers, it can't be him..." - and Alice went and hid herself just in case the real Black Smoker came along...).

No, the reality of a black smoker as it pours out its gases from the core of the earth is, in itself, awesome to contemplate, for here in its turbulence are some of the materials of which we are made and, indirectly, are the source of life as we know it. In particular, I want you to see the sulphur, for in its way it is so vital to our very origin and continued existence. Without the sulphur it is

LISTENING TO THE SILENCES

doubtful whether we would have rain. Back on the surface, and, could you see them, myriads of algae that continue the process originating in the earth's bowels, taking the sulphur and converting it into an organic and gaseous form, that then disperses freely into the atmosphere. And it is around the molecules of this gas that the moisture evaporated from the seas forms into droplets, into clouds and eventually rain. Without the algae and the sulphur - no clouds, no rain; no rain, no erosion of rock to make soil; no soil, no plants; no plants, no us. But the algae have other mysteries that have long puzzled biologists. Why are they equipped with anti-freeze? At last, and a paradox only recently explained. The algae need sunshine to survive and proliferate - but they create clouds don't they, so isn't that counterproductive, life threatening even, for sun-loving algae? But the clouds create storms and storms cause algae to be sucked up and carried to extreme heights where they might freeze to death - if it wasn't for the anti-freeze; and thus they are dispersed to other seas, other oceans. One of those incredible marvels of evolution, or a fantastic attention to detail of a prescient Creator, whichever you will.

In your imagination, can I take you even below the black smokers? The molten magma is oozing in mid-ocean, pouring through these gaps in the earth's crust, forming new edges to the tectonic plates, forcing them apart and under continents, creating the tremors and pustules on the earth's skin - the earthquakes and volcanoes. But even deeper, towards the centre of the earth, to the molten iron core. Without it you would never have been even a gleam in your father's eye. Without it life on earth would just not exist in the form that we know.

Thermal movement of the iron within the core effectively creates a magnet with two ends or 'poles' that we call north and south. The magnet in turn creates a magnetic field that, effectively, is our shield. The sun pours out the 'solar wind' in constant stream - a never-ending flow of electrically charged particles. Our magnetic shield diverts them, and mostly they flow harmlessly past. Without our shield, the planet would be 'scoured' by these particles and would be completely barren, as are the other planets that have no iron core. The particles of the solar wind arrive into our upper atmosphere at the poles, and create the magnificent displays of the auroras, while during peaks of sunspot activity they reach parts of the earth in quantity, disrupting electronic communication, and subtly altering the behaviour of sensitive people.

Take out a magnetic compass and unerringly the needle points to the north. Turn it on its edge and it will point down into the ground at an angle that depends where on the earth's surface you are - at my latitude it makes an angle of roughly 80 degrees with the horizontal; elsewhere it will be different. What it shows you is that always, everywhere, there is a magnetic field - a component of our evolution. But more than that, and unless you have special equipment you

LISTENING TO THE SILENCES

cannot see, it pulses with incredible regularity. There are various subtle low energies at frequencies of roughly one to twenty-five beats per second, but the prime one, and that linked by most researchers to the process of evolution and continued planetary life, pulses at 10 hertz (or cycles per second). It is part of the body clock that if it stops ticking or ticks to a different frequency can cause illness or even death in some organisms.

I have led you to contemplate, and I hope understand, just a minute few of the many elements that have been involved in the development and continued evolution of our lives and the other forms of life on the planet. Elements that are all pervasive and yet invisible - undetectable to the majority of us - yet without them we would become ill or die. But die we must - and what then?

Can we stay here on our lovely open shore without the noise, clutter and pollution of everyday life, and read or listen to some thoughts from a delightful book by Irish philosopher and poet John O'Donohue? I first heard them over the phone from a friend upon whom they had made an instant impression. Going into the local library later the same day, the first book upon which my eyes lighted was this self-same *Anam Cara - Spiritual Wisdom from the Celtic World* - and so naturally I brought it home to read, for my friend was quite firm when she said that it would be a long time before she loaned her copy, so entranced was she with what the book had to say.

John O'Donohue queries whether space and time are different in the eternal world, and writes:

"Time always separates us...Time is primarily linear, disjointed and fragmented. All of your past days have disappeared; they have vanished. The future has not come to you yet. All you have is the little stepping-stone of the present moment.

When the soul leaves the body, it is no longer under the burden of space and time. The soul is free; distance and separation hinder it no more. The dead are our nearest neighbours; they are all around us. Meister Eckhart was once asked, where does the soul of a person go when the person dies? He said, no place. Where else would the soul be going? Where else is the eternal world? It can be nowhere other than here. We have falsely spatialized the eternal world. We have driven the eternal out into some distant galaxy. Yet the eternal world does not seem to be a place but rather a different state of being. The soul of the person goes no place because there is no place else to go. This suggests that the dead are here with us, in the air that we are moving through all the time. The only difference between us and the dead is that they are now in invisible form. You cannot see them with the human eye. But you can sense the presence of those you love who have died. With the refinement of your soul, you can sense them. You feel that they are near.

LISTENING TO THE SILENCES

My father used to tell us a story about a neighbour who was very friendly with the local priest. There is a whole mythology in Ireland about Druids and priests having special powers. But this man and the priest used to go for long walks. One day the man said to the priest, where are the dead? The priest told him not to ask questions like that. But the man persisted and finally, the priest said, 'I will show you; but you are never to tell anyone.' Needless to say, the man did not keep his word. The priest raised his right arm, the man looked out under the raised right hand, and saw the souls of the departed everywhere all around as thick as the dew on blades of grass.
    Often our loneliness and isolation is due to a failure of spiritual imagination. We forget that there is no such thing as empty space. All space is full of presence, particularly the presence of those who are now in eternal, invisible form."

Lovely, and in some ways, comforting images. Perhaps an over-simplification. Doubtless, everyone reading this will have some view or belief of 'life after death'. Some will have beliefs shaped by their own experience; others will have entrenched views laid down within the unshakable dogma of their religion - sometimes comforting, sometimes frightening. Yet others will totally deny, and refuse even to contemplate, the possibility of continuing into a spiritual state. If you are one of the latter, yet nevertheless continuing to read of my actual experiences, I am at a total loss to know what, if anything, I can write to convince you, although truly, I can no longer concern myself whether I do or not. Perhaps, consciously or unconsciously, there is the unspoken belief that in acknowledging the existence of a spiritual state of being, you have to take on board all of the paraphernalia of a religion. A horror that you would have to go to some place of worship; that your life would be constrained by thoughts of 'sin' and 'damnation'. You may look at all of the human misery and turmoil, disputes and wars fought in the 'name' of religion - stoked by concepts of 'promised lands' or minute differences of textual interpretation - and curse all religions.

Believe me, you can accept the reality of the existence of a state of spiritual being without even remotely embracing any religion, or altering your way of life. But more important, much more important than your own enlightenment, you could use the knowledge and understanding so gained to achieve what I am so desperately trying to get you to achieve - the release from torment of people who are plagued by intrusive spirits.

Sometime, on a clear night, go out of doors, look at the stars, and reflect on what you can see. With your eyes or with the addition of your telescope, they are all there for you. They mean what you want them to mean. You do not have to be an astronomer to appreciate them, even to understand much of what you see. Although such devices as the Hubble telescope bring us wonders of vision, what you see is out of reach, out of touch. Some will look at, for instance, the Pleiades and imagine communication with Ascended Masters. Others will look for their future, and accept the predictions of astrologers who will interpret the 'signs'. Look at Orion and Sirius and reflect that, so we are told, the rulers of Ancient Egypt attempted a physical/spiritual union with these stars and that the Ghiza pyramids represent on earth a model of the constellation. In like wise, people try to give you a view of religion, of spiritual interaction - but reflect further, the only people who can tell you what it is like to walk on the moon, to travel and walk in space, are the people who have actually been there. So look at the stars, look at the planets, 'examine' the world of 'spirit'; take your own view of them all - but also remember that there are individuals who have had a different 'real' experience. Maybe they have something to tell you.

And before we leave the stars, reflect also that the light from the nearest star had already started upon its journey to you long before the first human, homo sapiens, had taken a single step upon this planet. Yet here you are, at the very forefront, the cutting edge of evolution; the very latest model. What do you make of yourself? My oft quoted Paracelsus could never have known how immense are the distances to the stars, but he, like us, must have looked; imagined; dreamed - and as he dreamed, so he wrote:

Roy Vincent

"…the human body is vapour materialised by sunshine mixed with the life of the stars."

Poetic? Mystical? Or very near the truth in the language and thought of his time? What do you think? Every atom of the material that makes up your body was there in existence when the stars were formed. Over millennia upon millennia they have been transmuted many times before they were assembled around the nucleus, the egg and sperm, that became you. Take the sulphur which inhabits every cell that forms your body; changed into organic form by the algae it is dissolved in the rain, and, on falling to earth, is taken up by plants that you eat, or by the animals that eat the plants that at second hand you eat - all the way from a black smoker. The calcium, so necessary for your bones and teeth, might derive from chalk or limestone - the compacted remains of myriads of tiny crustaceans, worms, algae, deposited in the seas over aeons. And virtually all dependent upon the action of the sun.

Evolution or Creation? It is not for me to decide for you. The records of the rocks show the remains of tiny mammals already in existence in parallel with the dinosaurs, which latter seem to engage the imagination of so many people. Is the source of the fascination the fact that they were extinguished sixty-odd million years ago and that people can let their imaginations rip, or be terrorised by someone else's imagination in Jurassic film epics? Is it because *big* is exciting?

LISTENING TO THE SILENCES

Twentieth century thinker Schumacher told us 'Small is beautiful', and there is something exquisite in the thought that, over the last sixty million years or so, that little fossilised mouse-like creature has developed into us. Species living in a coherent environment have little cause to change or develop - they are suited to their food or environment. But change causes change, adaptation and development and survival - always with the main imperatives of self-preservation, procreation and enhancement of the species. All imperatives that still reside within us. Our problem is that we have an intellect.

Fossil remains from over two million years ago show a transition from quadruped to hominid; from *homo erectus* and *homo habilis* to homo sapiens and *neanderthalis*, namely us, and our recently extinct collaterals. Did they die out, were they exterminated by our ancestors, these Neanderthal peoples, or did they and we merge, interbreed and become one strand? If only we could find out, we might derive some clues for the future destiny of the human race - after all, Neanderthals were around for 150,000 years, far longer than *sapiens* has yet existed. This is not a hypothetical, nor an allegorical question. Analysis tells us that they were eminently adaptable, as we humans appear to be. They adapted to changes that natural phenomena imposed upon them - climate changes, ice ages and the like. Will we equally adapt to the changes that we ourselves are imposing upon ourselves? Or will we drive ourselves to extinction? We are already doing a very efficient job of preparing ourselves for the latter fate. I do not mean by war, although we, with modern technology, can manage to eliminate considerable quantities of people at a stroke.

No: what I am getting at is that we are becoming very efficient at making ourselves ill. For as long as people have lived in societies there have been social diseases, the products of malnutrition, poor dwelling conditions, poor hygiene; but enlightenment and resource have eliminated many of these. (I am writing essentially about the 'developed' world - much has to be done to eliminate disease from the less developed people; a moral issue too vast for my consideration here). The diseases and illnesses that we are bringing on ourselves are those resulting from affluence and technology; diseases that are both physical and mental. But, perhaps with more and increasing relevance, we are imposing upon ourselves and others a range of traumas that result from ignorance of, or a refusal to acknowledge, the existence of a 'spirit' within each of us. And beyond that, a refusal on the part of many to acknowledge the existence of intelligent and independently acting spiritual 'beings'.

I have often wondered, and continue to wonder, how and when the concept of 'spirit', of an 'otherness', arose in the minds of developing humanity. To some, and particularly acknowledging that the spirit is always represented as 'speaking', it may presuppose the existence of a language in the culture of the 'hearer'. But this need not necessarily be so, for my experience has shown me that very potent communication can be established subliminally by the creation of ideas, concepts, feelings and moods, rather than by statements or instructions spelled out in actual words. As I have written earlier, in every part of the world and in every culture that has ever left a record throughout history, there has been an acknowledgement of a spiritual dimension and of the reality of invisible and independently acting spirits. It has also been perceived and acknowledged that within this dimension there is a source of knowledge and wisdom that far surpasses the knowledge and wisdom that may be developing as the result of natural observation and experiment. And knowledge and wisdom have always been represented as coming from the 'supreme divine', who, it was always believed, had the power to impose sanctions in the event of non-compliance with the divine advice or instruction which had become enshrined in religion and religious dogma.

Likewise, in each of these cultures, the *obverse* of the benevolent source of divine wisdom and protection has been acknowledged – namely the universal presence and action of spiritual *malevolence*. It is a source that appears to have in equal measure to the divine, knowledge and a perverted wisdom that are used to intrude into the minds, bodies and lives of sensitive and vulnerable individuals; intrusions that can encourage people into an actual *practice* of evil themselves, or which can undermine the mental and physical functioning of a person and lead to mental or physical illness, or both.

As I write, it is now twenty-three years since I began to experience the reality of what hitherto might have been speculation - the actuality of a spiritual state of existence, and the ability of spiritual 'entities' to influence the minds and bodies of humans. At this point, you might find it worthwhile to re-read the earlier section where I described the manner in which I first experienced intrusion into my mind and body. Nothing that has occurred during the intervening years has done anything to change my understanding of those events. On the contrary, everything that has happened to me since, all my experiences, have reinforced my certainty. *Every day*, in a variety of ways, I am reminded (*as if I needed reminding*) of the presence of the intruders. Gone, however, are the gross, obviously malignant, presences. No domination: no threats: no obscenities or salacious introductions into my mind. Everything that happens is at a more subtle level, almost unnoticed - would indeed pass unnoticed, if I had not gained an awareness of the whole process.

Let us hark back together to what I wrote earlier, to the thoughts of two men who have experienced the spiritual in life - *used* the spiritual: *invoked* the spiritual: *worked with* the spiritual. Men with such widely different backgrounds and antecedents - one an Irish poet and philosopher, the other an American-Jewish surgeon *and* philosopher. The first writes:

..."Often our loneliness and isolation is due to a failure of spiritual imagination. We forget that there is no such thing as empty space. All space is full of presence, particularly the presence of those who are now in eternal, invisible form."

The second, equally, has no doubt as he states:

..."As a healer I'm trying to get people to have faith in their own lives and in the whole process of life. You can act from that faith and make the rest of your life simple, or you can keep testing (the source of your faith) and make the rest of your life difficult... I counsel you to choose your direction, make the leap of faith and fly. Let the occasional spiritual flat tyres redirect your life. That's what survivors do. They don't have failures. They have delays or redirections. *Choosing spiritual guidance also helps you to see that people's minds and souls are interconnected in ways normally obscured from our everyday vision. The separatedness most of us experience is illusory, and seeing through it makes life even more meaningful".* (My italics)

It is here, at this point in the contact or discussions that I have with individuals, that I find myself running into sand. Minds are preformed. They may be preformed through the existing religious beliefs of the person - beliefs that may be set in stone and allow for no re-examination or interpretation. Minds equally set in stone may be those of individuals who, for whatever reason, are determined to resist completely the idea of the *existence* of a spiritual state or of individually acting spirits. I have had to make my own adjustments, and come to terms with the *reality* of my own experiences. One of the largest obstacles, points of disbelief, that many have, is with the traditional concepts of 'God'. God as creator of the Universe; God as an omniscient, prescient being, able to shape the lives of people and events on earth. On my computer screen when I switch on there is an image that came from the Hubble telescope, an image of the Whirlpool galaxy. I have it there partly for its intrinsic beauty, but more so to remind me of the *immensity* of the Universe, of the comparative insignificance of our sun and planet earth. On this earth I read of or watch almost daily the actions and behaviour of individuals and groups doing the most vile things to each other because of their varying and individual beliefs in 'God' - Who is, nevertheless, so it is claimed, the *same* for all peoples. I have a number of friends who are Buddhist, who, while having a deep and active spiritual life, nevertheless, have no belief in a 'God'.

Whenever I can, and from any available source, I acquire and study whatever is available relating to the evolution of the human species. Back and back, and yet further back they

LISTENING TO THE SILENCES

go, the palaeontologists, billions of years to 'the fish that walked': to the tetrapod that breathed air, that became a mammal and became us. Across the room on a shelf is a fossil trilobite that was alive four hundred million years ago, and elsewhere in the house a fossil ammonite from some time later - both species having been wiped out in one or other of the mass extinctions that have beset evolution. And thus and thus I try to face reality and shape my beliefs, for while my intellect and observation enable me to keep my grasp on what I can see with my own eyes, or take into my hands and accept as believable, I nevertheless have had the experiences that I have related.

I have had experiences that I have tried to describe as fully as my powers of expression allow, and have only held back when dealing with something that is spiritually and personally too deep and intimate to share. My experiences penetrate the interface between the visible and tangible and the 'ethereal' and intangible. I have felt the physical strength employed by a spiritual source in the manipulation of my body; daily I am aware of the intrusive movement of 'others' within my self and of the interactions within my mind. In the face of indifference and outright or unexpressed disbelief, I nevertheless continue to write, to explain, in the profound hope that *some* will accept, that *some* will profit. With the acceptance will, hopefully, come application - application of the knowledge in the care and 'release' of individuals who have been similarly invaded and who have, as a result, become disturbed and ill.

As I now begin to try to describe the reality of my current or past encounters with the 'intruders', I think that you may yourself realise that I am not recounting *religious* experiences such as one might find in the lives of the saints or the like. What I am, in fact, presenting is a series of ploys that have been used, continue to be used, to undermine my thoughts and actions and motives. You might recognise them as parallel experiences in your own life or in that of someone you care for. What I hope you will recognise are examples of what are commonly called the 'First Rank' symptoms of schizophrenia. What I also hope is that you will see that I have experienced them all, and recorded them in my own words - experienced and recorded some time before I had even become aware of such a list of symptoms. What I further hope to impress you with is the fact that *I have never been ill from this cause*.

To remind you, let me list the symptoms as given in *Schizophrenia Genesis* by Irving J. Gottesman:

1. Voices speak one's thoughts aloud.
2. Two or more voices (hallucinated - *his words not mine*) discuss one in the third person.
3. Voices discuss one's actions as they happen.

4. Bodily sensations are imposed by an external force.
5. Thoughts stop and one feels they are extracted by an external force.
6. Thoughts not 'really' one's own are inserted among one's own.
7. Thoughts are broadcast into the outside world and heard by all.
8. Alien feelings are imposed by an external force.
9. Alien impulses are imposed by an external force.
10. 'Volitional' actions are imposed by an external force.
11. Perceptions are 'delusional' and un-understandable.

Words such as 'hallucination' and 'delusion' are never my own choice, and I reject them and all their connotations *totally*. These are words used by the professionals in psychiatry and medicine, and imposed upon the 'outside' world in default of other more suitable expressions. But, and let us be clear about this, they are not words which would be chosen by those who actually *experience* the phenomena. By the time the latter have come within the orbit of psychiatry, they have often become so disturbed that they cannot describe rationally what they are experiencing, and, by default, accept what they are told - that they are hallucinating, deluded. By contrast, and as I have described, apart from the brief period at the outset of my encounter with 'voices' when I was deeply affected by what was happening to me - apart from then, all my experiences have come while I have otherwise been engaged in the *normality* of living. I drive to my local town; shop; borrow books from the library; travel to such places as the Hebrides, York, Scotland, on holiday. I have come to terms with my computer as a late starter - and you can judge my prowess for yourself. With its help I have communicated by letter or e-mail with a wide range of people including the Prime Minister and other major politicians, at least two retired consultant psychiatrists on matters about which I hold strong views, and received replies which indicate that my comments are welcome - indeed, one very well known professor of astronomy commented that he is always delighted to receive e-mails such as the ones that I have sent to him.

Thus a life - perhaps a bit more adventurous than many, as I indulge the privileges of my seniority - a life in which I am accepted as someone who has all his marbles; a life that embraces a wide variety of interests and a life through which I have, with success, tried to help, encourage, individuals who are disturbed in their minds. As you read, therefore, please remember, and remember well, that these experiences are not the product of a diseased or sick brain or one with a chemical imbalance within, nor of an aberrant mind. Everything that happened did so when I was wide-awake and doing, or trying to do, the normal things of life. Please remember also

ts
LISTENING TO THE SILENCES

that I am not writing on my own behalf, but as an advocate for the many who have similar experiences, who are rendered inarticulate or confused by them, who are labelled 'schizophrenic' and who suffer all that society throws at them because of the label.

Roy Vincent

LISTENING TO THE SILENCES

CHAPTER 10

I have been taught

by

dreams and

fantasies,,

Roy Vincent

LISTENING TO THE SILENCES

> I have been taught by dreams and fantasies,
> Learned from friendly and darker Phantoms,
> And got great knowledge and courtesy from
> The dead kinsmen and kinswomen,
> Ancestors and friends.
>
> Edwin Muir

A few pages ago I suggested that you should re-read the earlier part of my writing in which I described the events leading up to the moment in which I began to 'hear voices' and experience other phenomena. Recollect that I had not sought any spiritual contact, nor had I been seeking 'divination' or converse with the dead. I had simply followed what at the time seemed to be a logical progression from the reality of dowsing using bent metal rods, to a point where I had perfectly rational conversations in which I engaged silently within my mind and I received responses – *reasoned* and logical responses – via a pendulum and alphabet chart. Thus, 'characters' had emerged, one of whom was alleged to be a former, and now deceased, Buddhist priest. In 'conversations' with him I became aware of a separate phenomenon, namely that of 'ambience'. At those times, I was imbued with and surrounded by an inexplicable and indescribable feeling of the sanctity and spiritual demeanour of someone of deep personal spirituality.

By itself, this type of encounter did not totally prepare me for the experience of having my entire person intruded into. As I have described earlier, I sat in my quiet room, as had been suggested in conversations via the pendulum, and began to compose myself for a simple meditative stillness. Totally unexpectedly, and without drama, "…a presence moved from the space in front of me *into* me". From that time onward, I have never been free from intrusive physical presences – not manifest all the time, but frequently, and with potentially significant effect upon my demeanour and reaction. My older brother is an Anglican priest. Completely independently, and not discussed or even mentioned until I had my own experiences and described them to him, my brother has had experience of spiritual 'movement' within himself since his late teens. He has had a full and active prayer life since those days, and he related to me how, when composing himself for prayer, or during the Eucharist, he sometimes senses bodily activity. He simply says within his mind – "If you are from God, you are welcome: if not, please go".

LISTENING TO THE SILENCES

Not, myself, having my brother's spiritual acceptance, and he not having had the trauma of my experiences of spiritual malevolence, our reactions are markedly different. I do not *want* this type of activity within myself, from any source, unless I will it. Consequently, I view *any* intrusion with hostility and deep resentment. Over the years I have identified and recorded a number of 'ploys' used by intrusive spirits, and try in my accounts to describe the indescribable – often by analogy, as in the following:

It is all too easy to dwell upon the presence of the voice intrusions. Far more insidious, and possibly ever present, is the mute *physical* 'overlap'. Try to imagine a not quite exact 'fit', so that in every movement or reaction there is just the little bit of anticipation or lag; of speeding up when it is inappropriate; of not being quite in phase on a turn; of causing forward movement when there are obstacles to be negotiated – whether by deliberate intent or lack of 'skill' it is impossible to say. When the presence is continuous, or frequently in and out, it can become positively loathsome and one longs to be rid of it. If you have a copy, read in the *Thousand and One Nights* the story of the *Old Man of the Sea*. Sinbad, shipwrecked and alone as usual, stumbles across an old man who asks for his help to cross a stream. Sinbad, in his kindness, takes the old man on his back, and then, when the stream is crossed, finds himself in a stranglehold;

beaten about the head, made to go this way and that, by day and night, at the old man's whim; be-skittered and be-pissed all down his back and generally befouled. It is only ultimately by making some wine from wild grapes and getting the man drunk that Sinbad is finally freed, and one can sense the ultimate release as he crushes the man's skull with a boulder. *Many times have I wished for that boulder!* It is possible from one's own reactions to these presences to understand how it is that individuals will harm themselves in an effort to get at or get rid of this gross intrusion that is only reachable within their own body.

Next, a very simple but effective ploy – (in all of the ploys that I shall describe, '*they*' refers to the intrusion or intrusions – it is impossible to know at any time whether there is one or more involved in the current activity):

They can intrude physically and mentally into one's every moment, delighting in creating emotions or exploiting potentially emotional situations, until one realises that attempts are made to create laughter or tears where one is not in the least stirred up in either direction sufficiently to laugh or cry. Similarly, if the situation arose, *they* could create a feeling of anger and supply the words to go with it in a ready flow. *They* intrude into one's every thought and action, including the most intimate.

One just longs for an empty space in one's mind where one can think one's own thoughts, enjoy one's own emotions and reminiscences without these intrusions. One develops the most intense hatred of *them*. One result of this barrage is that one resents *any* intrusion or contact, thus rendering suspect those that might originate from a desirable spiritual source – *they* simulate these as well, so as to create animosity in one's mind to potential or existing spiritual helpers.

Another, and somewhat different, example of a mute but explicit physical intrusion occurred as follows:

On one occasion, a female friend who was visiting asked me to help her to accomplish something personal and intimate that she could not achieve because of the difficulties of simultaneously looking and reaching. Having been married more than once, and having brought up a daughter and stepdaughter, I have no problem or embarrassment with female anatomy or exposure, but while I was delicately preoccupied, I felt an intrusion, or more specifically, a subtle *insinuation* into myself. Almost immediately, I was suffused by *someone else's* embarrassment, and *female* embarrassment at that. 'Who' had been persuaded to intrude and by 'whom', and under what pretext, I have obviously no way of knowing.

Physical intrusions can and do occur at any time and the differing intensities and variety are so great that is difficult to be specific. One example can occur when I am woodcarving.

At these times there can appear within me a 'heavy' intruding presence with a 'working' mouth of concentration and with laboured breathing – the conclusion being that someone 'in spirit' is trying to experience what they did not achieve in life. There is also the implication at other times that someone formerly skilled in life wants to impart that skill. This can present one with a difficult choice. There are or have been many musicians, composers, artists, writers and others who have freely acknowledged that they cannot produce their finest work unless their 'Muse' is present within them, and many and great are the works that have been produced. (See *The Unknown Guest* by Brian Inglis; also listen to the accounts given by concert pianist John Lill of his own experiences of spiritual presences that have occurred during his own public performances.) By contrast, I do not want to be 'taken over' – I want to work out my own problems and then want the sheer pleasure of, first of all, visualising, and then, creating my own art or craft. I do not want to be the vehicle through which 'someone' operates vicariously and, in doing so, takes away the pleasures of my own originality and craft skills.

I once had a very good sculpture and carving teacher who gave advice on concepts and techniques, but did not attempt to influence one's individual expression; nor did he touch the work unless asked to demonstrate, but was always there with advice if asked. Above all, he inspired immense confidence, and could rescue one from the most depressing artistic disasters.

This, by extension, is what one would hope for from desirable spiritual associates. Having done much to my house by way of development, and not having had craft training or much DIY experience, I have, nevertheless, been given much help by inspiration, in ways and on occasions that are too numerous to detail. It, however, helps me to make the point that there is much support and knowledge available, but it is received at a much, much deeper level than the other phenomena about which I am writing – virtually subliminally.

There can be a very great danger in accepting a 'Muse' into one's person. It can often be represented or inferred that this is the spirit of someone who, for example, was formerly a well known artist or musician. The belief that one has been chosen by this 'famous person' can be very flattering, but if it became continuous, one could gradually lose one's own identity and capacity for originality.

Once, while working on my private water supply, which is isolated and completely hidden from view, I was caused to fall by a 'wrestle'*. This effectively demonstrated, and was confirmed by implication, that I could be made to fall and be injured anywhere, with no chance of summoning help (or to fall in a dangerous location e.g. in front of a train or vehicle). It was then impressed upon me that I should always plan where I was going and what I was going to do, and that if I was going to be alone in an isolated location, I should ensure that someone was aware of where I could be found. It was further impressed on me that I would get immense help and protection if there was forethought in all my actions – that if I wanted to draw from the spiritual help which is always available, I should prepare beforehand for such activities as studying or giving healing. Although the purpose of this incident was benevolent and aimed at informing me for my own protection, I have included it here because it illustrates more than one aspect of what I am trying to convey. Earlier in my writing, I related how my body was manipulated physically with great skill. I am recalling it now to reinforce what I am trying to convey, namely the physical powers and skills of the 'intruders', whether they be benevolent or malevolent. Secondly, during this and the earlier happenings, there was no mental 'voice' communication. Entirely and fully, all that flowed did so at the deep subliminal level of 'concepts'.

On another occasion, when I was walking between my house and workshop, I was physically 'gutted'*, for want of a better word. This was completely spontaneous and without explanation – none was needed, for the meaning was obvious. It was as if a hand had reached in and torn out my solar plexus. Physical recovery came quite quickly, but the mental shock and implication stayed with me for much longer.

LISTENING TO THE SILENCES

On yet another occasion, when playing a game of rounders or cricket in my field with some nephews and nieces, I was running vigorously for the ball, when, suddenly, my legs were 'kicked'* from under me and I fell heavily. It was equivalent to the most blatant foul I had ever experienced when playing rugby at school or in the Navy.

From time to time, I re-read what I have written, and I am always conscious of the number of times when I have been forced to place inverted commas around a word or phrase that I have used in trying to describe the indescribable – as in the three instances at *above. On no occasion was there a visible agent through whom the effects had been engineered, although, on the third occasion, my fall was very public and the result of what I can only describe as a vicious attack.

The experiences that I have drawn on so far, or that I shall go on to describe, have occurred over more than twenty years, and continue to happen in one form or another. Throughout that time, I have kept notes of events as they took place, and have them with me now. I hope that in my writing I have shown myself to be capable of lucid communication. People with whom I come into contact treat me as an intelligent, 'normal' person who has a wide-ranging intellect; someone to whom a number come for advice on a range of topics; someone who is regarded as a good communicator. Yet, in spite of these personal qualifications, I am having the greatest difficulty in describing my experiences in such a manner that I will succeed in convincing anyone – particularly the sceptical, the determined 'unbelievers' – of their truth.

> Truth came and knocked on your door.
> "Go away", you called, "I'm busy looking for the truth"
> ....and truth went away...puzzled.
> Robert Pirsig

I find that I can continue to write most effectively by the use of analogy and by drawing upon my own personal experiences, although, in this instance, they are experiences gained in everyday life and several years before the beginning of the 'voice intrusions'.

Some time after the collapse of my first marriage, I took the plunge again and married a widow who had two teenage children. By nature, I am an optimistic person, looking for the positive in a relationship, and, probably naïvely, not looking ahead to the possibility of incompatibility or of serious dissent. Thus the prospect of sharing my newly acquired home and its four acres of land with someone who had similar interests in horses and the development of a smallholding, seemed to have a lot going for it. With my guard totally down, I made my newly acquired family completely free of the establishment and facilities in an endeavour to let them integrate totally, and feel wanted. Without going into detail, in a short time I found myself overwhelmed. With their own lines of communication well established, I found that preferences were being decided and acted upon in a manner which excluded me from the process, with the result that gradually I began to feel submerged and almost an alien in my own home. Worst of all was to have one's every action observed and analysed, and possibly commented upon or reported back. Remarks such as "*I wouldn't do it that way*" began to intrude: "The person who taught *me* to drive..." or similar comments were delivered in a manner that always presumed the superiority, or personal 'omniscience' of the lady.

The result was that very soon I found myself, at almost all times, living in anticipation of some remark or action that reflected or rebounded upon what I may have said or done. I had the constant inward feeling akin to 'looking over my shoulder', in expectation of some sort of intervention. In extreme instances, it was possible to find oneself unable to think a plan through or to make a rational decision, and even, as a result, to come to a total and dithering stop. These and similar reactions (or lack of actions) might occur even when the antagonising influence was not actually present, but in the offing or about to return. I sought isolation and longed for the 'space' and independence for my own thoughts and actions, free from observation and comment; free from the intruding voice and presence.

Many individuals, either by choice, or unwittingly, place themselves in situations in which 'voices and presences' intrude into their minds and bodies – indeed, some actively *seek* the voices and presences. Reflect that, unsuspectingly, without guile, but gullibly, and without anticipating any adverse consequences, through the use of my pendulum and alphabet chart, I was completely taken over, and my mind and life were totally dominated - until eventually I was able to break free. What, initially, had appeared to be a desirable development in my life, soon became a dominating influence. I had not been seeking spiritual enlightenment, or any esoteric practices, whereas many individuals do have such goals.

The 'seeker' may, for example, join a workshop with the aim of becoming a 'channeller' of enlightenment and truth from 'ascended masters', and be delighted at the arrival within of an inner voice and presence. Another might enrol for instruction in Reiki, and receive 'empowerment' or 'atunemet' from some (presumed) spiritual source. Others may follow the directions given in the writings of the Simontons or similar authors and endeavour to find their 'inner guides'. Some might go through a process of 'past life regression' under hypnosis and emerge convinced that they have their former persona 'who' speaks through

LISTENING TO THE SILENCES

them. Yet others might seek the inner 'atunements' to be reached through deep meditation practices – indeed they might work diligently at the practices with the objective of achieving, or contacting *sidhis* (depending upon the meaning each might give to the word).

Some seekers are well integrated mentally and spiritually, and are introduced to their chosen practice with care and control. Others may be 'opened' spiritually in a rash or incompetent manner, and may become the victims of undesirable intrusions into their bodies and minds. (Once again quoting Dr. Elmer Greene when he writes of the perils of a hasty descent into the deeper realms of the mind: 'The persistent explorer in these realms…brings himself to the attention of indigenous beings…').

The arrival of the voice in the mind and the presence within the body, may be instant and very obvious, as they were in my case, or they may appear as if by subtle and gentle infusion over time, in such a way that the 'host' may never be sure *when* they actually arrived, or, indeed, whether they had always been present. With the awareness that there is, seemingly, a powerful spiritual or 'different' influence in ones life, it is possible that one feels flattered at being chosen, particularly as a feeling of 'warm solicitousness' may be being created simultaneously. As within the analogous situation of my second marriage, it is difficult to be certain subsequently *when* things began to change –

when the presence and association once welcome and sought, became so *un*welcome, aggravating and dominating.

Analogies can be taken too far, and then cease to be useful, yet, nevertheless, the changes that I have used my former marriage to illustrate, do occur, sometimes over a period of time – sometimes within the span of a day, as in the following example that I have recorded.

The moment of waking, or the time of gradually emerging awareness after sleep, is most crucial, for one is then at one's most vulnerable. One's first thoughts at these times are 'answered'; indeed, it might seem that one is already in a conversation. It is exceedingly difficult to avoid responding, and a dialogue can ensue from which it is hard to break free. There can be a feeling created on waking, a sense of being with very gentle spiritual people, warm, welcoming and caring. It is so easy to slip into this ambience, particularly if the rest of one's life is bleak or fraught.

But, as one is starting to feel 'cosy' and cared for, *they* start to imply that there are one or two, oh-so-teeny, defects that need correcting before one can be *truly* accepted and enjoy this ambience and ultimately be accepted into it after death. Gradually the emphasis shifts becoming more needling and ultimately threatening. One's defects become grossly magnified, one's sense of unworthiness exaggerated, and all the earlier warmth totally disappears.

LISTENING TO THE SILENCES

Sometimes an intrusion can be of such a cold, inhuman presence that one can feel oneself to be totally devoid of humanity, of love, of caring. *One could become either very ill or very evil.*

It is virtually impossible for anyone in this state to convey to another the sense of threat or terror that can be experienced at these times. This inability to communicate can so increase a person's sense of loneliness, of total isolation, that they can easily try to seek oblivion in drink or drugs or suicide - indeed, it is quite possible that in their mind they will be actively encouraged down some desperate or diabolical route.

It is some time since I experienced this particular type of ploy, although the memory never fades. While my own experiences were long ago and intermittent, I was once briefly acquainted with a woman for whom similar and worse ones were a daily occurrence. Married with two young children of school age, her days began inside the warm 'cocoon' of the mind and the ambience of a benevolent spiritual presence. With the husband at work and the children at school, the warmth and gentleness of the voices and presences changed significantly, and she was accused of being an incompetent and wicked mother whose children were in danger of being corrupted by evil. She was told that she should kill the children and then herself in order to escape from the evil that surrounded them, and to ensure that they all would be secure spiritually. Each day saw her cowering in a corner with the curtains drawn, subjected to constant abuse and torments, until about mid-afternoon, when the agony gradually ceased, the curtains were drawn back, and the children welcomed home. All would be peace – until the next morning, when the omissions of the previous day would be piled onto the long and growing list of her incompetences and inadequacies.

The person was an active, practising Christian, the minister of whose church lived less than fifty yards away, unable, seemingly, to help. I talked to him on one occasion when I visited a friend who lived nearby, and tried to interest him in my experiences, and their relevance to the situation of his parishioner. I might just as well have saved my breath, for like so many in the Christian ministry today, he had come under the spell of modern psychiatry and psychology, and believed all that was said about voice hearing, schizophrenia, and the efficacy of modern drugs in controlling the condition. Instead of asking, exploring, trying to learn more, this man was more interested in trying to analyse *me*, and in putting me in a 'category' that would explain *my* alleged experiences.

I can only comment from the standpoint of someone who has been a lifelong Christian, and can only speculate that people of other faiths might have their religious beliefs and observances used and turned against them as they strive for the perfections that their religion advocates. One fruitful hunting ground for

LISTENING TO THE SILENCES

intruding spirits is the highly charged, emotional setting of a religious gathering, where the charismatic appeal of the speaker can cause individuals to drop their inhibitions or controls and open themselves wide to a hoped-for spiritual manifestation, or 'conversion'. The huge appeal of the moment; the wonderful feeling of being 'born-again'; the dramatic reaction to being 'slain by the spirit', can all conspire to make the sensitive, susceptible ones believe that they have been 'chosen'. They can feel numinous presences within or around them, and rejoice at the inner voice that tells them that they are one of an elect band and that they will 'purified', and, when pure, will be allowed close and personal contact with the 'ultimate' – that, if pure, they may even be chosen to 'channel' wisdom and truths. In the joy of having been accepted into this inner circle, it is so easy for the susceptible to lose all sense of discernment and to immerse themselves completely within this newly revealed inner world.

      Undoubtedly there are many spiritual locations and gatherings from which people return uplifted, inspired and renewed – locations and gatherings where, often by long association, there is spiritual guardianship and protection. There are, however, undoubtedly others, where the speaker and venue are used to draw the vulnerable, susceptible, and where their weaknesses can be seen and exploited spiritually. I am fully aware that many have great difficulty even in accepting the reality of a spiritual state and of the existence of individually acting spirits. I am equally aware of the much greater difficulty that the concept of the reality of spiritual evil and of *intelligent*, individually acting spirits presents. I have long ago given up any attempts to convince anyone who is determined *not* to accept any of this; but even these readers, if they truly have the welfare of suffering individuals at heart, should consider what I am writing, and, if nothing else, use my experiences and observations as 'patterns' to be held against these individuals to see if any fit.

To return to ones who have been 'entered' and inspired, and who now believe that they are to be purified and 'used' – by whom? Do they question? *I* did not – I was gullibility personified – *because I had no reason to doubt what I was being told, through the pendulum, or in my mind*! Remember, I was alone, with no one with whom to share my experiences or from whom I might have received counsel and caution. Indeed, one ploy that might be used is one in which *they* gradually encourage isolation, advising that friends and associates are not 'worthy' to share in the new experiences, and that all inner voice contact would be better served by the hearer withdrawing into a more solitary life. Within the new world of increasing solitude and isolation, the victim, without realising it, is more vulnerable and open to suggestion. Thus, it might be proposed that a prayer regime should be established, which gradually might become more severe as an indication of inner piety – possibly involving waking and praying through the night. Different forms of asceticism, such as diet restriction, may be suggested strongly.

[Let me remind you of my earlier description of the arguments and propositions that were put to me, and let me also recall that at the time I felt no strain or overt pressure – all appeared logical and desirable, and it was all achieved *as the result of discourse in my mind*. This is what I wrote:

"… nevertheless, there was strong argument that I should become morally impeccable, but that I should not choose a philosophy or religious affiliation because it allowed a degree of moral latitude. It was put to me that as, at an earlier time, I had elected to be a Catholic, I should 'return to the fold', or, if not, then my rejection should be for sound reasons of belief, and not because I was looking for a path with less exacting moral standards.

I was encouraged to adopt a sincere prayer life and spent long periods in prayer each night…"]

With each acceptance of a new devotion or stringency, the victim is creating levers that may be used to torment him. If he should default on any of his commitments, *they* will seize upon and try to exploit even the most minor peccadillo, or even a supposed one, and make it become an obsession beyond all reason, while at the same time creating a physical ambience of censoriousness. *They* might even propose a more severe asceticism as a form of penance to restore his spiritual standing. The feeling created, of unworthiness and censure, can overshadow the brightest company or activity, almost as if there was a sentence hanging over one – reminiscent of when, in my past serious depression, there existed a feeling of 'gut hollowness' that totally prevented one's enjoyment and development, much as I imagine the presence of a cancer within one's body might do. Within the major religions, many do spend time in isolation, or engage in stringent ascetic practices, but they do so *within* a 'control group', having checks and balances and spiritual advisors, together with a long tradition upon which to draw, and an understanding of the potential dangers of such activities. (Recollect the 'Rules for the discernment of spirits' given by St. Ignatius of Loyola, the founder of the Jesuit Order, to which I referred earlier in my writing).

Within the context of self-purification, the hearer is encouraged to dredge his mind and to bring to the surface any – usually long past – events or thoughts of an embarrassing, shameful or similar nature, especially if others are involved. *They* will encourage recollection of incidents in which others – family, friends, - showed up badly, especially reminiscences about known or imagined (and usually, sexual) peccadilloes. *They* might next pretend that the persons themselves are present in spirit and are aware of the thoughts, and that one will be confronted with the consequences of these unnecessary revelations that should have been allowed to pass into history, when one dies oneself. In this context, *they* will insert into one's mind a name that is calculated to produce reminiscences from the past – often the name of someone with whom one has been close or intimate – always trawling the mind, encouraging recollections, particularly of a sexual nature.

Yet again, a 'heavy' presence, purporting to be a senior spiritual figure, may introduce the concept that someone (deceased) does, or will wish to apologise for lifetime's hurts. This is calculated to cause one to go over in one's mind the circumstances that led to the hurt, with the possibility that an old wound may be opened and that one could renew resentment against the 'person' who is alleged to be present, and aware of one's thoughts. All thoughts of apology to be given or received can rapidly disappear. One might also be encouraged to consider the apologies that one would feel it necessary to make oneself. This is another ploy aimed at inducing a further mind trawl, calculated to reveal incidents or thoughts that are derogatory of others or oneself.

Intent upon self-purification and spiritual development, the hearer may find himself being drawn closer and closer into contact with, and reliance upon, the voices in his mind and the ambient presences that are subtly intruded. Apparently proceeding in a manner that gives satisfaction to his 'mentors', he might find himself being rewarded with the presence around him of supposedly senior and powerful beings, and being told in his mind that he has been accepted, but at a junior level. Henceforth, he will be part of a 'team', but as a receiver of instruction and a neophyte. Yet another step has been taken along a road that may deprive him of his own reasoning and decision making abilities, and lead him into a state of dependence from which he may never break free, unless he receives skilled and understanding assistance.

He will become a 'listener' – listening within to his 'controls'; not focussing on the people and world around, but always within. You have perhaps been in a cocktail party or other gathering where there is fervent conversation going on in the groups all around, and you are trying to converse with someone who is directly in front of you, someone whose face is turned attentively towards you, but whose eyes are seemingly vacant, and certainly not focused on you. The conversation in the adjoining group, the little bit of gossip half heard, is *so* much more interesting, riveting, than your conversation. These are the same eyes and the demeanour of someone who is locked into the inner mind and communication; someone who is listening to current conversation within, or who is listening to the silence – waiting for the next contact, which has become more real than the people around. Still in this context, I am reminded of a woman who briefly passed through my group of friends, who, in a similar way, exemplifies what I am trying to convey. While, say, gardening and carrying on herself with what she was doing, she would say "Listen, Roy...." while she thought of something to say and hold the centre of attention, and, until I learned to ignore the call, I would stand in suspense, waiting for the next remark.

We still have within ourselves all of the instinctive, behavioural actions and reactions of our mammalian evolution. The automatic and autonomic functions are too frequently dismissed as 'flight, fight, adrenalin'. There are very many more reactions and interactions prompted by social and instinctive triggers. I have a book that provides instruction for budding cartoonists, and which shows a hundred stylised cartoon faces that are designed to illustrate an equal number of emotions and reactions. Each of the expressions, when on the actual face of a person, would be accompanied by a range of corresponding internal changes, involving sphincters, eye focus, blood distribution, muscle tensions and breathing, that are, mostly, too subtle to be observed or actually felt. A wild creature that hears a sound that might suggest a threat, adopts a 'listening' state. In this state, and simplistically, ears are cocked, breathing is almost suspended to enable the hearing to become more acute, genitals are tensed and anal and bladder sphincters are tightened, while the creature adopts a 'shoulder hunched' posture, possibly to create a low profile. In the animal, the changes last as long as the stimulus exists, and a quiescent state returns, or the creature reacts to the next and different set of stimuli.

For the perpetually listening human, there is no release, as the internal reactions become the norm. To the blank, listening gaze of the listener will be added the hunched shoulders and shallow breathing. Invisible, and probably unremarked, because it has become the norm, is the tight anal sphincter, which, in turn, is accompanied by a constriction at the base of the throat. The latter constriction is part of an internal mechanism that, in the threatened mammal, diverts blood supply from the digestive organs and brain into the muscles of response, preparing the latter for immediate action if the potential threat becomes real. In the human, the long-term diminution of blood supply to the brain must have many consequences that I am not competent to analyse. However, in the analysis of the brains of schizophrenics, note is often taken of local changes in brain structure, which are then considered to be among the *causes* of the schizophrenic state. To me, it is reasonable to question whether the changes within the brain are the *result* of a curtailment of the blood supply, and are themselves, in turn, a consequence of the perpetual listening.

        I am reminded of these phenomena as I sit at my computer in intense concentration and suddenly realise that *my* shoulders are hunched, *my* breathing is very shallow, while my thought processes are turning into treacle and a series of aches and tensions are created in various places. I am 'listening' intently into my mind and memory as I try to convert my notes and experiences into a coherent narrative. Until I learned various methods of preventing the results of my absorption from having these effects, I used to be concerned at the persistent shallowness of my breathing. At that time, my efforts aimed at restoring regular, deep breathing, produced only limited results. In an effort to induce natural breathing at all times, I went to visit someone whom I know who is a properly trained hypnotherapist, having the idea that it should be possible, under hypnosis, for her to programme me to breathe regularly and fully, even when in deep and persistent thought.

Having heard me through, my friend said firmly that her training would not allow her to do what I asked: she would need, over a number of sessions, to find out *why* my breathing was shallow, and *then* try to change the pattern. Disappointed, as we live some distance apart, I nevertheless accepted her offer of simple hypnosis aimed at inducing deep relaxation. In all, I am acquainted with five qualified hypnotherapists, three of whom are also G.P.s, and had then already experienced hypnosis induced by two of them. Among other motives, I was interested in comparing my friend's technique with that of the other two.

While I still remember that her approach was different from those that I had experienced previously, it is sufficiently long ago for me to have only a vague recollection of the actual details. What I *do* remember is going through a series of stages of 'induction' and becoming mentally detached, and on the verge of losing awareness. At this point, and yet still capable of thought, I experienced a strong physical, spiritual intrusion into myself, while my rational mind helped me to hold onto consciousness. Within my state of residual awareness, I had been able to realise that *had* I allowed myself to continue into deep hypnosis, there was a strong possibility that I would have been taken over and spoken through, as is a trance medium. This is not only my assertion. I formerly had many discussions with one of my G.P. friends, who, with the patients' permission, used to let me observe his technique at work. On one occasion that I remember, my friend had recently returned from a conference of medical hypnotherapists, and related how one of the speakers had cautioned members about the very things of which I am writing.

In increasing flow, Eastern religious, philosophical and esoteric practices have made their way westward – concepts of reincarnation, past lives, karma - almost, one might say, in a 'pick and mix' combination with aspects of Buddhism, yoga, martial arts, Qi gong and many more. I am not drawn into this world of belief myself, although I have many friends who have a greater or lesser interest, and some who are ardent practitioners, and I read much of what is accessible to the non-participant. There is a common thread that seems to link many, and that is a belief in past lives, reincarnation and the possibility of regression into a past life while under hypnosis. I do not intend to get drawn into a discussion about other peoples' sincerely held beliefs and practices; however, my own experience while being hypnotised makes me question most strongly the merits and reality of alleged past life regression. I see it as being fraught with danger for the vulnerable – and even for the apparently stable.

Several years ago, someone who stayed at my home for about two years, used to like to be taken to local group meetings of a national healing organisation. I did not stay for the actual proceedings, but returned for the social chat and refreshments with which the meetings ended. Almost the entire group of very delightful people believed that each had a persona derived from a past life. What struck me forcibly was that some appeared to be acting out a version of the personality that they believed that they once had. Of itself, this activity is for the individual and not me to choose. In the context in which I am writing I *am* concerned, for within this belief and practice there is the mechanism by means of which a person can be taken over and controlled. There is the distinct possibility that, under hypnosis, intrusion may have occurred, and that the perceived change in attitude and function may be interpreted as being a reflection of the character of the supposed previous incarnation. Often, the earlier status is presented as having been important or desirable for some reason, and the person is flattered and consciously or unconsciously adopts a new role and personality.

In time, the 'real' person, i.e. the one in *this* life, may become dominated completely by the inner, and unable to function normally.

The ability to hypnotise is easily achieved, but is not necessarily accompanied by the responsibility or awareness that should pervade the practice. The Web lists numerous courses, many controlled by responsible bodies whose aim is to produce competent medical hypnotherapists. However, the Web also lists others of dubious probity and responsibility, offering 'training and qualification' by distant learning, as indicated by the following extract from one advertisement:

HYPNOTHERAPY IS THE CAREER OF
THE FUTURE
NO EXPERIENCE NECESSARY

"It has really taken off in the last few years. Now is the time to get in, before it becomes strictly regulated. You too can discover the joy of taking control of your life, your future. If you are interested in enhanced income, life enjoyment, success, financial independence then this is the career for you! A qualified hypnotherapist can earn between $75-$150.00 an hour! Many practitioners working part time with 4 or 5 clients at their convenience, can earn an extra $350-$500.00 a week. Full time professionals are earning $75,000+ a year. With some reporting much higher earnings. You too can discover the

LISTENING TO THE SILENCES

joy of taking control of your life while promoting your own health and wealth. Jump-start your Career for the Millennium! We offer a no nonsense approach to education.

There is no previous educational experience required at this time to take these courses. Anyone with a desire to succeed and excel can enrol in our courses. We are only interested in your knowledge and ability in this field. You must however possess a positive attitude and a willingness to succeed, a test score of 75% or higher and a taped session to become *Certified*."

Reading the complete advertisement reveals that there is no personal contact between school and client – all is 'achieved' using books and tapes. And the 'examination' is similarly conducted – a written test paper and a video or audio tape of a 'session' being the only requirements necessary to gain the coveted certificate, and a series of convincing letters to place after the name! Such is the type of 'training' of some who offer, among other benefits, 'regression therapy' and N.L.P. (neuro-linguistic programming). The threat to the minds of vulnerable people is immense, and is added to in significant measure by the antics of the 'stage hypnotist'. A further advertisement on the Web offered 'the fastest training for stage hypnotists'. The public distortion of peoples' minds and behaviour for the sake of entertainment has, in my belief, the possibility of causing harm to the participants that may result in permanent damage to their personality.

In 2001, one member of the public featured in a lawsuit against a well-known stage hypnotist. The former had willingly and actively participated in a performance, only to find that, shortly afterwards, he began to 'hear voices', and subsequently experienced a complete change of personality. In court, he had a number of prominent psychiatrists and psychologists arrayed against him, who declared that he had undoubtedly been a latent schizophrenic, and that the actual manifestation of the condition had nothing to do with the stage participation. Naturally, the man lost his case. 'Naturally', because there was not the remotest possibility that anyone would even *suggest* that he had been the subject of spiritual intrusion. My experience leaves me in no doubt that hypnosis should be used only with caution – certainly not for entertainment - and with the constant awareness that, under its influence, vulnerable individuals may become the victims of intrusion.

Just as sharks know where food is most likely to be found, and just as they have highly sensitive detection equipment to inform them when something suitable has arrived: just as prey animals know of the waterholes where victim species are likely to be present and off their guard: just as vultures have the keenness of perception to detect from afar the potential meal – in like manner are the spiritual intruders equipped. It is not my intention to catalogue all of the circumstances and venues that lend themselves to spiritual intrusion, only to use a small number as illustrations.

One that readily comes to mind is the so-called 'clubbing' culture in which many simply want to get 'stoned' on drink, drugs, or both, and to end up with a quick 'shag'. No doubt there are many who remain in control, but there are undoubtedly many others who do not, and who risk damage to their lives and minds, and put themselves into situations in which intrusion is possible. The desire to use the latest 'recreational' drug or combination of substances to achieve a much-vaunted experience may induce individuals to pursue practices that, if they were to be examined rationally, amount to little short of self-degradation.

Many will have read the series of books by Carlos Castaneda, who sought 'knowledge and enlightenment' via mescaline and the 'spirit' of his own peyote plant, which 'revealed' itself to him in the desert. I read the first book on the recommendation of friends who were raving about it. All that I saw was someone who was prepared to degrade himself in the pursuit of some supposed goal of inner enlightenment and power. To crawl around on all fours in the guise of a dog, and to vomit uncontrollably in the desert night, does not suggest itself as an ideal preliminary to spiritual development. While reading the book, I was reminded of the story of one young woman, a committed cocaine addict, who went into a public lavatory in order to give herself a much-needed 'fix'. Her trembling hands dropped the powder on the toilet floor, and she came to her senses to find herself on all fours about to lick it up, so desperate was she for the drug. The shock of seeing herself in such a state of degradation was sufficient to drive her away from drugs.

Others are not so fortunate, and having, in their mentally weakened state, become the victim of an intrusion, have their desires and degradation turned on and off at the whim of the intruder. There are many other potential sources of personal degradation than drugs that I do not intend to catalogue, but, rather, will leave it to you to compile your own list. One unfortunate consequence of a degraded lifestyle is imprisonment. Once in prison and 'banged up' for possibly twenty-three hours a day, the mind of the prisoner can become a happy hunting ground for intruding spirits. With endless time at their disposal, *they* gradually enter the thoughts of the incarcerated and can produce untold torment that may ultimately lead to self-harm, suicide or mind destruction. Many who have been convicted of the most degraded or despicable crimes are advised to accept solitary confinement to keep themselves away from other prisoners who might attack them. Within the solitude, the captive mind can be toyed with and 'bounced' between a seemingly endless variety of voices, or 'harried' by a duality of voices in the manner of greyhounds coursing a hare.

LISTENING TO THE SILENCES

A person can find himself or herself persuaded into wrong-doing by warm, 'companionate' voices, that may have become part of their normal thoughts, and accepted almost as an 'inner counsellor'. This can become the lot of an intelligent, imaginative and, possibly, isolated person. Such a one can become used to the inner discourses that may be a part of the normal process of mentally teasing away at a problem or argument. A separate inner voice may be truly indistinguishable from ones own thoughts, and yet become a source of deliberately, yet subliminally, intruded thoughts. Such a voice can become companionable to the solitary person and apparently share memories and reminiscence. Such a voice can pour the balm of solicitude on the hurts and injustices of life; can become a permanent, trusted friend, and yet, withal, keep the resentments stoked, and suggest ways of getting one's own back. Such a voice can, almost as a joke or game, propose an action such as shoplifting. 'The coast is clear, go on, I'll keep watch'. With the first attempt a success, the joint venture is set to become a constant game and, between them, the person and the inner voice devise new and ingenious strategies, until, possibly at the urgent prompting of the voice, the person believes that he can accomplish something daredevil – and is exposed.

I sometimes wonder whether this was the fate of a well-known person – a regular broadcaster, magistrate and author – who was detected shoplifting, sentenced, and, in her shame, committed suicide. It was revealed that she had devised an ingenious topcoat, with numerous inner pockets designed to receive the booty. Personally, having experienced the persuasive ways of the voices, although not in this particular context, I find it easy to believe that this person had been tricked as I suggest, and when exposed, had been hounded to suicide by her 'friend and companion', the inner voice, which had now turned against her, and mocked her in her humiliation.

Does this seem far-fetched? Does the concept of friendly encouragement, support, and reliable and close companionship that turns into, or exists as a cover for, deceit and malevolence, seem far-fetched? It can happen at the human level. Do the names Burgess, MacLean, Blunt and Philby resonate with you? Perhaps you are too young to have known. Three were highly placed in British Intelligence, having access to much secret and extremely sensitive information, while the fourth was greatly regarded within the world of fine art, and occupied the position of surveyor of the Queen's pictures – he having also served in Intelligence during World War II. All lived lives that were apparently impeccable, and fully integrated into the society and government of their day – and all were traitors of the vilest kind, working in the closest possible way with the then Cold War enemy, the Soviet Union, and being, amongst other things, betrayers

LISTENING TO THE SILENCES

of many British agents, sending them to torture and death.

Of many ploys adopted by the intelligent intruding spirits, one is to become the inner voice of someone who lives a life of utmost probity, who is highly regarded, and who develops a reputation as, for example, a 'channeller', a giver of 'readings', a 'trance medium', a clairvoyant. Providing accurate, and perhaps comforting information, and, seemingly, giving excellent advice, the inner voice can, nevertheless, operate in one of the classical ways of espionage. This particular ploy succeeds when, within the confident and believable delivery, a 'weasel' word or piece of advice is slipped into what may otherwise be genuine and sound. Can I recall to you the events that I related earlier, when, following the recommendation of a then associate, I went to see a woman who, it was said, was deeply spiritual and full of insight? I had no particular need of any sort of so-called 'reading', but, as with many things that I do, I went mostly out of curiosity.

As I have written previously, she was a most delightful person – open and welcoming. For almost two hours, with a break for lunch, I listened as I was fed words of presumed wisdom – words that I began to realise were of no significance, and meant nothing to me. However, within the inconsequential discourse, certain ideas were planted, which took me several years to discard. 'I give you X and Y', said she, mentioning two names. 'You will write a book in collaboration with someone who is already established in your field and, consequently, your writing will get a much needed boost'. Whenever, subsequently, an X or a Y came into my orbit, in spite of myself, I wondered 'Is this the X, or the Y whom she meant?' Likewise, when I became acquainted with someone new who appeared to have suitable writing talents, inevitably I would speculate about whether this was to be my collaborator.

Rather more serious and insidious was the statement: "You will have teaching dreams". As well as intruding into the mind and body while a person is awake, it is evident that intrusions from spiritual sources occur during sleep. I do not intend to become involved in a study of the many instances when individuals through history have claimed to have been warned or given prescience during dreams. To do so would divert me from my main task. I do not doubt that it is possible for an individual to be influenced in this way. Had I, myself, been so gullible as to accept this proposition, and believed that I would be fed esoteric knowledge during my sleep, and then had been naïve enough to incorporate the knowledge into my thinking and everyday practice – what then? With my experience of spiritual intrusion, I was able to see the ploy for what it was, and essentially, thereafter, have tried to apply all my growing alertness and discernment to an understanding of the sometimes weird world of my dreams. Someone *without* my experience might have been flattered to think that they were to have communication from – perhaps an

LISTENING TO THE SILENCES

'Ascended Master', to use the current glib jargon, or 'The Source', to use another frequently used name – but who can say what the source might be, or how they have been influenced subsequently?

On a much bigger stage, a well-known American woman journalist developed a talent for automatic writing. She was fed such informed and corroborative detail relating to her personal life, that she doubted not that the sources of her writing were 'all-seeing' and infinitely knowledgeable. The latter identified themselves with ideograms for 'Donkey' and 'Lily' – claiming that if they disclosed who they had *really* been when alive, the author herself would be overwhelmed at being chosen to channel from such eminent people. Over the course of her first book, *A Search for the Truth*, the author, Ruth Montgomery, passed on the 'wisdom and insights' from – *whom*? How can anyone possibly know? She interlaced her chapters - first one from the 'sources', then another, into which appeared apparently corroborative words from major American political or other well-known figures. Then back to the sources, and so on through the book – a book that, to some minds, gave the author credibility as a vehicle for 'channelled' wisdom.

A second book followed, inspired again by the 'sources'; a book called *Strangers Among Us*. Without giving a lengthy description of the contents, I shall summarise two key ideas through which the book could be calculated to influence the vulnerable or gullible. The first is the concept of 'walk-ins'. This applied to individuals who may have become so desperate at the distressfulness of their earthly situation, that they would, by spiritual means, be offered the chance to exchange with 'someone', now in spirit, who had so learned to match them that a 'seamless' change could be made. The body would continue with its new 'occupant', and the 'dispirited' one would proceed, spiritually, to another plane of existence. The gullible, deceived by this seemingly desirable strategy, would, after a time, and still in the same body, believe that they actually were the 'walk-in'. So believing, an individual would thus continue in life, but in a state of being controlled totally by – *whom*? This ploy may seem even more far-fetched than some others that I am describing. Having, effectively, been 'shadowed' spiritually, and, at one time, been aware of the presence of an invisible *doppelgänger* paralleling my being, I have no doubt about its reality and feasibility.

Many people have scant scientific knowledge, and know very little about the planet upon which they dwell. This state of ignorance can easily be exploited, as exemplified in the second strategy that I have taken from the book. 'There will be a nuclear holocaust within a specified number of years'. 'The earth will wobble on its axis, or even flip right over, causing huge sea waves which will swamp coastal areas, allowing only those inland and on high ground to survive'. Such were some of the predictions of the 'sources' - predictions that many would accept unquestioningly because of the apparent authority that the author had built up through the merits of her first book. Well, the specified number of years have long come and gone without, as far as I am aware, there having been a nuclear holocaust, and the earth has not wobbled nor flipped! (Although it *does* have precessing movements involving its orbit and axis, movements that are well know, but are capable of being mis-represented to influence the uninformed). Both of the quoted predictions were aimed at people who were gullible, and who, in their gullibility, were somehow made to feel that they could be among the survivors who would be required to repopulate and restore the earth. Strong in their beliefs, many formed small communities in isolated areas and learned basic survival crafts, ultimately losing touch with reality, and becoming disillusioned when the earth was not devastated and did not flip. This is a very limited summary, but one that, I hope, will serve to illustrate the ways in which an author, full of self belief, can be used unwittingly to influence and unsettle many individuals.

Before leaving the topic, I must recall an earlier period in my story when I was myself living in a state of total conviction that the 'Other' who were in my mind, and fully in my life, were real and had a *right* to question and pressurise.

Looking back, I *know* that they were *real* and were neither hallucinations nor delusions, but *how* they came to have such authority and dominance, or how I *allowed* them to, I shall never be able to recall. All I know now is that they did, and that I allowed them. How else would I even *consider* the proposition that they made? This is what I wrote earlier:

"More and more the theme of the 'Second Coming' of Jesus was developed, and then, quite bluntly, it was put to me that He would return in a more mature person than was generally expected, and that I was a suitable candidate within whom He could manifest Himself. I cannot remember exactly how I declined such an offer that, it must be thought, no one could refuse. I do remember that I declared that I was too much of a coward to be able to accept such a high profile role."

Someone well known in the world of football who, in accepting the proposition, achieved fame or notoriety depending on how one views the events, was David Icke. Convinced by a series of seemingly inexplicable coincidences, and accepting what he was told via the direct 'channelling' of a well-known medium, David went public and proclaimed himself a 'Son of God'. He subsequently published books whose contents also arrived through 'channels'. '...I have communicated almost daily with Rakorski, the one known as Lord of all Civilization, who is directly responsible for the changes the earth will

LISTENING TO THE SILENCES

undergo...' '...I was led to many psychics in Britain and other countries, and through them the Godhead and other beings of vast evolution have unveiled to me the mysteries of life. All have told of the same events to come in this decade, the great geological upheavals that will bring an end to the pain and suffering, anger and conflict that have taken this planet to the brink of non-existence...'

As was the case with the prophecies given by Ruth Montgomery in her book, David Icke's decade also has passed and the geological upheavals that he foretold have not happened either. His books are read by some as if they contain genuine prophecy, by others as the outpouring of a mind whose balance is questioned. Innocuous as they may seem, to me they provide the openings through which the minds of susceptible individuals may be entered and eventually dominated.

'...I hope that by the time you have read this book you will appreciate that communication with such beings on other levels of Creation is the most natural thing in the world.... Every time we think we create energy, a *thought-form* as it is called...A thought-form sent out by an Italian will be decoded by an Englishman into English, by a Frenchman into French. In this way thought-forms sent to us by the Spirit of the Earth or a being from another part of the universe can be decoded into spoken words by someone with psychic gifts which, indeed, all of us possess. This is called *channelling*...This decoding can manifest in many ways, not only through the spoken word. The thought-forms can be turned into written words, and this is known as *automatic writing*...It is also possible to hear the thought-forms as a soft gentle voice inside your head. I call this method 'getting it direct'. On a more limited level it is possible to communicate through *dowsing*.'

In my mind I yell with horror that such ideas are so gullibly spread to other potentially gullible people. The whole purpose of my writing is to *warn* the sensitive, the susceptible person of the dangers inherent in all these practices. If such people actually accept as genuine what they read, and if then they are persuaded by the books and their contents to try to communicate '...with the one we know as Jesus, the Spirit of the Earth, and many others...' they are in great danger of having their minds entered and taken over as was mine before I realised what was happening. I have written before of the need for discernment by the readers of such books and proclamations. Many individuals are prevented from exercising any form of discernment by their very ignorance of anything remotely scientific, and by an amazing lack of curiosity about themselves, how they function, and about the planet upon which they live. Within this ignorance, many can be persuaded to believe the most outlandish propositions that are represented as coming from the 'Ascended Masters' or similar. '...the body has changed and adapted itself as it

LISTENING TO THE SILENCES

has risen up and fallen down the frequencies. Since Atlantis it has changed from taking in energy externally to digesting energy from food internally. The light levels have had to step in to help here and there, but...'.

There are many such allegedly channelled books and other literature in the catalogues, offering the 'truths' from the 'Ascended Masters', who channel under a variety of names ranging from Aldebran to Zed. Some are a collection, or collage, or heterogeneous mixture of existing philosophical or religious concepts. Others pretend a science such as the one from which I drew my illustrations. All hold the potential of influencing vulnerable minds. Some books have an inexpressible ambience that may be sensed even before they have been opened, almost as if they come with an attachment for good or evil. I have just talked on the phone to a friend who agrees entirely with what I am trying to convey. My friend has a daughter who trades in second-hand books, and many pass through the house, or come in from the library, for she is herself an avid reader. Only recently, my friend told me of two books that she had borrowed from our local library and which she could not wait to return. It was not that intrinsically the two purveyed evil; rather that, comprehensively, they seemed to embody it within their total and indefinable ambience. On the other hand, certain books on her shelf seemingly draw the eye, and in themselves are inspirational.

Roy Vincent

Undoubtedly there are books that have been inspired from evil spiritual sources, although I cannot imagine that their authors would claim that this was the case. Evil itself works by being surreptitious and underhand – even by parading itself in the guise of good. On the other hand, there can not be many books more blatant than those of such authors as Aleister Crowley; books which, by their very challenge to orthodoxy, draw a readership – some sceptical and intent on debunking, others perhaps curious but open to the evil associations of the books and authors. And so, possibly touching just a few who are most vulnerable and clouding their minds to reality, the books and the original sources achieve their aim. Certain books about vampires and the cult that they inspire had a most profound effect upon a young man who this week has begun a life in prison. Influenced to the level of derangement, he murdered an elderly widow, cut out her heart, and drank her blood. I find it hard to believe that there are those who will not accept that the youth was evil and had been inspired by evil. But evil succeeds by pretending that it does not exist, and by persuading the 'sophisticated' that such concepts are mediaeval and not 'politically correct'.

Those who should speak out are often silent because, perhaps, they fear derision. It is possible that they also – they who, by virtue of their position within their culture or faith, should warn of what has been proclaimed in every region and at every time since the earliest – that they have been persuaded that 'evil' is something arcane and passé. Someone of eminence within the Catholic Church, who had, by omission, adopted such a position, was Cardinal Suenens. He admits such when he writes…

"I confess that…I have not sufficiently stressed the reality of the Powers of Evil at work in our contemporary world, and the necessity of the spiritual combat we must wage. It is difficult to row against the tide and not succumb to the spirit of the times…This, too, must be said, even at the risk of offending those who obstinately place their trust in the natural goodness of man and the myth of 'Progress'."

I am currently reading a book that was published very recently, and which takes the reader as far back in the history of religion as it is possible to go, there to find the first recorded statement of the belief in the existence of the conflicting spiritual powers of 'good' and 'evil'. The book, *A Search for Zarathustra* by Paul Kriwaczek, traces the author's quest to find the continuing influence on all subsequent religions, of the faith proclaimed by the prophet Zoroaster/Zarathustra. The point that I am making now, have made before, and will continue to make is this: whether one believes in one religion; whether one acknowledges the validity of a number of them; whether one rejects totally *all* religions and religious thought – how can anyone completely reject and ignore the one theme that runs through every faith – namely the existence of spiritual good and evil and their influence upon individual people?

In my efforts to bring the argument in to the present time, I have quoted the late surgeon and Psychiatrist, Dr. Kenneth McAll, and from his book, *Healing the Family Tree*; I have drawn from Clinical Psychologist, Wilson Van Dusen, and from his widely quoted chapter "*The Presence of Spirits in Madness*". Thus, from the earliest times to the present, there has run a consistent thread that just cannot be ignored. If you deny its existence and refuse even to think about the implications, just ask yourself whether you are one of those who are completely out of step, and whether you are denying those in your care the potential root of understanding and the relief of their suffering.

In writing from so strong a personal conviction, I must ensure that I do not fall into the trap that Cardinal Suenens so ably revealed in his book of the nineteen-eighties, *Renewal and the Powers of Darkness*. Written at the peak of the then highly popular and influential 'Charismatic Movement', in which individual Christians felt the upsurge of a revitalized recognition of the 'charisms' or gifts of the Holy Spirit at Pentecost, the author cautioned against some of the excesses that were becoming manifest. One of these was a growing belief the *all* mental illness was the result of malevolent spiritual influence, a belief that created a consequent growth in individual attempts at exorcism – sometimes bringing harm to the participants – something that should be borne in mind by those who are engaging in the increasing practice of so-called 'Spirit Release'.

The fact that this path is difficult to find and to follow should not, nevertheless, deter anyone from attempting to follow it, bearing in mind that it is not a path that one should wander down alone, nor without thought and preparation. Before I move on myself, I shall describe the real experiences of someone whom I know, which might add further illumination.

'Ruth' used to work in a music shop that I visit from time to time. As I became better acquainted with her, I learned that she is epileptic – a condition that is obviously well controlled by drugs and an appropriate lifestyle. In time, Ruth told me that earlier she had had two types of fit. The first type is the one that she has had since her teens, and is controlled by the drugs. In the second, she experienced great distress as she was assailed by a 'vile hag', who would try to drag her away or snatch the child from her womb. A reading in Church one day reminded Ruth of the account of Jesus curing an epileptic by driving out an 'evil spirit'. Prompted by this reminder, Ruth was prayed for within her Church community, and, during the same day, she experienced an immense relief within herself, and has since had complete freedom from the hag.

Roy Vincent

Sometime afterwards, someone in the Church decided that there must be many who have experienced what might be called 'mini-miracles', and invited such people to contribute to an intended publication. Ruth wrote her story, but, even before the accounts were published, her family home was invaded by a poltergeist. Among its varied activities, the latter would stamp around in first-floor rooms with such vigour that the light fittings in the ceilings below would shake. The noise of the stamping could be heard by neighbours at times when the family were not at home. It also startled one of Ruth's students when the latter was in a ground floor room during a piano lesson. Once, when the family had been on holiday, they found on their return that a collection of ornamental bottles, normally kept in the bathroom, had been thrown and smashed into the bath. The torment finally ended when a service of exorcism was held in the house, and, speaking on the phone to Ruth a moment ago, she assured me that, one year on, the creature has not returned.

CHAPTER 11

A Message In a Bottle

Roy Vincent

This insert has absolutely nothing to do with my book,
but is here to take advantage of the possibility of
wide coverage through the circulation of the book –
To publicise a potential method of
Controlling Malarial Mosquitoes.

To examine an alternative link between the injection of
vaccines and both
Gulf war syndrome and autism.

To publicise the use of Comfrey (Symphytum officinale)
as a means of controlling infant diarrhoea and dehydration
in the developing World –
Comfrey in Africa

If ever you have tried to promote what you yourself consider to be an original thought within the fastnesses of any of the major professions, it is possible that your experiences will mirror mine. There is an invisible intellectual barrier through which the ideas cannot penetrate. It is obvious from the responses, or, more likely the failure to respond at all, that one's proposition has sunk without trace. Any reply beyond the polite acknowledgment reveals a slight amusement similar to the one that I have experienced when trying to float an idea with a certain type of G.P. – humour it and it will go away!

So, in the hope that *someone* will see some merit in my proposals, and that they will at least give them a second thought, then, if feasible, promote them, here goes:

CONTROLLING MOSQUITOES

My starting point with the mosquitoes is the successful campaign that has virtually eradicated fruit flies from American fruit farms. Fruit flies are hatched in captivity and then subjected to gamma radiation, which sterilises the males. When released, the males breed naturally, but are infertile.

Such a method is obviously too impractical to be able to influence the wide-ranging presence of malarial mosquito. My plan is that the males should be sterilised in their own location in the following manner:

Female mosquitoes seek a mate at dusk, and fly to a particular height where they emit a buzz at a frequency peculiar to their own species. Males hover in clouds above the female, and one eventually mates successfully; the female then goes in search of blood and lays her eggs.

It should be possible to fabricate slim unclimbable pylons of, say, carbon fibre, of appropriate height – the height at which the target species hover. The pylon would have at its top a unit that would contain a radioactive source in a shield of suitable design allowing radiation to 'shine' upwards. The unit would generate the female hum at a frequency of the chosen species, and would be turned on automatically at dusk. If the plan works, males would hover above it and be sterilised.

There would be no radiation hazard at ground level, and a full education programme would be needed to enlist local support. Units could be arrayed in batches around villages, or could be on mobile facilities.

When one considers the colossal cost in human suffering, and financially in terms of the loss to local economies and the provision of health care, I would think that *any* idea should be taken forward, no matter how far-fetched it may seem at first.

LISTENING TO THE SILENCES

AUTISM AND GULF-WAR SYNDROME

In considering the second 'big idea', i.e. the possible connection between inoculation and Gulf War Syndrome, and possibly autism, it is necessary to understand a little about acupuncture.

As I describe at various points in my main text, there are many acupuncture points distributed over the total body and head. Any particular point may have a wide repertoire of ailments capable of being treated from that point. The ailments are not specifically local, and can be very diverse in nature. It is well known that if one causes damage at the site of an acupuncture point, one risks provoking the very conditions that one would use that point to treat. Normally one considers the damage caused by physical trauma – fracture, surgery – or similar.

The essence of my speculation is this: does the injection of a noxious substance, i.e. a vaccine, *into* an acupuncture point produce any adverse reaction elsewhere within the body and head?

Most inoculations in adults and in infants above a certain age are given in the arm, and specifically in the deltoid-V. In *exactly* the same place is a point on the so-called 'Large Intestine' meridian, namely Large Intestine 14. In expressing my certainty, I had confirmation of both locations from a Senior Nursing Sister and an acupuncture practitioner of many years experience.

The point does not have a large repertoire listed in the textbooks, and the acupuncturist says that she hardly ever uses it in treatment. However, over the years I have devised ways of self-experimentation, and can confirm that stimulating L.I. 14 may generate unspecific reactions within my head. I had further confirmation of some link when I had my flu injection in autumn 2002. Normally I ask the nurse to inject away from the acupuncture point, but on this occasion I let her proceed as normal, and she hit a bulls eye. Within half an hour I began to develop unpleasant sensations in my head, similar to those at the onset of a severe headache, and on the same side as the injection. These persisted for about 8 hours, when they slowly subsided.

The 'cocktail' of drugs used by the armed forces contains many substances that are foreign to the body's normal functioning, and only serious research will determine whether I have found a 'missing link'. In considering any link with autism, my speculation would only apply to infants who have an arm injection, but, my G.P. informs me, this happens at the age when autism usually shows and so a link such as I am postulating would be difficult to prove. Confirmation of the connection could only be achieved if *all* infants were injected in a neutral location.

LISTENING TO THE SILENCES

COMFREY IN AFRICA

During the nineteen-eighties, I maintained a regular correspondence with a member of the 'White Sisters' religious order (Missionary Sisters of Our Lady of Africa). Marie was in charge of a bush dispensary in Uganda, and was trying to restore its function after the overthrow of Idi Amin, the Ugandan dictator. They were desperately short of money, and at one time she wrote to say that they could not get medicines, even if they could pay for them, could I help? My former employer, British Nuclear Fuels, gave generously of material from the local works' dispensary, as I pondered what I could do myself.

At the time, I was making a personal study of herbal remedies, and had become impressed with the efficacy of comfrey (*symphytum officinale*), particularly as a treatment for a variety of skin conditions and for wound healing. With no further thought, I sent off my existing supply of comfrey ointment, and awaited comments. When they came, I could not have been more delighted. The ointment had been used to treat a large ulcer on the leg of an old man who had walked for three days to reach the dispensary. Marie reckoned that such an ulcer would take upwards of a fortnight to heal using conventional remedies. The ointment was applied on a Friday, and by the following Monday, new pink skin was developing around the ulcer, which then healed rapidly.

With the help of Lawrence Hills of the Henry Doubleday Research Institute, several kilogrammes of ointment were shipped out, as were some seeds that Mr. Lawrence obtained from seedsmen, Thomson and Morgan. The ointment rapidly acquired a reputation as a 'cure all' for skin problems. I also sent a copy of the book *Comfrey*, written by the indefatigable Lawrence Hills. In the book was a photograph of a lady who regularly bought at cattle markets, young calves that were 'scouring' – i.e. had diarrhoea – and which no one else wanted. These she took home, and fed with milk in which she placed chopped comfrey leaves. The scouring soon ceased, and the calves thrived.

One of the Sisters in Uganda saw this, and thought that what cured the calves might also work on African infants. Dehydration following persistent diarrhoea is one of the killers of infants in the developing world. To the delight of the Sisters – who surprisingly found comfrey already growing in their garden - the strategy was successful, and infants began to thrive, where previously they might not have done.

I then lost contact with my White Sister friends, and so I have no way of knowing whether they developed the further use of comfrey, and whether they informed a wider world.

At one time, comfrey became suspect as a potential cause of liver cancer, and has been largely removed from sale for internal use. The 'research' on which this view had been based had involved a high dosage in rats, and was itself suspect. Commenting purely from my own experience, I rate it very highly for all skin ailments, and particularly burns and scalds. I also employ it internally in an appropriate manner, with no harmful effects after twenty-five years intermittent use. Used properly as a medicine and not a *food*, as some were doing, it has high value, particularly in its role as internal vulnary.

And there they are my three 'great ideas', and just like the proverbial message in a bottle that is thrown into the sea, I am hoping that mine will arrive on a 'beach' somewhere, and be opened by someone with a mind like mine – and at least *give it a try*.

Roy Vincent

CHAPTER 12

Still as they run

They look behind,

And hear a voice

In every wind.
Thomas Gray

Roy Vincent

LISTENING TO THE SILENCES

Rocks, rivers and lakes as smooth as glass...

So wrote William Wordsworth, a man completely familiar with Lakeland, this my chosen home for more than fifty years. Travelling south from this house, I come, in turn, to two stretches of water. First, I arrive at the estuary of the Duddon, a river that the poet fished and wrote about. Then, after a short journey, the upper reaches of Morecambe Bay come into view. Both are inlets of the sea and respond to the surges of the tides. At full tide, the expanses of water are extensive, and, if I travel on a sunny day, the sight is spectacular as the sun on the water gleams and sparkles at me when I look down from high points of my route. Low water creates equally stunning views as the sands and mud are exposed, and the water diverts into a multitude of channels, creeks and runnels.

Upon the walls of this room hang two paintings of the Duddon estuary, created by local artists now dead. The smaller is a keepsake given in memory of a friend on her death – a gentle view, done in Jane's unique style. The larger painting, by a man who was 'unique' in a variety of different ways, captures the scene with a wildfowler's eye and brush – a wild waterscape with scudding clouds, and the mud banks and saltings favoured by the wild geese and widgeon in the winter. Both estuaries have been a source of bounty for the hardy gatherers of food in times past. Even today, the sands of Morecambe Bay yield food for sale, and an income for the 'harvesters' of cockles and fluke – the local name for a variety of flatfish.

The saltings and sand look benign and approachable, especially in summer sun, and the maps show the red broken lines of the routes that would lead one from shore to opposite shore. Foolhardy would be the one who ventured out to gather a few cockles or tread for fluke. Reckless would be those who set out to cross the sands guided solely by the red lines on the map. The history of the area lists many who have perished in both types of venture. The summer just ending adds a father and son who were isolated by the sudden descent of a mist and drowned – just a short distance from, and in earshot of the shore, on what had been a bright sunny day.

The greatest source of danger is quicksand. Ever changing, apparent only to the trained eye, the sand first holds and then overwhelms. The cockle gatherers and fluke fishers are experienced and know the signs, although there are numerous records of horses, carts and tractors having been trapped and abandoned. As the numbers of experienced people diminish, their lore will be lost irretrievably. The guide who even yet escorts parties across the Bay sands is old and has no trainee to follow him – his experience of the daily changing conditions is irreplaceable.

At the outset, I linked the quicksand of the shore and the 'quicksand' of the mind, with the dire, lonely peril of the one who is lost in the latter. I offered myself as a guide on the merit of my experience of becoming trapped and nearly overwhelmed, but I am not immortal, and I am training no one. Sometimes I think that I am continuing to write in a vain hope – a hope that my experiences will truly influence the way in which individuals classed as 'schizophrenic' are treated and actually helped to regain control of their minds and lives, and not just to be subdued by mind-altering drugs. In the medicine of the body, many practitioners have encountered personally some of the conditions that they set out to treat. Lucky is the one who, arriving at early adulthood, has not had a variety of infectious illnesses, fractures or sprains. Such is not the case in psychiatry or psychology – essentially the practitioners are theorists, never, except in a small minority of instances, having experienced the mental conditions that they yet feel competent to diagnose and treat.

    As you read my accounts of the various ploys, I would ask you to recollect that I am, or have been, aware of them because I was aware and observant from the very beginning. Not having been made ill by the 'invasion', but, nevertheless, having experienced times of disturbance, I have been sensitive to all that has been worked within me, and have recorded much. As you read, then, I would ask you, further, to try to put yourself in the place of someone visiting his G.P. for the first time. Aware that all is not in control within mind and, or body, and yet not sufficiently articulate to be specific – does he end up with an anti-depressant or tranquilliser just to give the impression that something is being done? Should he return for a second consultation, he might not even see the same G.P. – but, by now, he has some sort of label.

In my own case, a non-nervous illness (*Cryptosporidia* infection) was misdiagnosed as an anxiety ailment, and I began taking Librium. After two years continuous use, an involuntary addict, and exhibiting many of the acknowledged side effects of the drug, I was referred to a Consultant Psychiatrist – who saw me as a 'garrulous hypochondriac' (albeit of above average intelligence!). Changing the Librium to Tryptizol overnight, and giving me 'cold turkey' in the process, my bizarre reactions were put down to an 'idiosyncratic reaction' to the replacement drug, not to the sudden withdrawal of Librium. In his next communication to my G.P., and discussing the hitherto unrecorded reactions, the Consultant writes - "The same quality of description is, alas, also seen in schizophrenic psychoses in this sort of person. I am beginning to lean towards the latter diagnosis although I have nothing definite to confirm it. Meanwhile, hedging my bets, I have put this man on Melleril 25 mgms. T.d.s…" Melleril is an 'anti-psychotic' drug, and has a large and frightening list of side effects, including 'drowsiness, apathy, pallor, nightmares, insomnia, depression, agitation…blurred vision, cardiovascular symptoms (assorted)…' - need I go on?

LISTENING TO THE SILENCES

In the short space of time between 22nd November and the 7th December, I had progressed from having a mis-diagnosed 'anxiety state', to being a suspected 'schizophrenic psychotic'. In spite of that, and with no credible reason given, the Consultant (who admitted in correspondence to "...lacunae in my training...") yet prescribed Nardil – a potent anti-depressant, having the usual range of most undesirable side effects, among which are '...psychotic episodes with hypo-manic behaviour, confusion and hallucinations...'! I will not continue; all of the heart-breaking details are covered in full at the beginning of my opus. I am reprising them here simply to make the point that a person can be made very ill as the result of wild and unstructured interventions. I would make the further point that *no intervention* other than understanding and support may be the best course of action for many who are experiencing non-specific mind disturbance.

It can be comparatively easy to describe the most overtly serious, threatening and obscene intrusions. Far more subtle and insidious – and arguably more effective in disrupting one's life and thought – is the intrusion that itself appears to be an extension of one's own thoughts. I have already written about the ambience that can be created in the moments of first consciousness after waking. Unless one has established a personal 'drill' aimed at excluding any responses that one may be tempted to make in one's mind, it is exceedingly difficult not to respond. The semi-automatic and instant reaction closely resembles the interchange that can take place between couples who have shared their lives for many years. A stage can be reached when it can appear *rude* not to respond in ones thoughts.

This ploy is one that frequently is used at the start of what promises to be a productive day in whatever activities one plans to be engaged. As one begins to address one's mind toward the first task, *they* will put forward a pressing alternative. Then, if that is rejected, another, and another, and so on, inducing a feeling of panic and the thought that nothing will be commenced, the whole lot aborted, and the day completely wasted.

In time, it will be realised that this particular ploy is often used, and used most effectively, when the meteorology is such that a woolly brain is being induced. By 'meteorology', I do not mean wet or dry, hot or cold, windy or still. Instead, I must refer you back to where I wrote about the Föhn wind and the effects that may be induced in sensitive individuals. I wrote that while we in Britain do not have named winds such as the Föhn, Chinook, Santa Ana and the rest, we do have movements of air across the country that can provoke reactions in people similar to those produced by the notorious winds. The property of these winds that is replicated in those that blow across Britain, is the excess of positive ions over the more desirable negative ones.

LISTENING TO THE SILENCES

It is so relevant that one should consider the effects of all winds and other ambient influences that I believe it to be worth repeating the quotation from the book *The Ion Effect* that I included earlier:

"The search for information that led to this book actually began in 1970 as an attempt to prove to myself that I was neither a manic-depressive nor a hypochondriac. For ten years I had lived and worked in Geneva, and almost from the moment I moved there from New York I suffered totally inexplicable fits of anxiety, depression, physical illness, and the kind of bottomless despair that at times even led me to flirt with the idea of suicide. Neither doctors nor a psychiatrist could explain what was happening to me, but when one said vaguely that it might be "something electrical" in the air of Geneva I seized upon it as a possible explanation and spent five years travelling through Europe, the Middle East, and North America meeting scientists and amassing an awesome pile of scientific literature.

I made three discoveries. The first was that in certain places at certain times – in Geneva, in a large part of Central Europe, in southern California, alongside the Rocky Mountains and in at least a dozen other parts of the world – the air becomes sick not because of the pollution we all know about, but because of imbalances in the natural electrical charge of the air…"

In archive material that I obtained from the *Boston Globe* newspaper, I found interesting corroborative comments:

Folklore has the so-called devil winds bringing out crazed behavior among Californians. In her essay collection "Slouching Towards Bethlehem," sixth-generation Californian, Joan Didion, calls the time of the Santa Anas "...the season of suicide and divorce and prickly dread, wherever the wind blows."

While Raymond Chandler wrote: "Meek little wives test the edge of the carving knife and study their husband's throats".

In the main, the winds across Britain do not blow for long periods at a time, certainly for insufficient time for them to acquire a name or a 'character'. It is undoubtedly one of the benefits of our rapidly changing weather pattern of which the majority are unaware. However, because the changes are so frequent, and because there is a lack of awareness about the *quality* of the winds, their effects upon the behaviour and mental health of individuals are largely ignored.

The wind most favoured by the originators of the ploy that I am describing comes as a mild, warm south westerly. It flows from the Azores 'high' and traverses many mid-Atlantic miles. Perhaps the most noticeable effect, and the one frequently remarked upon, is the ability that it has to activate every source of ache or

LISTENING TO THE SILENCES

neuralgia that exists in someone's body. (To anyone who doubts that the weather can induce such effects in people, I must refer to one of the many Websites devoted to weather, and to one that I use that shows a map of North America indicating where it is anticipated that individuals will suffer 'aches and pains'. The forecast is based on the predicted levels of temperature, humidity, wind chill and other factors, and divides the country into areas of anticipated severity.)

In the context of my ploy, it is the second effect that is most exploited by *them*. Unless one has identified the effects and consequence in oneself, it is difficult to envisage them in others. As I mentioned earlier, brains turn to cotton wool, the ability to think coherently vanishes, and a sensitive or vulnerable person is potentially at the 'mercy' of the intruders. Into the mind that is made sluggish, inert or confused by such winds, *they* will introduce a controversial topic, a topic that is skilfully aimed at provoking one into response. Just as stupid and pointless domestic arguments can develop out of nothing, and go on and on with no resolution until one party recognises the futility and waste of time, so can the inner controversy. Looking back at the times when I have been drawn by *them* into such stupidity, I can recognise those occasions when it has happened and when I have been about to make something that requires precise measurement or neat fitting, and acknowledge the frequency of the times that the result has been a cock up. Either material has been wasted, or I have had to waste time in a 'rescue' operation. In both such cases, one can end up feeling exactly the same as I did when I had the 'know all' partner of the second marriage, who always seemed to be about when anything went wrong.

Dramatic images downloaded from NASA satellites have provided me with a wider understanding of the effects created by the next two winds. I have to emphasise that often it is not a 'wind' in the accepted sense, but rather an air movement or gentle breeze. The first of the two also arrives from the southwest, but has a different origin from the previous south-westerly. The drought-ridden regions of North Africa are shown from space, and from them huge dust clouds appear, clouds that then ride the air streams. From the Western Sahara, Morocco and Mauritania the clouds of dust stream out into the Atlantic where they are caught up in an air flow that skirts Iberia and France and floods over Britain. By virtue of its origins, the air has already been deprived of its negative ions, while many of the remainder attach themselves to dust particles and become ineffective.

There are a number of individuals who make regular contact with me and ask my advice about these phenomena. To a person, the comments describing the effects of this wind are the same. No longer are there neuralgic aches, but a feeling inside the head as if someone is trying to restructure it from within. Adding to the confusion that this can cause, eyes become difficult to focus and lose the cleansing effect of blinking, resulting in the effect of looking through a distorting glass. The inability to focus the eyes parallels the inability to focus the mind, a situation that is exploited by *them*. The day is often warm and the air can feel 'electric' as it might do prior to a thunderstorm, effects that are made worse when a person wears clothing that incorporates a high proportion of man-made fibres.

Even further confusion can be caused within locations such as a supermarket by the mass of fluorescent lighting and the electrical fields created by all of the display cabinets. The person who is already plagued by voices and presences can find himself harried and 'jostled' to such a degree that confusion can be piled on confusion and mistakes can be made that may result in accusation of shoplifting.

The air that makes up the third wind also has its origins over North Africa, but this time from the area of Libya. Satellite pictures show vast clouds of dust that delineate the course of the wind as it sweeps across the Mediterranean, over Italy, Greece and the Balkans, swings in a big arc across Central Europe, and arrives over the British Isles from the *southeast*. As this air passes over Austria, Switzerland and South Germany, it becomes the notorious Föhn wind with its destructive powers both to the physical landscape and to the human mind. Even as I write, (15.11.02), the European news bulletins show pictures of huge swathes of trees and mountainside homes, blown down, destroyed by the Föhn that is still blowing. The weather charts for the day illustrate dramatically the exact weather conditions that I am trying to describe. It is, however, the *electrical* properties of the wind that create its well-known and frequently acknowledged qualities. The effects that are created by these characteristics may be observed in Britain by certain sensitive individuals, although the consequences are markedly different between males and females. It would be invidious to identify any particular woman; instead, I will present a conglomerate of all observed behaviour. A loss of a sense of immediate reality is accompanied by a continuous tirade in which all of the partner's alleged defects and misdemeanours are meticulously rehearsed and added to. Depending upon the partner's response, the tirade is often the prelude to a physical attack.

The male might, in the meantime, have a type of headache that has a gnawing, aggravating effect, which may provoke either of two responses. In the first, he may simply endeavour to remove himself – a move that might further infuriate. In the second, he may respond in kind – either verbal or physical, with possibly devastating consequences. This is a situation that *they* seize upon and exploit with immense skill, stoking anger, 'feeding' the words that accompany it, and subliminally encouraging violence. I have noted reports of several spontaneous and seemingly inexplicable domestic killings that, weather wise, appear to fall into this category.

LISTENING TO THE SILENCES

One bizarre sequel to the whole sequence of events is that, assuming no actual physical damage, the female emerges from the conflict with, seemingly, no recollection of the events, or possibly exhibiting a slightly sheepish demeanour. The male, thankful that the storm has passed, usually, and wisely, lets it pass without comment.

In case anyone should suggest that I am presenting a fictional picture, let me assure you that female *animals* also exhibit odd and frequently observed behaviour when such a wind blows. This will be apparent to anyone who has ever kept mares. Mine used to live in a field that I can observe easily from my kitchen. She used to prance stiff legged, back and fore along the eastern boundary of the field, tail arched over her back, snorting and then backing into the wind and behaving exactly as if there was a stallion in the next field and she herself was in season. Quoting the poet Virgil when he wrote "The mares to the rugged rocks repair and with wide nostrils sniff the western air, when, wondrous to relate, the parent Wind, without the stallion propagates the kind" illustrates one of the many primitive beliefs that foals were sired by the wind.

Female animals obviously experience interesting internal frissons. I have never been bold enough to enquire further about those experienced by the human female. Repeating what I wrote above, this behaviour and these reactions are understood and exploited fully by the elements that intrude into the bodies and minds of individuals, often with devastating effects upon the lives and behaviour of the latter. As I have written before, will write again, and will continue to write and declaim, one is dealing with 'beings' of inordinate intelligence, which understand and exploit many aspects of the human condition, for what purpose, one can only guess.

During the normal change of the seasons, the prevailing *courses* of the wind flow move north in the spring and back south in the autumn. These changing times coincide with some observed peaks in the behaviour of individuals with nervous and psychiatric conditions. A colleague obtained for me a graph that plotted psychiatric 'incidents' among a wide population of individuals who were under the charge of 'Care in the Community'. The graph showed two pronounced peaks – one in May-June, and the other in October-November, both of which coincide with the seasonal shifts of the air movements that I noted above. The peaks were also mirrored by those that appeared in a graph that recorded incidents of personal injury, possibly resulting from confusion and resulting accident, although it may be reasonable to suggest that some may have been inflicted by self or others.

Finally - and this really *is* a wind! From the east, emerging from a Scandinavian or Siberian 'high', usually in late February or early March, it arrives in Britain from across many frozen miles. Every drop of water has been frozen out of the air and every available particle of dust has been sucked up from the land. The possibility of any negative ions surviving in such an airflow is minute. More than that, the friction of the air over the frozen ground creates additional positive ions that add to those already present and combine to create a wind that is antagonistic to human mental well-being. My notes record many instances of the reactions of myself and others during these times – my own records showing many comments about the nature of the intrusions that I have experienced, and describing a number of the ploys that I am trying to illustrate. Incidentally, this is a wind that here has a name – possible just local to the area. In Kendal and district particularly, it is known as the 'Helm' wind, and is notorious because of its effect upon people in such ways as I am describing.

I make no apology for dealing at length with these causes and effects. Until there is a greater understanding of the electrical nature of living things and their interaction with their electrical ambience, many triggers of mental ill health will be ignored. Many researchers have recorded a variety of triggers and reactions within the field of body function, but there appears not to be an appreciation and understanding of the need for the body and mind to be treated as an electrical totality, nor of its interaction with its *total* electrical environment. While not specific to my chief concern with the 'schizophrenic', let me consider someone who is manic-depressive. So manic-depressive that she is a 'world expert'. She is a professor of psychiatry in the United States whom I heard in a radio programme, together with her insistence that lithium, lithium, lithium was the only treatment for the condition. Following the broadcast, I obtained and read her book – mainly autobiography.

Spending most of her pre-teen years on the east coast of North America, she did not show any apparent signs of manic-depression until the family moved to Los Angeles, *home of the Santa Ana wind.* She spent one of her undergraduate years in St. Andrews, Scotland, with its robust North Sea climate – where she was not affected. In her immediate post-graduate years, two sabbaticals took her to London and Oxford, where again her problem diminished considerably. She had many desperate years coping with manic-depression and lithium, until her career took her once again to the east coast of the U.S., where her condition improved. Significantly, the life and career of her father disintegrated after the move to California – a career that had taken him to a number of locations worldwide with no apparent harm to his health.

There are aspects of manic-depression in certain individuals that parallel many peoples' conception of 'possession' by intrusive spirits. Harry, the former G.P. who used to stay with me, told me of many of his escapades undertaken when he had been 'manic'. They were so bizarre that they confounded the rational mind – and Harry's mind when *he* was rational. The thought of 'possession' never entered our discussions, but many of his remarks and descriptions unconsciously paraphrased the state. The word was actually used in connection with the behaviour of someone with whom I once had contact. An artist and sculptor, his appearance naked in church wielding a sword at the candles and panicking the congregation, earned him a period of 'sectioned' confinement. It was his partner, a sensitive and perceptive woman, who used the term and speculated about it.

Someone whom I had known for a number of years of struggle with this same distressing condition was a highly intelligent man who was establishing himself most successfully in his career. He had no need financially to shoplift; yet, in one strange aberration, he did and was caught. I am simply speculating, never having discussed the events with him, but it was so out of character that I find it easy to believe that he had been prompted in his mind to behave in that way.

If one stops to analyse the spontaneous behaviour involved in certain events, it is possible to speculate further that many who have no psychiatric problems nevertheless respond to an inexplicable prompting and behave out of character – often with unfortunate results, as happened to two men whom I know.

The first man worked near my house, and every day went home by the same route. Yet, one day, for no reason that he could afterwards identify, he chose an alternative route, met a speeding car on a narrow bend, crashed, was injured, and wrote off his car. The second normally cycled to his work. He is a man who is completely engrossed in what he does, and freely acknowledged that as soon as he got on his bike, his mind went into 'automatic' as he began to think ahead to the tasks that he knew were waiting for him. He rode a cycle with dropped handlebars, and I can just visualise him, head down, engrossed in his thoughts, as he powered along eager to get to work. One morning, for reasons that have since baffled him, he took his son's baseball cap from its hook on the back door and put it on to cycle. Riding along a fast straight stretch as he neared his work, vision limited by the peak of the cap, he suddenly found himself on the back seat of a stationary car, blood pouring from his face and neck, having entered the car through the rear window. The driver, being early for work, had parked and was reading his newspaper. My friend, also, cannot account for the sudden impulse that induced him to take the baseball cap. I have never suggested to him that he might have been prompted in his mind to do so, but, with my own experience of being aware of injections of thoughts into my own mind, I can believe that both men were incited by malevolent external intrusions.

Having arrived inside a car, albeit by an unconventional route, it will be profitable to stay there and analyse some of the simple, yet effective ploys that can be used to influence a driver. If you yourself are a driver, try to recall the instances when, having been driving for some time, suddenly your eyes seem to focus, and you say to yourself 'How did I get here?' Like my friend on his bike, you have been on automatic pilot. One part of your mind has been driving the car while the other has been – where? Only you can know – or perhaps you cannot recall. The mind, or the part of it that is not driving, has been in free-fall, possibly continuing the row that you have left behind at home; possibly ahead, mentally conversing with a difficult customer/boss; possibly – *anywhere*!

The mind in free-fall is easily entered and manipulated, and the isolation of the driver makes the process even easier. The resentment that has been simmering against someone, or possibly over an injustice, is suddenly switched on, and you are in the middle of an aggressive dialogue in your mind, unaware that it is being fuelled and fanned skilfully. Totally engrossed, back on automatic pilot, suddenly around the corner there is a badly parked vehicle, or a driver stupidly overtaking and on your side, or – any one of the possible driving hazards. It is a 'classic' ploy that can be triggered in any one of a number of situations, and not only when driving, and not only by resentment or dispute, for a salacious thought can be introduced just as easily, and stoked with recollections. Then, if you were guilty of doing something ill-judged or stupid yourself, even though there was no accident, a perception can be created around you similar to that that would exist if there was a back-seat driver actually in your car. You may find yourself feeling hangdog, head down, low profile, as the nagging 'ambience' persists around you – and your driving may be affected and erratic.

Remaining with the car and driving, *they* will attempt to build a camaraderie, pretending to be, in my case, my father who taught me to drive. *They* will often insert thoughts and feelings about other road users and their styles of driving, all the time trying to develop reliance upon *them* and *their* opinions or advice. The relationship might develop to such a degree that a subliminal suggestion that it safe, say, to overtake is accepted. Often it *is* safe, but woe betide the one who relies unthinkingly upon this 'advice', for, with guard dropped and not taking normal precautions, the time will come when one has been 'set up', and the inevitable crash happens. Fortunately, I recognised the ploy for what it was before it could become effective, but recognition of this or any other ploy does not confer immunity from attack. There is only one safeguard, and that is constant vigilance.

The same ploy involving the building of confidence in the apparently inspirational source can be used in other situations in which the unwitting can be set up. The gambler can be fed impeccable advice, and, seemingly, every bet can be a winner, until, with confidence at its height and a belief in personal infallibility in place, 'all' is staked on a 'certainty' – and all is lost. Hounded by creditors, life in ruins, persecuted and tormented in the mind, suicide is often presented as the only escape – escape into what, one can only guess.

While one may be congratulating oneself on the recognition and avoidance of a particular ploy, there can 'appear', as at one's elbow, an entirely new character, representing the cynical, 'seen it all before' individual who attempts to build on the mood of self congratulation and tries to develop a fellowship. It is quite easy to fall into this trap and warm to the 'smooth', cynical recognition and association, just as in real life, one may warm to someone who can see through the deviousness of politicians and advertisers, for example. Many of the ploys and their variants are devices by means of which one unconsciously accepts a subliminal 'companion' and in doing so, indirectly, and ultimately completely, loses one's capacity for original thought and self-determination.

Always it is the solitary mind that is easily entered. The solitude does not have to be that of physical isolation. Many are intellectually isolated, but are, nonetheless, working in company with others. Someone whom I know well spends much time welding complex structures. Although he works in a busy workshop, nevertheless, with his welding mask down and his ear-protectors in place, he might as well be on Mars for all of the contact that he has with his mates. I have known him for over twenty years and have had many deep and long conversations with him, and never cease to marvel at the scope and intricacies of his thoughts. At times, I have been struck by the way in which some of the 'exchanges' within his mind when he is isolated resemble those of someone who, if they lost control, would be classed as schizophrenic.

Solitary, isolated, often for many hours at a time, are the artist and sculptor, the author and composer, and the solo performer. Many have acknowledged the existence of a 'muse', without whose presence they are unable to create their best work or even perform at all. (I have already mentioned *The Unknown Guest* by Brian Inglis, a book that explores this phenomenon). Many unconsciously accept the input of the muse into their work without specifically realising that there is an 'other' within their personal equation. The subtle intrusion, accepted and used, but not recognised for what it is, can often become a dominating presence, and eventually take over full control.

Two who owe much to acknowledged spiritual inspiration are Rosemary Brown and John Lill. The former received through direct 'dictation' within her mind, music that was alleged to come from deceased famous composers. A competent pianist, Ms. Brown wrote down music that has been assessed by many others who are experts in the field as being well beyond her undeveloped ability as a composer. I have just been re-reading the sleeve notes of a recording on which she plays music that she has received, allegedly from the specified composers. The sleeve has many comments from

LISTENING TO THE SILENCES

eminent people – performers and musicologists, and from Sir George Trevelyan, a man of acknowledge spirituality and insight who actually sat with her as she received and wrote down music. All recognize her honesty and integrity, while the specialists agree that the music could well pass for that of the designated composer.

I also have a recording of renowned concert pianist John Lill O.B.E., although it is not of his actual playing. My tape is of a broadcast programme in which he freely and lucidly describes his awareness from when he was as young as three – awareness of an inner compulsion to play the piano, and of an innate ability to play with a competence well beyond that of his age. My reason for recording the broadcast – of *Desert Island Discs* – was in expectation that Mr. Lill would describe what happened when he was in Moscow to compete for the Tchaikowsky prize – a prestigious accolade for pianists. His parents were not well off, and he desperately wanted to win in order to help them out of their poverty.

The evening before the competition, and while he was practicing, and in his own words: "The surprising thing was I had a very strong vision…and you could call it a ghost, but it was more real, and it said quite strongly and quite clearly 'You are going to get first prize'. Then I thought 'This has to be. If I *do* succeed and get first prize I shall have to reconsider this' - for it was such a strong material force. That has happened many times in my life, and when I am playing, there are times when I feel inspired – inspired means 'of the spirit' – and I have often seen myself playing from *outside* myself, and feeling disastrously reluctant to go back to that dank earth shell at the end of the concert. That to me is inspiration. It doesn't often happen, but when it does, you never forget."

"I saw a person in old clothing, smiling in a strange way – unmistakably Beethoven. I thought that I was imagining things, for I was working a bit hard at that time. But when the message came across that '…you would absolutely win first prize, and let that be a reminder that we are working through you…', it meant a lot to me…it was very strong thought transfer. The words weren't English, but the meaning of the thought transfer was unmistakable, and one of many I have received before from different sources …and during concerts. It is often the case that I am talked to by other forces…(By other composers?) Yes, and by other people. It is not something unique; it is not just for you. It is like your (Sue Lawley's) own voice now going out over Radio 4 – you can be heard all over the world. It is not geographically confined – it is virtual spiritual help; it is always available; it is always there for all people."

(Inevitably, people will think that it is very mystical…)

"Yes, I have learned that you can't talk about it. It is a very personal, private thing. Although I have been given a great musical gift, my greatest gift is the evidence that I have had that there is no death; that the mind *does* continue; that the spiritual soul *does* carry on. I have learned that it is wrong to talk about it. The only way that I can prove the experiences that I have had is to do better what I have done before."

I would dearly like to be present as a fly on the wall if someone was to tell John Lill that he is deluded, hallucinating. Yet that is what happens to many other individuals, is it not? Not everyone has the standing and prowess of a world-renowned concert pianist. Not everyone is as articulate, nor yet has the understanding that his own personal experiences and convictions allowed him to achieve. Thus if someone describes visions, voices and presences – phenomena that are overwhelming and disturbing to them – what then? Do you recall something that I wrote much earlier? I described how a former parish priest would deliver homilies based upon the experiences of someone, undoubtedly saintly, who had achieved marvels at the behest of voices and visions, and yet how he inevitably concluded with "If any of *us* hear voices, we should consult a psychiatrist". I also described how someone had compared the visions and ecstasies of Teresa of Avila with those described in the diary of an anonymous female schizophrenic. If you can recollect, the descriptions provided by both women were virtually identical. Saint Teresa had the support of a religious community, and had spiritual advisors whom she consulted regularly if she had any doubts about the origins of the 'locutions', as she called them - doubts about whether they came from a desirable or undesirable spiritual source.

Many people accept without question the presence of an inner voice and do not find it disturbing. 'Everyone hears voices', said one friend when I described some of my own experiences. Another friend made an interesting remark after she had joined a prayer group into which I had introduced her. After several visits, she said 'Now I know to whom I have been talking in my mind all my life – it's God', and was delighted at her discovery. Yet another had been aware of voices and visions or presences from the age of three, when she had 'seen' her deceased grandfather. This friend accepted without question, and, apparently without discernment, all that came from 'them'. I remember well an occasion when she stood in front of me and began 'They say...', and went on to describe what 'they' said about my inner state of mind – how my calm exterior supposedly hid an inner turmoil. The assessment was totally incorrect, and in my mind I was formulating words to describe what I thought of 'them' and their opinion, words that were far from complimentary. What surprised me was that 'they' did not appear to pick up this adverse commentary, and she went on at some length undeterred.

This particular friend worked untiringly through a variety of complementary therapies in her endeavours to alleviate suffering.

LISTENING TO THE SILENCES

However, she also gave 'readings' derived from 'them', and, no doubt, by virtue of her intrinsic personal goodness, the content would be accepted by the recipient without question, providing, as I have illustrated before, potentially life-changing influences. I know a number of individuals who 'channel' in addition to giving unstinted help to many people through the therapies that they practice. What alarms me, and especially so in the context of my writing and its attempts to describe the variety of ways in which vulnerable and 'accepting' individuals can be influenced, what alarms me is the way in which channellers appear to accept without question the 'source', the 'guide' and what is fed from them.

        Referring back to my own development and enlightenment: Initially I had been led to believe that I had four attendant named 'guides', until, as I described subsequently, I was shown, and shown without equivocation, that henceforth *all* communication within my mind deriving from desirable sources would be entirely anonymous and not from any named and identifiable 'individual'. Harking back to those naïve beginnings, I cringe at the recollection of my supreme gullibility. Feeling the vibrant presence of 'an other' within me, and imbued with a strong sense of being 'chosen', I gushed out virtually any crap that was fed into my mind. That is now twenty years behind me, twenty years in which I have fought shy of passing on *anything* that has come spontaneously into my mind. In all of that time, there have been at most ten occasions when

I have felt confident enough to tell a person what has come to me, and what seems to be directed to them. Two of the ten stand out in my memory. I have already described how Judith literally thumped me in the back as she urged me to tell her mother that, following her early death, she was now happy within her spiritual environment. On the other occasion, I was inspired with words and a healing touch that went to the core of a mother grieving so desperately for a daughter just in her twenties. Only a few days ago, I came across the letter that the mother subsequently wrote to me, asking me to recall what I had told her and what had so moved and comforted her, a letter that evoked so many poignant, yet happy memories.

The latter occasion was instantaneous and spontaneous. At all other times I have pondered at length before finally speaking. As I gained experience and became aware of what was being attempted within my mind and thoughts, I recorded some of the different ploys. I have already described several: in this particular context, I wrote -

"When composing in my mind what I intend to say to someone, *they* will 'offer' a suitable word where an alternative exists; it is often the most obvious or best choice, but *they* will try to create the impression that it is *their* choice. This can lead to a situation or continuing state in which one becomes reliant on being fed the appropriate word or sequence. If one has not had cause to question the source, but indeed believes it to be 'genuine' and benevolent, one can end up waiting to be 'inspired' and believing that one is a 'chosen channel'. Indeed, when one is writing or speaking, possibly promoting an idea or cause, they will invade the mind and/or body, creating an impression of excitement and implying that one has been 'chosen' to channel words from an 'exalted' source. In the euphoria of believing oneself to be so chosen, it is possible to lose any critical or common sense analysis that one would normally apply, and to let oneself be used solely as a mouthpiece, often destroying one's credibility in the eyes of those whom one is trying to convince."

My brother, as I have mentioned, is an Anglican priest, though now on the point of retiring. He was ordained late in life, but from the time of his late teens, he has preached, and was often in demand in South Wales as a preacher. From the outset, my brother has always acknowledged that much that came into his mind at those times was by inspiration, but always knew that he, himself, had the ultimate power of censorship over what actually issued from his mouth. As I have mentioned before, but it is worth repeating, he has always had a dedicated prayer life, and recognised that many times, as he settled to his private prayer or approached the moment of consecration in the Eucharist, his body was entered physically and spiritually – if that does not appear to be a contradiction. Always my brother's mental response has been the same – "If you are from God, you are welcome. If not, please go".

For some time many people have chosen to reject traditional medicine and to enter the expanding world of complementary therapies. Concurrently countless others have moved away from the spirituality of traditional and mainstream churches and sought an alternative spiritual focus in their lives. Many of the latter believe that their own 'hot line' to the world of spirit supersedes the seemingly outdated and sterile one of 'religion', and they are drawn into the world of 'channelling'. They might even buy a book that I found advertised on the Web:

"CHANNELLING - What it is & how to do it"
by *Lita de Alberdi*

Lita de Alberdi is a gifted spiritual teacher who has taught hundreds of people in the UK to channel their guides. In this accessible and practical book she explains how to contact and channel your own spirit guide.

In this book, Lita includes channelled material from her guides and answers the many questions that people ask.
If you want to learn to channel successfully and safely and if you want to learn from an experienced channel and teacher, this is the book for you.
Full of easy to follow meditations and exercises based on her successful courses. Channelling will enable you to:

LISTENING TO THE SILENCES

- Shift your awareness to an expanded state of consciousness.
- Work with guides and angels. Use psychic protection effectively.
- Channel to receive help with health and past life issues.
- Conduct channelled readings. Enhance your confidence and creativity.

As with the hypnotherapy advertisement that I quoted earlier, there is no personal contact between the teacher and pupil. Always, I am concerned with the vulnerable. Having read about and practiced such techniques, and no doubt willingly accepting the desired contact within the mind, the aspirant is wide open to mental intrusion from any source. The blurb promises instruction in how to "use psychic protection effectively". I squirm inside as I read, and think to myself... "How can authors be so insensitive to the dangers that they are creating for readers, and how can readers be so gullible as to believe that they can somehow weave 'psychic protection' around themselves". As I have noted several times, all of the main religions have well tried and tested systems of induction of the novice. All are aware of the dangers that threaten the 'opened' mind, and all have experienced novice masters to give guidance and support. There is none of this in the 'do-it-yourself' readily available book or weekend 'workshop'.

By today's post, I received my regular update of a catalogue of books on a variety of alternative and complementary practices and life-styles. Glancing through it, I responded as I usually do – with a sense of wonder that so many books can be written about so many techniques and practices and beliefs. In the various categories there are numerous volumes of introduction or instruction covering virtually every form of 'divination' that one can think of – I Ching, Tarot, dowsing in its varied forms, to name but three. It is also possible from the same catalogue to buy, for example, a set of Celtic Wisdom Sticks '…a powerful divination tool drawing on the ancient memory and wisdom of the trees and the Celts…Further advice is given for phrasing questions to the Oracle and interpreting the responses given…'

Many individuals will, probably light heartedly, have tried such devices as an ouija board or planchette, and moved on equally light heartedly. Some, and often the most open and vulnerable individuals, will have been influenced, become 'hooked', - and even disturbed. I reflect how easily I became so obsessed with the contacts that I was making by using a pendulum and alphabet chart. I began so innocently and naïvely, not seeking 'divination', and initiated a most dramatic change in my life – a change that subsequently has influenced more than twenty years of it, and now ties me to my computer to write this, and, hopefully, warn others of the inherent dangers.

Responding to the ever increasing demand for alternative and complementary therapies and therapists, the catalogue reveals the extent to which the demand may be met – at least, through the medium of 'how to do it' books. One therapy that, more than others, has come to the fore in recent years is Reiki. Of itself and originally described by its modern founder, Dr. Usui, reiki is a simple and effective therapy, differing very little in practice from other forms of natural 'hand-healing', touch therapy. The chief difference lies in the 'atunements' that a potential practitioner undergoes, and in the acquisition of 'symbols' and 'mantras', leading the aspirant into a world of mysticism and contact with 'others' – so-called Ascended Masters and the like. It is possible for someone who is prepared to spend £260 and two days, to become a certificated Reiki practitioner, and for a further £290 and two days, to become a Reiki Master. With this 'training' and possibly little actual experience, it is now open to the Master to 'train' more aspirants, provide them with mantras and atunements, and links to Ascended Masters.

I am not seeking in any way to deride the dedication and desire to heal of many practitioners. What I am seeking to illustrate is yet another route along which vulnerable individuals can be 'entered' by intruding and unwelcome 'entities'. The whole process of their Reiki induction is aimed at an opening up to – to what? Information that I receive describes courses that, ultimately, lead to "…channelled and psychic and spiritual techniques. Communicate with spirit guides, learn astral travel, clairvoyance, psychometry, how to see auras…". Nowhere in the literature or course descriptions can I find any reference to the possibility of any adverse psychic experiences occurring. Undoubtedly, many who participate in these and similar courses, whether as aspirant or instructor, are completely unaware of these possibilities

There is a danger that by continually listing and describing some of the hazards and pitfalls that may be encountered in a variety of practices and life-styles, I may be overshadowing many of the *benign* activities of the limitless, desirable spiritual sources. As I have written in earlier sections, I have had considerable help and received much enlightenment "…and got great knowledge and courtesy from dead kinsmen and kinswomen, ancestors and friends". Even though I repeat myself, in the main these interventions are and have been anonymous – for which small mercy I am infinitely glad. Always I have resented unsolicited intervention or comment, and so the thought of 'Grandad' overseeing me and making comments would be more than I could tolerate!

Not always anonymous, though. I once had a friend who was a long time a-dying from an inoperable brain tumour. David was nursed at home until that became impracticable. As time went on, he became obsessed with imagined problems involving his catheter. Many times during a visit, he would disappear beneath the bedclothes to check its function, and had an array of tissues that he named 'dabber, mopper and wiper'. On the day of his funeral, I arrived early at the crematorium and sat looking at the burnished brass 'catafalque' that awaited his coffin. It appearance made me think of some ancient priestly altar, and as I sat musing, I distinctly 'heard' David's unmistakable voice in my head, saying portentously "O Ra, O Osiris!", and chuckling. Then, as I made sure my handkerchief was easily accessible to staunch the inevitable moisture in the eye, again I heard his distinctive voice say, "Have you got your dabber, mopper and wiper?" And finally, as the coffin came in – "Have you got the regulation lump in the throat?" Then there was Val, who had been my secretary at work and who was also a very good friend. Val's spine had become twisted as the result of illness in her youth, and one day, while turning her head to see to reverse her car, she had blocked the blood flow to her brain and died. Someone else who died too soon in a seemingly unjust world. Val also had a distinctive and unmistakeable voice, and a few days after her death, as I was shaving, I 'heard' it saying – "Can't catch me, I'm a bumble bee!" – and no doubt revelling in the untrammelled freedom after release from her twisted body.

I have already told how I rolled about laughing at the comment that accompanied my efforts to drain a hot water cylinder. Recalling the incident acknowledges the fact that droll comments can be made in the mind that are so apposite that one is bound to laugh. Recently I rode my bike, and on the outward journey went easily down a long and gentle slope. On the return, however, the slope no longer seemed gentle – long, yes, but not gentle – and I carry excess weight! As I put increasing effort into my pedals, I heard a friendly voice in my head saying, "You need a banker". The meaning was immediate, and I laughed as much as my breathless state allowed. But only meaningful if one knew a little railway history. In the days of steam, express trains from London to Glasgow used to stop at Tebay, at the approach to the notorious Shap hill, in order to connect a 'banker' – a supplementary engine to assist the train up the bank. And yes, I needed a banker!

Again, very recently, I searched the Web for an obscure CD that I could not find at my usual suppliers. It was probably my first attempt at an on-line purchase, and seemed to go very smoothly. As I put away my credit card, I reviewed in my mind the skill with which I had negotiated the various hurdles, and was congratulating myself, when I distinctly 'heard' in my mind just one word – "Cool": but 'said' with all of the savvy of the culture of today.

Constantly, as I write, I am aware of the ultimate purpose of my writing, although, as I weave through the convolutions of my story, it would be very easy to lose sight of the goal. I am reasonably content with the way in which I have covered the first part. This has been to create an understanding, with all of the writing skills that I possess, that the intrusions that create the voices

LISTENING TO THE SILENCES

and other phenomena within the bodies and minds of individuals are of spiritual origin. My greatest difficulty is with my current task – namely the 'how to do it' bit. How to avoid attracting the intrusions in the first place: how to recognise them for what they are: how to cope with them when they are active: how, ultimately, to eliminate them.

There are times, as at this moment, when I feel as must an expert rock climber who is engaged in trying to write a manual of rock climbing. He can write and describe all of the skills and preparations that a climber will need. He can describe hand-holds and belays and such, and can even provide minute detail of 'classical' routes up well-known pitches. What he cannot do, however, is to *climb* on anyone's behalf. The novice climber can read and read, and mentally picture individual situations, but the reality is on the rock face. Success or failure will depend upon so many factors, the range of which I shall leave to your own imagination. I have described earlier how, in my teens, I read avidly anything that I could find about small boat sailing, and how, when I finally took the helm of a boat, I recognised every factor and effect about which I had read. My reading and study did not, even so, prevent me shortly afterwards from allowing a dinghy to capsize because of not observing a fundamental precaution.

In writing for the person who is disturbed and whose life is out of control, however, I am conscious of the fact that such a person cannot tackle the rock face of their life alone. The novice climber is roped securely to someone who leads, fixes pitons and belays, and always secures the rope. Who will lead and secure for the disturbed individual who cannot go it alone? 'Individual' is a most appropriate word. No two climbers are alike. Height and reach, weight and its distribution, size of foot even – all, either alone or in combination, define the unique person on the rock face. Within small limits, the rock is the same for everyone and predictable.

Would that there was some degree of stability and predictability in the world of the voice hearer and the way each, he or she, is understood and helped. To continue the climbing analogy, it is as if each has to begin climbing from scratch, with no training and with no foreknowledge of *where* to climb, and to climb in shackles and loaded with extra weights. The shackles are the drugs that suppress and subdue someone's natural abilities and resources. The extra weights are all of the preconceptions that exist in the world of psychiatry and psychology. Physical illnesses have recognisable and measurable symptoms and, within reason, predictable outcomes. Temperatures and pulses can be checked, bowel movements studied, breathing deficits analysed and blood pressure taken. In all probability, the physician and medical staff will have experienced various forms of physical illness themselves and will have a degree of understanding. How many workers in psychiatry can say "I have experienced such-and-such, and can understand and sympathise with you in what you are going through". How many?

Within the last week, I have listened to radio programmes devoted to the phenomenon of synaesthesia. "Synaesthesia is an extraordinary condition in which the five senses mingle. (The programme)...discovers how it is changing our understanding of neuroscience and explores the world of synaesthetes who experience flavoured words or coloured letters, or see music as patterns and colours." As the programmes unfolded, I listened with growing surprise as speakers described what they saw or tasted in response to the various stimuli. The one, for example, who told of her problems when young and learning to write. She could not form the letter 'R'; then realised that it was simply a 'P' with an added stroke. As she added her stroke to her P, the colour of the letter changed to what has since become her 'R' colour, entirely different from her 'P' colour. Or the one, an artist, who would lie back and listen to music, and from the colours and patterns forming in her minds eye, she would compose her abstract paintings, which were much sought after.

There were numerous contributions to the programmes from psychologists and psychiatrists. None had experienced the phenomena themselves, neither could they offer any positive explanation of how they occurred. All believed that the descriptions given by the synaesthetes were real as the latter saw them, and all were excited at what a coherent study might reveal in the future concerning unknown reactions and responses in the human brain. I repeat: to a person, the psychologists and psychiatrists said "I have not experienced the phenomenon: I do not doubt what you are telling me: I do not know the cause."

If only – *if only* - psychiatrists would have the courage to say those same words to the individuals who experience inner voices and other unseen phenomena! Whereas the synaesthetes were engaged in lively discussion and their descriptions of their experiences listened to intently, voice hearers are told that they are deluded and hallucinating, and no one engages them in a discussion of equals with the intention of actually finding out what is in reality happening to them. That has already been decided; it only remains to decide which drug or drugs will suppress the voices and render the individual 'manageable'.

'How to avoid attracting intruders in the first place', I wrote a few paragraphs ago. Apart from realising and acknowledging that the 'intruders' really do exist, what do you actually *tell* a young person? Most of today's Western young would probably laugh uncontrollably if they heard the word 'restraint' mentioned. 'Square', 'uncool' are two of the milder epithets that would be used. One has only to witness the way in which young people who choose to remain virgin before marriage are regarded to realise that they are considered to be some sorts of freak. From their earliest years at school, youngsters are warned and counselled on the subject of illegal drugs, to such an extent that not one of them should have reached their teens ignorant of the dangers to health and the problems of addiction. Today, (24.11.2002), a report has been issued that states that in the last three years amongst 14 – 15 year olds, cannabis use by boys has increased from 19% to 29%, and by girls, from 7% to 25%. Of all drugs, the teenagers believe, cannabis is the least harmful, and less harmful than tobacco.

"Cannabis is the least harmful". It is unlikely that the young will read or care about a report in the British Medical Journal of three days ago. "Early use of cannabis can lead to schizophrenia and depression", is the bald summary. The report analyses three papers, a short extract of which follows:

The increase in use is of concern because cannabis may be a gateway to other drugs, and it may cause psychiatric illnesses. The link between cannabis and psychosis is well established, and recent studies have found a link between use of marijuana and depression. Does cannabis cause these conditions, or do patients use cannabis to relieve their distress?

The explanation most accepted is that cannabis triggers the onset or relapse of schizophrenia in predisposed people and also exacerbates the symptoms generally. Establishing direction of causality is difficult and is most appropriately assessed in non-clinical samples, but a low incidence of the illness and the fact that most drug users take other drugs in addition to cannabis create methodological problems and explain the dearth of reliable evidence.

The study often quoted in support of the causal hypothesis examined the incidence of schizophrenia in more than 50 000 Swedish conscripts followed up for 15 years. It showed that use of marijuana during adolescence increased the risk of schizophrenia in a dose-response relation. Questions have, however, remained about the validity of the diagnosis, the possible causal role of other drugs, and prodromal symptoms of schizophrenia that might have led to the use of cannabis, rather than cannabis triggering the psychosis.

A longer follow up and reanalysis of this cohort published in this issue confirms the earlier findings and clarifies that cannabis, and not other drugs, is associated with later schizophrenia and that this is not explained by prodromal symptoms. In a similar vein, a three year follow up of a Dutch cohort of 4045 people free of psychosis and 59 with a baseline diagnosis of psychotic disorder showed a strong association between use of cannabis and psychosis. Length of exposure to use of cannabis predicted the severity of the psychosis, which likewise was not explained by use of other drugs. Participants who showed psychotic symptoms at baseline and used cannabis had a worse outcome, which also implies an additive effect. In a New Zealand cohort, individuals who had used cannabis three times or more by age 15 or 18 were not more likely to have schizophreniform disorder at age 26, although they showed an increase in "schizophrenia symptoms" (but not schizophrenia). The meaning of "schizophrenia symptoms" requires clarification to interpret these results.

LISTENING TO THE SILENCES

Earlier in my writing I made a facetious reference to the "longitudinal study of 50,000 Swedish conscripts, and 2,000 neurotic soldiers". Imagine my surprise when I saw that they have surfaced in one of the papers cited, having been followed for 15 years of further study. As I read, I reflect upon the task that I have set myself, and the constant uphill struggle and intense frustration. Knowing, as I do, that what is called 'schizophrenia' results from the intrusion of spiritual entities, and knowing, as most intelligent people know, that cannabis, mescaline and similar hypnotics are used by such as shamans and other 'ecstatics' to induce a suitable condition for the entry of the controlling spirit or spirits - is the result of the use of cannabis not obvious?

The shaman is born to his role... he does not become a shaman simply by willing it, for it is not the shaman who summons up the spirits, but they, the supernatural beings, who choose him. They call him before his birth. At the age of adolescence, usually at the period of sexual ripening, the chosen one suddenly falls into hysterics with faintings, visions, and similar symptoms, being tortured sometimes for weeks. Then, in a vision or a dream, the spirit who has chosen him appears and announces his being chosen. This call is necessary for the shaman to acquire his powers. The spirit who has chosen him first lavishes the unwilling shaman-to-be with all sorts of promises and, if he does not win his consent, goes on to torment him. This so-called shaman illness will anguish him for months, perhaps for years, as long as he does not accept the shaman profession.

The Encyclopaedia Britannica from which that is taken does not qualify the entry in any way that throws doubt on the intrinsic belief that the shaman and 'medicine' man or woman is controlled by, and is the mouthpiece of, a spiritual entity. The fact that the same beliefs are held world wide – from Oceania to Siberia to North America and beyond – should say something to the sceptic. Part of my frustration lies in the seeming inability of researchers in the field of mental health to make the connection and accept the link between the mind opening properties of the drugs and the subsequent intrusions.

I doubt very much whether anyone seeking the effects of cannabis includes amongst the desirable 'benefits' the ability to communicate with spirits, nevertheless, the door to intrusion is wide, wide open. I doubt whether many of today's young think about the consequences of drug taking, or *any* of their actions. The dramatic increases in the prevalence of sexually transmitted diseases in the young, and in the numbers of teenage pregnancies, are indicators from another field of activity where the pursuit of instant gratification, or 'peer pressure', are the driving forces. Among many there appears to be a total contempt for their body and mind. The only purpose for having them seems to be as vehicles for hedonistic 'pleasure'. Every source of substance abuse is used, every means and orifice for sexual abuse is used, and every available surface is tattooed and pierced, while the delicate brain is subjected to loud and violent forms of head-banging 'music' and movement.

"...the human body is vapour materialised by sunshine mixed with the life of the stars" wrote my much admired Paracelsus. Fanciful, I know, but surely a more inspirational way of looking at this ultimate product of evolution than the vacant shell that is many a human life. "The body is the temple of the spirit", declares many a religious text. Unfortunately, I have learned to recognise that this is an area of thought into which many are reluctant to go. Apart from an instinctive shying away from anything with a 'religious', 'spiritual' tag attached, it is an area where interpretations are as numerous as the interpreters, and words and concepts acquire meanings that depend more upon the origins and experiences of the interpreter than those that derive from dictionaries and documentary sources.

With reason did Humpty Dumpty say, "When I use a word, it means exactly what I want it to mean, no more, no less". I thought of Humpty when I read part of the report quoted above:

"...In a New Zealand cohort, individuals who had used cannabis three times or more by age 15 or 18 were not more likely to have schizophreniform disorder at age 26, although they showed an increase in "schizophrenia symptoms" (but not schizophrenia). The meaning of "schizophrenia symptoms" requires clarification to interpret these results."

The report queries the exact meaning of 'schizophrenia symptoms'; I would add 'schizophreniform disorder'. Just as it is not possible to be 'just a little bit pregnant', so one is hearing voices or not hearing them; experiencing physical intrusion or not, and so on. Earlier in my writing, I quoted from a radio discussion on schizophrenia that I had recorded, and how the definition might vary depending upon from which side of the Atlantic it came. Surely, when the mind and sanity of individuals are at risk, the necessity of precise definition must be paramount. Yesterday I watched EuroNews and a report showing from the air extensive floods over Italy. The woman presenter made me sit up when I heard her say "The floodwaters are spreading mayhem over Northern Italy". 'Mayhem' is used frequently in a variety of contexts, and I decided to find out from the dictionary exactly what it means. Imagine my surprise when I read, "The crime of maiming someone to prevent them being able to defend themselves" – and figuratively. I have just asked the genii within the computer for synonyms of 'mayhem', and was fed the following: chaos, disorder, confusion, turmoil, havoc, pandemonium, bedlam, and anarchy. I will not even begin to try to disentangle the linguistic twists that have so changed and distorted the original meaning of 'mayhem', just as it would be impossible to follow the sequence of changes that have, for example,

LISTENING TO THE SILENCES

transformed 'Alzheimer's disease' from its original definition of 'pre-senile dementia', to just about any form of senility that besets an *old* person, and which would, in the past, simply have been called 'senile dementia'.

Throughout I have tried to be precise and specific in an imprecise and non-specific region of thought and activity. Only *I* have experienced the events and incidents about which I am writing: the moment and action of my initial 'intrusion' are as clear to me and as potent at this moment as they were initially - now more than twenty years ago. Twenty years in which I have experienced and recorded all of the 'first rank' symptoms of schizophrenia – yet I am not, nor ever have been ill: I am not 'schizophrenic'. I wrote that just to remind myself where I have come from, and to remind you of my status. Constantly I am aware of intrusive presence and the subtleties of potential influence, but only aware of them because I have 'grown up' with them.

While my initial event was obvious and, in its way, dramatic, many initial intrusions may be so subtle as to be unobserved, and to be exerting influence before influence is even noticed or becomes commanding and dominating. Increasingly we are informed of the way in which the Internet is being used by paedophiles to 'groom' unsuspecting youngsters. Unwittingly the latter are gulled into believing that they are chatting on line to someone who is just what he says he is – young, possibly interesting and amusing, maybe a bit provocative or cheeky – all the time just edging towards sexual innuendo and excitement and the potential meeting and what may follow.

No matter by what route or mechanism the voice intrusion into the mind may arrive, it can be accomplished so subtly that it may seem always to have been there. The gentle sharing of thoughts and opinions as with a constant companion may become as natural as breathing. With this in mind, I wrote the following:

'*They* maintain a constant delivery of good, impeccable advice and an ambience of support, which, at first, is comforting. However, it persists into every act, or thought of an act or plan, to a degree that it becomes obsessive, by which time one can have reached a state of dependence and find difficulty in detaching oneself. But more than that, this can constitute a form of 'jamming' which can cause one to reject the desirable counsel that may come from a good source.'

Always, I return to the concept of 'ambience', and seemingly have come full circle, in that I began my sequence of 'ploys' with the silent creation of moods, influences and ambience. Unique to the person at the centre of the experience, it is the most difficult concept to describe, and, as I set out originally with reference to a former marriage, only really explicable by analogy. Over recent weeks, I have felt undermined and depleted as the result of natural phenomena that are currently in train. I am reassured by the fact that numerous comments and queries from friends show that others are equally affected. One result that is relevant is that I have been experiencing difficulty in collecting my thoughts sufficiently to make them coherent and continue my writing. My own natural frustration has been compounded by the creation around me of an unspoken 'atmosphere' such as I might have experienced within that former and unlamented marriage.

My personal frustration is supplemented by the feeling of physical inertia that is often a feature of life in November. The arrival within of the desire to begin 'comfort eating', and one's own commitment to resist it, provide even more openings through which the intruders can work. Nothing has to be said – the unspoken comment or anticipation of – what? Nothing is specific, but there is sufficient going on to induce the hunched 'if I keep my head down it will go away' posture. The fact that such a reaction reduces even further the ability to concentrate compounds the frustration, and many an hour, or even day, is lost in futile attempts to get something, *anything*, achieved.

Once again I have found it necessary to return to 'natural phenomena'. To those who have never experienced the effects that I describe, I might equally be trying to describe central heating to a Bedouin tent dweller in the Sahara. Much earlier, I quoted Paracelsus when he wrote "…a doctor must seek out old wives, gypsies, sorcerers, wandering tribes...and take lessons from them". Any suggestion that people may be influenced by the presence or phase of the moon is usually, and with contempt, dismissed as an 'old wives' tale. Think again, O ye scoffers! Ask yourselves why mammals have a circadian rhythm of 25 hours. If isolated from any perception of day and night, the sleep/wake cycle of mammals becomes 25 and not 24 hours. The one natural timepiece of planet earth that has a cycle of approximately 25 hours is the moon. The passage of the moon determines the rise and fall of the tides. When the mammalian 'body clock' was set ticking, the mammal was, in fact, a fish, for which creature the *tides*, and hence the moon, are of greater importance than daylight and darkness.

To those who may dispute my analysis by saying that *birds* by contrast, have a circadian rhythm of 23 hours, I suggest that the body clock of birds began its function when the earth had a faster speed of rotation, and when the length of day was, in fact, 23 hours. As the life of birds depends upon the presence of light in order to look for food, their daily cycle must inevitably be that of visible daylight and of darkness. The evolution of fish into mammal, and the gradual slowing down of the earth, have happened over such long periods of time that there has never been one significant moment when a step-change in the circadian timing could feasibly have occurred, and so daily we and the birds reset our inner workings to our respective ways of responding to the current *daily* cycle. *But the moon is still there.*

Those who dismiss the potential influence of the moon and also of other planets as old wives tales, are abandoning a whole realm of knowledge, albeit one that has not been studied systematically by people with open minds. I do not subscribe to astrology in any way, and regard the 'predictions' derived from the 'stars' with as much enthusiasm as I would those derived from an examination of the inside of a chicken, the flight of birds, or the shape of a piece of candle wax that had been dropped molten into a bowl of water. I arrived at a realisation that there *are* such influences pragmatically and from first-hand experience.

Other than making my home in a tent, I could not dwell closer to the living earth than I do. My house is constructed of the natural granite boulders that have come from my immediate neighbourhood and which can be seen in the many dry-stone walls nearby. In fact, the construction of the house walls is similar, only more precisely built; over two feet thick and rendered or plastered inside and out. The boulders – or, locally, 'cobbles' – rest without foundation upon fifteen feet depth of clay, the result of outflowings from the glaciers with which the area was once covered. Looking south now I can see, just two miles away, the mountain that was once a volcano, while on some occasions, when I take water from my deep borehole, I see traces of iron that was mined just half a field away in a primitive manner by long dead miners. Free from industrial, noise and light pollution, I have become finely tuned to my environment and to its subtle changes.

I did not choose to live here with any 'back to nature' motive in mind. As I have related, I bought the property over thirty years ago because I kept horses and was fed up having to rent land and buy in hay. Having lived here for so long, and being free from all of the influences and stresses of an urban environment, I have become finely tuned to subtle variations in the 'ambience'. Nevertheless, I did not set out to analyse myself, or compare myself with dwellers in polluted and less tranquil locations, nor do I sit navel-gazing and speculating 'about life, the universe and everything'. I simply observe, record and analyse, and try to relate feelings, reactions, mood shifts in myself and in others to *anything* that at the time may have had an influence.

I do not intend to describe in great detail the manner in which I first became aware of the influence of the moon, other than to say, as I did in an earlier chapter, that, having begun to wear vari-focal glasses, I became conscious of the fact that from time to time I became irritated by them, and by the frequent need to keep readjusting them on my nose. After about six months of this, I began to realise that the irritation coincided with the new and full moon. People are often express surprise when I mention the new moon, commenting 'but it's so *small*', and forgetting that the moon is there in its entirety, but

LISTENING TO THE SILENCES

that only a little of it is *visible*. There is another factor that determines the apparent location and size of the moon, and that is the tilt of the earth on its axis. In mid-winter the moon is almost overhead when full, and appears very large in the sky, while the new moon is low and seemingly insignificant. Conversely, in mid-summer it is the *new* moon that is almost overhead, while the full moon is low in the sky. However, because the new moon is not visible when it is at its most potent, i.e. midday, its presence and effect are never considered amongst the influences that may contribute to the behaviour of a person.

For almost twenty years I have obtained copies of the ephemerides of the moon and other planets in order to keep track of them. I am principally interested in what is called the 'transit time' – i.e. the time when the planet is at local south. (I also use what I call the back transit to refer to the point when the object is due north). I include all the planets, for in time I began to realise that alone or in combination they all appear to exert an influence.

Now I come to the bit where I have to describe central heating to a desert tent-dweller! First, let us observe others. Television provides innumerable opportunities for studying human behaviour when the subjects are not aware that they *are* being studied. At times, I like to watch snooker, indoor bowls and, less frequently, tennis - games in which the participants are functioning as individuals and not as part of a team. When one has seen players in action over a number of years, it is possible to acquire a knowledge of their game and mannerisms. I can think of one very well known snooker player who seems to be particularly affected, whose game will fall off for several frames, during which, and when sitting out, he may be seen massaging his forehead between the eyes, and looking ill at ease. Looking at my tables is almost unnecessary, for at that time I realise that I, also, have an imprecise 'discomfort' in my head – not a headache, but an unquantifiable unease, almost as if attempts are being made to restructure the head from inside.

In all probability, the tables will reveal that there is coincidentally a transit of the moon, possibly in conjunction with other near or major planets. There is a further probability that I will get a phone call from one of my 'controls', asking me what, if anything, is happening. With indoor bowls, there are often two or three scrappy ends when both players have gone off the boil and, again, it will usually be found that they could be responding to an external influence that is disturbing their concentration and judgement. These and similar events have occurred far too many times for them to be the result of coincidence, and as they are not happening to me but to the players, there can be nothing subjective about my observations.

There is nothing subjective about dying, nor about the actual time of dying. Several years ago, and using the obituary columns of the Daily Telegraph, I plotted on a year-long graph the number of deaths on each day. It soon became apparent, even before the year had ended, that the numbers peaked at the new and full moon, with higher peaks if the moon should happen to transit simultaneously with one or more of the nearer planets. What was even more remarkable was that of the deaths reported as 'sudden', more died at these times than at others. Listening also to reports on radio or television of the deaths of well-known individuals, likewise it will often be found that the death happened at these key times. The bodily stresses experienced, and however they are caused, appear to determine the actual time of release, especially after a long illness. Someone whom I knew died at such a very strong conjunction, and in the hospital the staff remarked that they had never known so many deaths in such a short time.

On one occasion that I remember, and just after a major grouping of planets, I rang a friend who is a night nursing sister on a ward that is close to a cardiology ward. She told me that while her ward had been comparatively normal, the ambulances were busy all night attending the other. Someone else with whom I am in regular conversation works in a major psychiatric hospital and, as much as protocol allows, she is able to tell me of the ups and downs of admissions and 'incidents', and nearly always tells of significant increases. The psychiatric hospitals appear to have abandoned the practice once used at Bedlam Hospital, of beating inmates for a week before full moon just to 'compose' them. Although on reflection, the beating probably had a shorter lasting and less damaging effect than E.C.T. does!

I have mentioned above how the head can feel 'as if it is being restructured from within'. Random effects within the body having no apparent cause can also become noticeable. The busy person with a full life to get on with will probably work through such events with help from a suitable analgesic, and as the events are transient, they will hardly merit a comment. For the person already troubled in the mind and already experiencing inner voices, there is a different story. At such times, it is possible that the tormentors will assert that *they* are the cause of the physical distress, and that the effects are part of a process of the destruction of the brain, and even of the creation of cancers over which they have control.

Many of the moon-induced effects are created around midnight and shortly afterwards, say, until 3 a.m., when often waking is frequent anyway, and the mind is a racetrack for worrying and alarming thoughts. There are occasions when sudden awakening so early in sleep is accompanied by a form of paralysis, when the body will not obey the mind. At such times, the half awake mind and the unresponsive body may be exposed to even greater torment. These are often times when the tales of incubus and succubus arise.

Whatever tales and myths are attached, the physical influences of the moon and close planets are real. I have no means of determining how the effects are produced. I can only speculate on the possibilities of changes in gravity induced by the pull on the Earth of the other planets, and potential changes in the electrical and magnetic ambience that their proximity might induce. My difficulties in describing and quantifying cause and effect are magnified manyfold by the fact that each individual person is just that, individual and unique, and that the range of effects created by the external influences is wide, but also unique to a particular time and location. One can only deal in generalities. But do not let that stifle understanding and prevent research, for in so far as *I* am having great difficulty describing these phenomena and reactions, how very much greater are the problems of a disturbed person trying to describe something that is intangible and ephemeral?

I am not generally given to making predictions, but in this field I do. Frequently I assess the locations of the planets from their ephemerides stored on the computer, and note their respective transit times. If from this information I see that a major conjunction is impending, and I believe that certain individuals will be affected, I send out a warning, giving days and times. Feedback that I receive tells me that my forewarning is usually correct and appreciated. I have a good friend whose former partner was grossly affected, especially if the planet Mars was involved. I used to send him a 'hard hat' warning, for his partner frequently became violent.

Is it not curious that the Romans named that planet after their god of war? Not, as is commonly supposed, because the planet is red, for in parts of the world where red is *not* associated with war, the name used is often that of the local god of war, pestilence, famine, disaster, death and terror. The Greeks even went so far as to name the two satellites of Mars, Phobos and Deimos – Fear and Terror. The reason for the naming can be deduced from an examination of Mars' behaviour. It has an eccentric orbit, which can greatly increase or reduce its distance from the Earth (56 > 400 million kilometres). The close approach to Earth is called the perihelion. From time to time, the perihelion and the opposition of Mars coincide. This means that the planet is at its nearest to Earth, but is also on the side of the Earth away from the sun. At such a time, not only is Mars at its closest, but also is at its most visible. It is comparatively huge in the night sky, and its presence is obvious.

For whatever reason, people are disturbed by the physical proximity of Mars. They are disturbed as individuals and as groups and nations. Disturbed individuals, governments and nations are frequently joined in conflict at these times, as history shows. Was it coincidence that Hitler's invasion of Poland, and Nasser's seizure

LISTENING TO THE SILENCES

of the Suez Canal that precipitated the 'Suez Crisis', both occurred within six weeks of the perihelial oppositions of 1939 and 1956, respectively, or that Napoleon's ill-fated invasion of Russia happened within the 'sphere of influence' of the one in mid-1813? I have no way of knowing, and leave it to more fervent students of history. However, as individuals, people are already declaring themselves to be undermined and disturbed in advance of the *next*, which will happen on August 28th, 2003. Between nations the events in Iraq have already appeared directly on cue, while at an individual level, many human tragedies and family murders are almost daily occurrences.

Recollecting that the ancients linked Mars with famine and pestilence, the coincidence of the Irish potato famine with the perihelial opposition of 1845, and the present outbreak of the so-called SARS virus should provide food for thought.

Nonetheless, it is the effect upon individual people that concerns me in my writing, and upon which I shall continue to concentrate, although the added uncertainty being created by world events must inevitably have its effect upon those who are already stressed in their minds. Yet again, I must make the point that the spiritual sources of intrusion into vulnerable minds are intelligent and appear to know how to exploit these periods of disturbance. The fact that there are being created *physical* influences on our planet, which in turn generate effects in sensitive people, will most probably be see as the latter react to the same physical stresses that are already increasing the numbers and magnitude of earthquakes and volcanic eruptions worldwide. Was it, in fact, coincidence when a most devastating earthquake in Armenia occurred very shortly after the September 1988 perihelial opposition?

We all are human mammals and must be seen and understood in our total milieu, and not in such artificial settings as consulting rooms, laboratories and hospital wards. The effects of which I write are not respecters of people and locations: a white coat does not confer immunity, nor a building, protection. All, whether patient, consultant, researcher, are within the range of influence: some, simply, are more sensitive than others are.

Something as simple as living in a different part of the country can affect some responsive individuals. I have known four such who, having grown up on the east coast of Britain, became depressed when marriage or work took them to live on the west coast. One woman described graphically how her depression lifted as she travelled east on visits, but was felt almost as a physical burden descending as she came back into the Lake District. In the general sense, she was happy in her marriage and everything else associated with her life in the west. One good friend of mine was born and grew up in Essex, where she frequently suffered from hay fever and asthma. These ailments vanished when she came to live in the northwest of England. However, her hay fever returns immediately when she pays visits to East Yorkshire, only to clear the moment that she crosses the Pennines on the return journey.

From anywhere in the world that one cares to look for examples they are there, where ambience or milieu influences strongly the mindset and behaviour and bodily functions of those who are sensitive. A one-time friend had worked as a nurse in Australia, in a remote north-western town called Fitzroy Crossing. I still recollect her vivid descriptions of those who at certain times in certain local conditions went 'troppo' - a graphic word for an easily imagined condition that affected 'strong men' as well as wimpish Poms.

Staying in Australia, the experiences of one young woman are relevant to my total story. Robyn Davidson set herself the challenge of crossing the desert at the heart of the continent alone, with camels as her pack animals. Properly trained in the management of camels and in desert lore, she nevertheless arrived at a situation where everything that could go wrong did. Sick camels, waterholes that had dried or were not where the maps said they should be, and nebulous tracks that petered out or went off at a tangent. In the graphic account in her book *Tracks* she wrote:

"…Some string somewhere inside me was starting to unravel. An important string, the one that held down panic. I walked on. That night I slept in the sandhills...The hour before the sun spills thin blood colour on the sand I woke suddenly, and tried to gather myself from a dream I could not remember...There were no reference points, nothing to keep the world controlled and bound together. There was nothing but chaos and the voices.

The strong one, the hating one, the powerful one was mocking me, laughing at me.

'You've gone too far this time. I've got you now, and I hate you. You're disgusting aren't you? You're nothing. And I hate you now, I knew it would come sooner or later. There's no use fighting me, you know, there's no one to help you. I've got you. I've got you.'

Another voice was calm and warm. She commanded me to lie down and be calm. She instructed me not to let go, give in. She reassured me that I would find myself again if I could just hold on, be quiet and lie down.

The third voice was screaming."

I have written elsewhere myself:

"Sometimes very vivid dreams are followed on waking by a deliberately fragmented conversation, often with the suggestion that one's mind is being taken over at a deeper level. If one is gullible, one can be convinced that one is losing one's mind, or that this is part of a process by means of which one will become integrated into the 'spirit mind'."

LISTENING TO THE SILENCES

Robyn Davidson recovered her composure and control by going into 'automatic', following established procedures, and staying in touch with what was visible and tangible – "…just one step and another, that's all I have to do. I must not panic", and after another trying day, there came the night and - "I slept deeply and dreamlessly, woke early and rose easily and cleanly as an eagle leaving the nest". She went a very short distance further and came to the abundant water that had eluded her.

I was once acquainted with someone whose philosophy and 'life skills' rested on strong foundations laid down in her youth. Jean Cooper had been born in China, and had lived as a Taoist all her life. The simple pragmatism of the Tao - the 'Way' - she said, equipped her to face most of life's situations. Jean 'stayed in touch with the visible and tangible'. She had no time for long periods spent in silent 'meditation': her very concentration on 'the moment' and with what she was meant to be filling it was meditation enough for her. Thus: 'I am going to fill the kettle'. That was the focus, not, while on the way to the tap - 'Oh that plant looks as if it needs water'; 'The dog needs a walk'; 'I must address that envelope' – and so on, in the way that many of us behave, be-straggling our tasks along so many side alleys and byways and inconsequential deviations.

There, in the behaviour of the two women, the one a reaction to an overwhelming situation, the other responding to the conditioning of a lifetime's belief and practice – there one can find clues to the ways in which individuals can be helped when they are in the grip of intrusive voices and presences. Jean Cooper's 'Way' had been a feature of her life from childhood, and had provided her with markers and references, both in the mundane daily functioning, and in the spiritual understanding and interchange. Robyn Davidson had resource and resilience, the accumulation of experience from upbringing on a Queensland farm, to her most recent tuition from an Afghan camel man. The two women coped unaided, having the core anchorage and stability of training, experience and belief.

Essentially, they were able to cope with all that their circumstances threw at them because, in their different ways, they were single minded and they had a direction and focus. I was reminded forcibly of the need for focus and single mindedness earlier today when out in my workshop. I am making something in wood that requires intricate curves to be cut on my band-saw. This type of saw is probably one of the most dangerous of all of the powered tools used in woodworking. Guiding a curving cut can bring ones fingers very close to the fast moving blade. To make the cut accurately and avoid the need for a lot of subsequent cleaning up with files and sandpaper, one has to be focused totally on the point where the curve that has been drawn on the wood meets the saw blade. The mind has to be emptied of unconnected thought – in fact, it has to

LISTENING TO THE SILENCES

be emptied of *all* thought. If all one's preparations have been appropriate, the wood will pass smoothly through the saw, and the cut will be near perfect.

One fundamental part of the preparation is disciplining oneself in concepts and practice of safe working. If it has not already become an instinctive part of one's working practice, the cut has to be planned ahead so that the wood can be held and moved securely without bringing one's fingers dangerously close to the blade. It is also necessary to anticipate difficulties and make so-called 'escape cuts' – i.e. cuts made up to the intended line at which the main cut can be halted safely and intelligently without losing the continuous flow.

If an instinctive safety strategy is not rigorously planned and cultivated, if thoughts are allowed to stray, one can become a sitting target for 'intruders'. As with the strategies that are used to divert the car driver into folly, so *they* have similar ones to distract the woodworker or anyone operating dangerous equipment, with resultant and potentially serious injury. Likewise with a chainsaw. I also used one of these today, and many of the same considerations apply – the inculcation of safe practice; the focus and planning of tricky cuts; the added dangers of electricity out of doors, and of branches and small trees that might fall differently from the intended direction. The possibilities of distraction and diversion are greater here even than in the workshop – the robin that always appears, the snowdrops that might be crushed – and *they* are always on hand to exploit any lapse with, perhaps, a sudden interjection into the mind, or a reminder of some topic that has been filling one's thoughts earlier in the day.

Returning to the band saw, I would like to remind you of the earlier occasion when I wrote about it. You may recall that I was making a shelf with a different curve at each end, and that, having attempted one cut before breakfast, I had bodged my work, and left it in disgust at my clumsiness. At that time I had an active prayer life that was more specific than now; then the target for my 'work prayers' was Saint Joseph, patron of woodworkers. After breakfast I returned to my saw and the other curve. When I started, I was held physically and mentally in such a one-pointed focus that, even if I had deliberately willed differently, *I would not have been able to wander from the line of the cut*.

Time and time again, and as now, I have to write by analogy. Potentially, the 'life encounters' confronting an open and vulnerable mind can be as hazardous as those facing one's hands when working a band saw, or one's whole self when using a chainsaw. Many of the same 'safety strategies' may also apply. Likewise, and essential, is the need for establishing a personal mind discipline. Importantly – and probably of much greater relevance – is the need to understand that vulnerable individuals will have the greatest difficulty in establishing safe mental 'working conditions' on their own. There is an overwhelming necessity for them to be supported and 'held in a one-point focus' - supported by others who have a complete understanding and belief in what I am writing.

In many lives, none of these prerequisites have ever been established, or, if once there, have ceased to exist. Self discipline; self control? Increasingly, hedonism is the driving force. Discipline, control – definitely not part of the vocabulary of many, where 'cool' is everything. As I have repeatedly pointed out, I am not writing from the standpoint of any religion, or of religion in general. However, all of the world religions have something in common which is worth reflecting upon. All promote a way of behaving that minimises wrongdoing and which promotes a standard of thinking that discards the obscene and reprehensible, while encouraging what is normally regarded as 'purity of thought'. Further, all of the faiths recognise the existence of spiritual good and evil, and of the contrast between the availability of the former, if invoked through such as prayer, to provide support and encouragement within the challenges of life, as against the deliberate intervention of spiritual evil to intrude and undermine through any weakness of behaviour and thought.

Unfortunately, purity of thought and intent do not always guarantee protection, and the vulnerable may still be defenceless. Someone with whom I am well acquainted lived an impeccable life within a well-integrated and loving family. Entry into university and living away from home in the isolation of student accommodation created a situation within which she was subject to vile and undermining intrusion. She had not followed any of the irresponsible practices that I am trying to illustrate, nor indulged in any form of 'divination', or other spiritually dubious activity. The intrusion was completely spontaneous.

My friend tried to get help through the 'usual' mental health channels, but soon realised that there was remarkably little understanding from those responsible for student welfare, and marshalled her own resources. She ploughed a very lonely furrow for much of her professional life, subject to frequent and unpleasant intrusion, until a unique spiritual awakening gave her the resource to combat and eliminate what had plagued her for so long. 'The isolation of student accommodation ' may seem to be a contradiction in terms, but for someone who has not mixed outside school and family, who is not outgoing, student accommodation can be a very lonely place, and an imaginative mind can provide easy entry for intrusions that are determined to plague and torment.

LISTENING TO THE SILENCES

CHAPTER 13

My

Only Enemy

Roy Vincent

LISTENING TO THE SILENCES

> This stranger holding me from head to toe,
> This deaf usurper I shall never know,
> Who lives in household quiet in my unrest,
> And of my troubles weaves his tranquil nest,
> Who never smiles or frowns or bows his head,
> And while I rage is insolent as the dead,
> ... and (is my) only enemy.
>
> Edwin Muir

(The Private Place)

The problem of trying to describe the indescribable in terms of the effect of spiritual intrusion is matched equally by the difficulties inherent in trying to answer the question – 'who' are the intruders, and where and how do *they* originate? Frankly, if I could answer that question with complete certainty, I would be the very first to do so since the question was first posed, since humanity had its first philosophical thought. Many individuals, organisations and theologies believe that they have answers, and, from within the answers, a perceived core of similarity emerges. All presuppose the survival after death of the 'soul' or 'spirit'. The quality of life and the manner of dying are credited with having an effect upon the 'destination' of the released spirit. Death in accident, trauma, suicide and battle are alleged to create a so-called 'earthbound' spirit. Such are believed to stay close to the location of their dying and to be unable to realise that they are, in fact, dead. Some, it is said, attach themselves to living people and become, in effect, an inadvertent intruder, still hopelessly lost.

Those who die at home or in hospital may, by the very nature of their previous life, be strongly attached to individuals, places or to particular activities, and may, in death, seek an appropriate place or person. Alternatively, the very act of dying may leave them so isolated that they attach to the nearest living person, whether adult or newborn infant. In time those in the latter two groups may realise that they are able to utilise the mind and faculties of their 'host', and that they can create thoughts, desires and emotions. It is quite uncanny and a revealing commentary on the generality of humans, that just as a new method of communication is invented, so it is swamped by individuals or groups intent upon perverting it. The invention of photography and cinema soon were followed by the pornographic picture and 'blue' movie. Printing gave an open channel for erotica. Citizens' Band radio was swamped rapidly by the intrusive obscenity and worse, while the Internet – yes the Internet.

The Internet provides an ideal analogy of the spiritual link into the human mind. As I have become more confident and fluent in my ability to access the Internet and e-mail, so much more comes to light than I had anticipated. With e-mail comes 'spam'. Many will have experienced having their mail in-box flooded with these unwanted intrusions. In my case, it appears that the Server that I use has had its lists of subscribers entered and circulated widely, (assuming that the Server itself has not sold the information). Now, every time that I open my in-box, I find that there are several entries from totally undesirable and definitely unwanted sources. Do I want to enlarge my penis? Almost daily there are offers of products guaranteed to accomplish this. Do I want to see college girls masturbating, or having lesbian encounters? Just enter. Do I want to get in touch with bored housewives, all apparently ravening for sex? Sign in for contacts. Do I want to watch live action of farm girls copulating with animals? Why, enter in. There is no area of indecency and depravity that is not available. And this is just on e-mail spam.

So it is, by analogy, the way in which the human mind that has been opened and somehow entered is flooded with 'spam' by the spiritual equivalent of the human providers of obscenity and pornography. If the offers by e-mail of access to what are euphemistically called 'preteens' are taken up, will this be the route that some follow towards the land of the paedophile? Temptation is strewn before the curious and vulnerable. Some, it is true, will have made an active search for web sites that offer access to their personal predilections. Others will be drawn in having been titillated by the images sent with the spam. Whatever the trigger, the die will be cast when the signing–in page has been completed with its all-important credit card information.

Major religions affirm that the 'stain of sin' is always present on the spiritual image of a person, and cannot even be washed away by confession and penance. Only time and one's ultimate death will reveal whether or not this is true. For the seeker after pornography and paedophilia, there is no going back once the 'Enter' button has been clicked. Indelibly there for the Cyber police to discover is the evidence of web sites accessed and paid for. The 'stain of web sin' cannot be washed away! Whereas it was always supposed to be GOD who saw all and meted out justice, now it is the Cyber police and the courts.

With the creation of the Internet, a new dominion of access into, and torment of the vulnerable mind was created and immediately colonised by the fomenters of spiritual evil. The solitary persons, believing that they are having surreptitious access to hitherto undreamed of images and contacts, were nevertheless subjected to an enveloping ambience of guilt and titillation –

the one source urging in the mind that the site should be opened, and the other heaping on an atmosphere of disquiet verging on shame and self-disgust. When, with the sudden revelation that all was not secret between the persons and the web site, and that high profile prosecutions were in train, one can imagine the panic at the thought of discovery, and simultaneously, the driving condemnation coming from the spiritual tormentors, taunting at the shame that was about to arrive. Certainly a number have been known to have committed suicide.

How many computers were abandoned or how many hard drives were changed, we shall never know, but still the stain of Cyber sin remained in credit card and phone details, and who knows what torment from unknown spiritual sources. Many, I am sure, were the excuses or reasons given for having had access to images of the young. The most blatant seems to have been 'for study purposes', or 'research for my new book'. The rest I'll leave to your imagination, though to come back to the human world and leaving briefly the Cyber spiritual, I suddenly recalled from the back of my memory an example of how the study of pornographic images changed the life progress of one student.

It is some time since I read *A Narrow Street* by Elliot Paul. Set in Paris in the 1930's, Paul relates an episode where a young habitué of the Street, a student, had virtually abandoned his work in mathematics and spent much time at 'Le

Pannier Fleuri' – the local brothel. There he became absorbed in studying the volumes of photographs kept to titillate and stimulate the clients. In time the student became so enthralled at the numbers of permutations and combinations of men, women and animals engaged in copulation that he was inspired to return to his mathematic studies! Perhaps this might be a flavour of the 'reasons' given for 'studying' sites portraying paedophilia!

Yet another introduction of a means of communication that has been ingeniously infiltrated by 'spiritual evil' is that of 'signing' for the deaf and dumb. Although there has long been a hand language using signs to represent individual letters, the more recent signing strategy has introduced a greater fluency and speed. At first anecdotal, and subsequently authenticated, have been the instances when individuals who, having been completely deaf and dumb since birth, have been taught signing and have become 'verbally' fluent. Some have reported that their new 'world' has been intruded into by visual images of 'people' signing the usual unpleasant, obscene and disturbing propositions that have been experienced habitually as intrusions into the verbal minds of vocal people. As ever, I find it so hard to try to come to terms with the motives of the malevolent 'who' flood obscenely and disturbingly into the new channels of communication almost as soon as they are created. It is even more heart rending to learn of individuals who, when thus

LISTENING TO THE SILENCES

disturbed, have abandoned their new skill, and gladly returned to their silent inner tranquillity.

As a side issue stemming from that, one might consider briefly the practices employed by those who deliberately choose a silent life. I refer to certain of the monastic orders of various religions, where to be in silence is the chosen mode of living. There has long been an awareness of the reality of adverse mental intrusion, and one method of blocking that has been the practice of mentally verbalising chosen prayers. The 'Jesus Prayer' is the one most frequently discussed:

"Jesus Christ, Son of the living God, have mercy on me."

- and shortened versions, even to the simple repetition of the name 'Jesus'. Others in the Christian tradition frequently use the rosary as a means of praying and maintaining inner tranquillity. Buddhists favour their own repetition of:

"ôm mani padme hum" – Hail to the jewel in the lotus

- while many techniques of meditation and routes to inner tranquillity use their own 'mantras' or chosen words or phrases. There is much to be learned from well established meditation practices that can be used to still the minds of individuals who are plagued by 'intruders', too much for me to include, and only capable of being referred to in passing. Always bearing in mid the constant caution that I repeat and repeat, and find in my frequent quotation from Dr. Elmer Green, when he warns of the hasty descent into the deeper realms of the mind, and the dangers of there encountering 'indigenous beings'.

An isolated life that does not revolve around the twin practices of prayer and meditation is that enjoyed by the dedicated computer addict or avid player of computer and play-station games. The computer screen and the play station become the bounds of the world of these individuals and the divisions between reality and fantasy become blurred or non-existent. Within the realms of fantasy that the screens project, and away from the balancing human contact, the mind can lose its powers of discernment and become fruitful soil for the intruders to establish themselves and flourish.

Returning to the condition of someone who dies in explosion, fire and panic, in all of the time that I have been subjected to voices and intrusions, I have experienced - or been duped into believing it - the access of friends and shipmates who died when our ship was mined. Trapped, asphyxiated, fragmented, incinerated, literally within feet of me - where, I wonder did their spirits go, and in what state were they? Cleaning some items in my workshop, I disturbed some dry and finely powdered rust, and as it floated as an orange-brown cloud in a shaft of sunlight, I saw a hint of the flame-lit cloud of cordite smoke that filled my eyes as I regained consciousness after the explosion. I could not have had a more potent reminder – potent even though it happened nearly sixty years ago.

Geordie – a frequent companion - 'broke his duck' in a brothel in Nice. Not my personal predilection, but, in the first year after the war, a good place to sell perfumed toilet soap and supplement our meagre pay. I left him to his particular choice – a young and attractive woman – and his one and only experience. 'Beaucoup de soleil' she had said as she looked at him. From time to time, using suitable mental cues, for example 'Beaucoup de soleil', my mind is directed to those times and to him. Maybe 'Scrumpy', the Leading Cook, who produced all of our regular daily roasts, and sometimes made bread in the galley where he sweated and sweated in the mid-summer Mediterranean heat. I remember him particularly in a stone hut on Mount Troodos in Cyprus– somewhere cool for a change – where we had been taken for a few days leave. He had dragged in some green branches and tried to burn them in a pot-bellied barrack room stove and talked into the night in his Cornish voice while we choked on the smoke. It requires only one key word to bring him vividly to mind. Is he there 'in person'? I have no way of knowing, but there is some sort of 'presence', and it only takes the insertion of one word – 'rabbiting' – into my mind for it to manifest. I could go on - to Dennis and 'Straker', who with me sailed the ship's sailing dinghy at Haifa and Famagusta; Lofty, who bought his sister a vivid pair of pyjamas from a bumboat man in Grand Harbour, Valetta; the Chief Telegraphist, with whom I sometimes 'walked' in the dog-watches - thirty paces up to the torpedo tubes, turn and thirty paces back to the after deckhouse, turn... He was a 'regular', due for discharge at the end of this particular commission, and already full of plans for his impending retirement. They all have their verbal or visual triggers.

It never ceases to amaze me how, even in a comparatively short time, but in the close confines and enclosed community of a small ship such as a destroyer, individuals and personalities can be indelibly imprinted in one's memory, and how easily they can be brought to mind. It never ceases to amaze me how, by a single word injected – and I mean 'injected' – into my mind, these and others can be brought to such vivid memory. It does not have to be an actual word. From the world of the 'twitchers' – the birdwatchers - comes the word 'jizz'. The jizz of a bird – the essentials of shape, flight, call and colour that are imprinted on the mind of the experienced birdwatcher – is all that is required to alert the watcher to the presence of the bird. *People* have jizzes, and the 'flash' across one's mind of the jizz, as of a bird momentarily seen, can bring the person totally into mental view, together with many well remembered details. On numerous occasions when this has happened I am left wondering whether the person was actually present in spirit, or whether the memory

LISTENING TO THE SILENCES

has been used to develop another mind-trawl, aimed at uncovering yet more information about each of us.

Have no doubt; *all* of one's five senses can be activated in the creation of the essence of a person, location or event. The jizz of someone can be created in minute and exquisite detail, even to the quirks of speech and accent. Likewise, all of one's emotions can be stimulated and used to console, recall or provoke. When, at the outset of my own experiences, and I went through a major spiritual awakening, I was subjected to a rigorously searching catechism in my mind, and emerged feeling as if I had been skinned, so vulnerable and exposed had I become. I had not questioned the right of this particular numinous presence to probe and expose every facet of my life as it was then, and in years past. I was reminded of these events recently when I watched a television programme about the experiences of individuals who had been declared clinically dead, and yet were resuscitated. No mention was made of anything 'spiritual', but the programme achieved its aim, which was to explore the continued function of the mind while the brain was effectively dead and not functioning.

Several of those who had had the near death events, described what has become a common feature of these experiences, namely the encounters with the spirits of deceased family and friends and the mind-to-mind communication with them. Especially did they comment on their encounter with a 'luminous presence', and the way in which every aspect of the life that they had lived was scrutinised, not with judgement and possible reprimand, but with open minded love and understanding. Following their return and ultimate recovery, all reported a significant change in their way of life and a total loss of fear of ultimate death. I did not have a near death event when I had my own spiritual catechism, but the *result* has been similar in my own understanding of life and death, and in the purpose of my own remaining life.

The continuation of memory through and beyond the actual process of dying is a concept that can lead to much speculation and controversy. Someone whom I know very well had three brothers - twins, A and B, and the third, C. One summer when the twins were about ten years old, all three were swimming in a creek near the local small docks. Suddenly, a sluice was opened to fill one of the locks, and C was sucked down. A went to the rescue of his brother, ensured his safety, but drowned himself. When B was in his early twenties, he emigrated, eventually married and had children. One of the children subsequently drowned in a swimming pool in circumstances for which there was no explanation. Another, a boy, as he was growing, would ask about "My other mother, the one with red hair". The mother of the three brothers, A, B and C, and my friend had striking red hair – no one else.

Reading that, some will accept 'reincarnation', others, 'transmigration of souls'.

LISTENING TO THE SILENCES

Unfortunately, there is never consensus about exactly what such terms mean. For myself, I, as usual, adopt the simplest explanation, such as that A, in spirit, attached himself to B, his twin, and subsequently to one or other of B's children. I have not the slightest concept of how such would happen in practice, but it is an explanation subscribed to by many and from numerous different philosophies. Any 'spiritual' explanation flies in the face of those who, with dogged determination, are resolved to 'rationalise', and who will proffer alternatives that, when fully analysed, are much more far-fetched than the simple spiritual concept.

There is a genre of radio and television programmes frequently presented in Britain where the inexplicable experiences of individuals or groups are examined. The greater part of the programme is devoted to interviews with the people involved, and with reconstructions of actual events. In the majority of cases, the explanation that would be accepted by many is that, in some unfathomable way, there has been 'spiritual' involvement. However, part of the programme is inevitably given over to a psychiatrist or psychologist, whose rôle, again inevitably, is to offer a 'rational', 'scientific' explanation of the phenomena, and to pooh-pooh the concept that, not even in the remotest way, could there have been *anything* of a spiritual nature involved.

Without going into the details of any of the programmes that I have seen, one salient fact emerges, namely that these specialists in one or other form of mind medicine, claim a *universal* expertise in all matters scientific and practical. Thus in one programme the psychiatrist became an instant expert in house fires and the potential for the creation of an explosion of such precision that it could propel a child through a window without it suffering any harm. In another, the psychologist had never driven a tractor, yet knew exactly how a runaway tractor would behave as it trundled down a slope, positive that it would be deviated randomly by grass tussocks, sufficient to avoid running over groups of picnickers, and to pass safely by. These are but trite and inconsequential examples, but they serve to illustrate the wider and exceedingly dangerous premise – namely that a specialist in one particular and narrow field of medicine can be accepted without question as being an expert in a whole range of unrelated specialities.

A gross example of such 'global' expertise has just been exposed in the High Court, and in the media. The case concerned a woman who had been given two life sentences for the murder of two of her infants. The most telling evidence against her came from a renowned paediatrician, who kept repeating that the odds against two cot deaths occurring in one family were 73,000,000:1. As well as his claims of knowledge as a statistician, this man also, by virtue of his comments, claimed expertise as a toxicologist, in a branch of human psychology and in an area of law. He was not trained in any of these specialities; yet, by weight of his demeanour and presence, he was able to influence a jury against the power of all the other evidence. In another era, before the abolition of the death penalty, it is possible that the woman would have been hanged before the evidence that saved her came to light. Fortunately, the woman was released on appeal.

With increasing frequency over the last several years we have seen instances of individuals who, having been wrongly convicted of murder, have been released after spending as long as twenty-five years in prison. Again, had they lived in earlier times, they would undoubtedly have been hanged many years ago. By a combination of deceit, inadequate defence or the superior forensic skills of the prosecution team that can overwhelm a jury, many innocent individuals have gone to the gallows. Every prosecutor in years gone by wanted to be a Sir Bernard Spillsbury, by whom every jury seems to have been mesmerised, and whose aim in life appeared to be to obtain a conviction, irrespective of the *justice* of the prosecution case.

Another renowned prosecutor, and later judge, was Christmas Humphries, one of the leaders of the expansion of Buddhism in Britain. I once heard a broadcast interview in which he described his life in the law courts. He explained at length that he chose to be a prosecutor rather than defence lawyer, because he did not want to use his skills to obtain the acquittal of someone who was palpably guilty. However, through the interview, there came an almost arrogant certainty in his ability as a prosecutor. There was no apparent recognition of the fact that his forensic skills may have resulted in the innocent being hanged. I recorded the broadcast – *My Brother in the Dock* – principally because I wanted to hear in his own words how he came to espouse Buddhism. I listened to my tape a number of times, and each time I became more aware of his 'self-certainty', almost to the point of disliking the man.

Some time after I began to hear voices, and could distinguish the various 'levels' from which my communications appeared to come, and by the use of certain key words from the tape, I began to comprehend that I was being led to an understanding of a significant concept that I had never ever addressed in my thoughts. I was not 'told' in the sense that I received 'verbalisation' in my mind, but rather I was presented with a totality – a full and instant appreciation of what was being conveyed – the real meaning of which is this:

Acknowledging, as one must at some time, that the 'essence' of a person continues after the death of the physical body, one must also acknowledge that memory, character and intent survive intact and are absorbed into a general spiritual state from which it can continue to function intelligently. In the context within which I am writing, the continuity of function assumes a living human mind that is capable of being influenced. Without a broad acceptance of this, what is to me, fact, much of what I am writing will disappear into the minds of a certain category of reader in a similar manner to a river vanishing into the sands of a desert, and be totally lost. Which would be most unfortunate, for *continuously* I experience the practical expression of what I am, with acknowledged difficulty, trying to share.

Having, in their new found state of being, acquired a full realisation of the effects of their actions while in life, many are shocked to realise the extent to which their personal arrogance, professional tunnel vision and other self-inflationary traits have had a damaging effect upon the lives of those for whom it should have been their professional responsibility to care. In the case of the legal prosecutor and judge that I am citing, there may come a recognition that in his blind pursuit of the goal of obtaining a conviction, he may have done so in ignorance of the fact that evidence may have been fabricated, that vital evidence may have been withheld from the defence, or that a defendant may have been 'stitched up' by the police, and that he may have contributed himself to the execution of an innocent person, or to the long-term incarceration of others.

The effect of this clarity of 'vision', my insight tells me, is a strong desire to educate, inform and reform through the minds and responses of receptive individuals. Even though reparation for the wrongs inflicted upon individuals may not be achieved, - for how could one compensate someone whose life had been drastically shortened in a most terrible way - by helping to change a climate of thought and somehow being instrumental in inspiring reformers, judicial arrogance and culpability may be lessened.

In other fields, notably medicine, and most particularly mental health, there dawns the awful realisation that much harm has been done to 'innocent' healthy minds, sometimes resulting in the premature 'death' of these minds or in long periods of incarceration of their owners. With awakened comprehension and understanding of the involvement of intruding spirits into the minds of vulnerable individuals, comes the strongest desire to disseminate this awareness and to minimise the further harm that inevitably will be visited on the defenceless minds through the continuation of many of the current practices. I have come to a firm conclusion that I am one of the 'receptive individuals' who finds himself in this particular unsought and, at times, completely unacceptable rôle.

There have been numerous times over the last twenty years when I have concluded that I am on an 'assault course with live ammunition'. In all battlefield training, members of the armed forces are subjected to situations where the bullets flying overhead are as lethal as those that will be encountered in genuine conflict. When I joined the Navy and was issued with a service gasmask, we were all given the ultimate demonstration of the efficacy of the mask. In

LISTENING TO THE SILENCES

groups we were confined in a small chamber that, we were told, was then filled with tear gas. After some time, during which we were able to breathe freely in our masks, we had to remove them. Anyone who had had any doubts about the actual presence of the gas was soon disillusioned as the disabling tears flooded our eyes.

In a similar manner, I am constantly subjected to the experiences and ploys that I have recorded and am describing. Often, when I have yet again fallen for a ploy that I should have seen coming a mile off, or when, gullibly, I have been taken in by a new strategy, and when, thereby, I have gained more experience and understanding, I receive in my mind a quiet, but unmistakable and imperative request to 'write it down, write it down'. Mostly I have done so, and you are reading the results. There are other times when I have been so pissed off at having had my day disrupted as I have gone through a real time experience, that I let my feelings be known through violent imprecations within my mind, and curse the intruders in the forceful language of the lower deck. Many will have seen on television the gruelling jungle, desert and arctic training endured by service personnel. The heat and cold are real, likewise the leeches and thorns. The sleep deprivation cannot be simulated but has to be experienced to be understood; the forced marches with heavy packs have to be endured, and then kit and weapons have to be cleaned before sleep is allowed. And all of the time, the urging, goading instructors will have been hated and cursed.

Roy Vincent

No amount of classroom theory, rôle playing or simulation can prepare anyone for the actual environment. No exercises with paint-ball guns can act as a substitute for the close proximity of lethal ammunition. Awareness and instinctive reaction can only be achieved through a recognition of the presence and modes of attack employed by an enemy. Recent conflicts such as the Falklands campaign and the Gulf Wars revealed a plethora of armchair commentators and strategists. Every TV and radio channel, and every newspaper had its interviewers, reporters, analysts and strategic experts. Apart from a few notable exceptions, all were inexperienced in any field of combat. But most seemed to have mastered the jargon, acquired a flak jacket and intrepidly gone to war.

But war is not a game or something that can be interpreted by the onlooker and commentator. It is very real, but the true reality is only experienced by those whom it is affecting directly. Likewise, the 'war' that is going on in the mind and life of someone who is invaded by spiritual intrusion is only capable of being understood fully by those who are in the conflict. Just as some of those who are directly affected and may be victims of the international conflicts are rendered speechless, 'shell-shocked' or incoherent by their experiences, so those directly affected by their own battle in the mind, may similarly have great difficulty in communicating the reality of their own inner conflicts.

LISTENING TO THE SILENCES

Inevitably I return, as I shall always return, to the paradox that is thrown up by the situation of the voice hearer, the person who is dubbed 'schizophrenic'. In expressing it I want to do so without intentionally causing offence to all of the medical professionals who sincerely believe that they understand the actual inner mind of someone whom they are they are putting in this particular category. Expressed simply, the paradox is this, namely that with a few rare exceptions, the professionals have not experienced any aspect of the phenomena that the voice hearers are trying to describe. It should be obvious by now that even though I am drawing upon the experiences of more than twenty years, and though I have all of my communicating skills, nevertheless, the problems that I have in conveying the reality of it all are immense. It is no wonder, then, that when faced with the variety of bizarre experiences described by the hearers, the professionals themselves arrive at such a variety of interpretations. 'It's the two sides of the brain talking to each other'; 'It's the product of the bicameral mind'; 'They are illusions'; 'They are delusions'. Words such as 'schizoid', 'schizophreniform' and the like pepper the dialogue and writings of the commentators.

With a wide variety of definitions and explanations crossing and re-crossing the Atlantic and Pacific oceans; with the legacies of Freud and Jung and their successors holding minds and closing minds over the years, wouldn't it be wonderful if suddenly there came the 'Eureka' answer that all desire? In another field I saw recently a superb example of such an answer to a universally posed question. For as long as it has been recognised that humans evolved from apes that began to walk upright, the mechanism and the reason for the upright stance have been endlessly analysed and debated. 'Savannahs developed and the apes had to leave the trees, and eventually stood upright'; 'Without the shade of the trees, the apes exposed less of their body surface to the sun by standing upright' – ignoring the extension of this 'logic' that would have all equatorial animals standing on two legs; 'Lifting the head higher above the ground would bring it into a breezier, and hence, cooler region, and benefit the brain'; - and many more attempts at explanation, each attracting its core of adherents. The 'Eureka' moment that produced illumination came to those who were filming in Africa for the recent BBC 'Life of Mammals' series. Apes were being filmed in a swampy area, and suddenly *there* was a female carrying its young and wading upright and waist deep through the water *exactly* as would a human in similar circumstances. Paleontological and geological analysis of the era when upright walking is judged to have begun, confirmed that extensive swampy areas and lagoons formed in the territory of the apes, and that wading and hence walking, would become the norm. The sight of that female ape wading is one of the most potent that I have ever seen on television.

LISTENING TO THE SILENCES

How I hope that from within the volume of my writing there will be that which will cause some in psychiatry to echo 'Eureka'!

That it is going to take a huge leap of faith I have no doubt, faith that is going to insist that everyone is treated wholly as an individual, and not, as apparently in the Swedish study of cannabis use among conscripts, 50.000 human clones. I have group photographs taken at various stages of my naval career, and I defy anyone to find a much more diverse collection of *individuals* drawn from the Britain of the time.

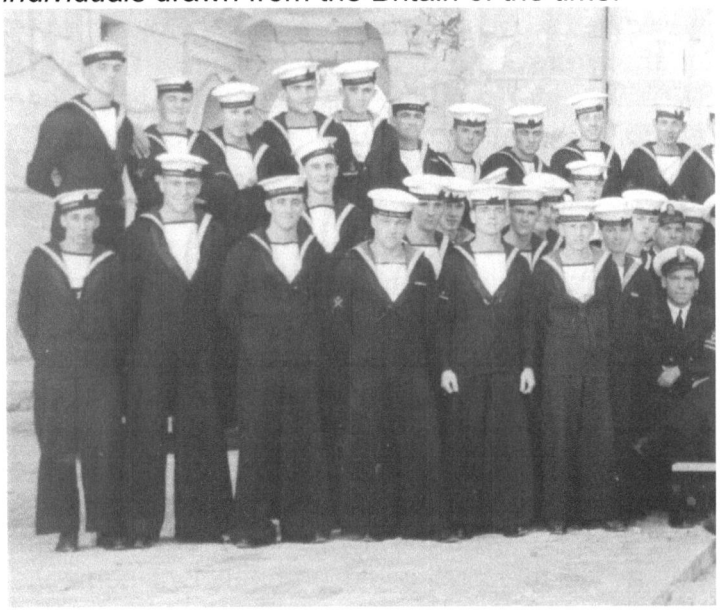

Roy Vincent

Here is a portion of the ships company from a photograph taken in Malta several weeks after our ship had been mined, and shortly before we made our way to Britain, crossing France by train. Just study them as a group and then as individuals. Approximately twenty-five, a mixture of 'regulars' and 'hostilities only' ratings who are equivalent to just one two-thousandth of the Swedish study. What image is conjured up for you at the thought of '50,000 conscripts'? Do you think of 50,000 Swedish look-alikes, all dressed in field grey, all called Sven, or Jan, or Per, or Bjorn? I can look at my group and see Cornish, Welsh, Devonian, Irish, and Scots. Not the full range of 'British', for we were a West Country ship, and such were normally crewed from those regions. There are two who, as orphans of seafarers, had been brought up in the *Arethusa* tradition of caring for such boys, and who had been enlisted as boy-seamen at an early age; then two others who had been to top public schools. I can see some who didn't 'draw', were 'temperance' – i.e. they didn't draw their daily tot of rum, whereas the majority would be 'grog' and would 'draw'. Until the daily tot was discontinued in about 1970, the 'grog' ratings had an extra currency with which to reward favours. "Come around at tot time" was the invitation to receive payment – 'sippers', 'gulpers', 'half a tot' were the normal level of repayment. For a 'full tot', one could probably get someone murdered! I see some for whom a 'run ashore' meant time spent 'down the Gut', if in Valetta, and in the many bars. For others it could mean time

LISTENING TO THE SILENCES

spent at "Aggie's" – the Missions to Seamen founded by Aggie Weston. And then there is one man whom I never saw go ashore, but who spent his free time making pegged rugs from discarded naval uniform clothes,

There are men in the photograph who had soon acquired the naval jargon, or had it ingrained after more than fifteen years at sea, for whom 'avast' and 'belay' still had everyday meaning, and who knew what to do with soojie-moojie, baggywrinkle, and a pusser's dip. Men who were in a sense cloned by their surnames – if you were Walker, you were 'Hookey'; if Williams, 'Bungey'; if Martin, 'Pincher'; if Miller, 'Dusty'. Rhodes was 'Lonesome', and Carpenter became 'Chippy', while Wright was 'Shiner', Green answered to 'Jimmy' and Grey, 'Dolly' and every Wilson became 'Tug'. Like every other Welshman, I was Taff, while every Cornishman was Jan. I can see able-seamen and gunnery ratings, torpedo men, stokers and 'bunting tossers' or signalmen. You can identify yourself the ones who would be 'Lofty', and which, 'Shortarse'.

Multiply such a group by 2,000, and then try to imagine a study that would give meaning to the consequences of one particular activity such as smoking cannabis, a study that was continued over ten or fifteen years, and from which conclusions are being drawn about 'schizophrenia'. And then look back at the accounts of my own personal and actual experiences, and the results of my observations and records covering well over twenty years. I look at myself in the full photograph of the ship's company, and reflect that I, also, was very much an individual. One of a small number of electronic specialists, I lived in a seamen's mess, because in a small ship there wasn't enough room in an artificers' mess. My upbringing had defined and pre-conditioned much of my behaviour and choice of activity. I didn't smoke or drink, and at the time, and from my background, 'teenage sex' was mostly in our imagination, so I didn't frequent the brothels or accept the invitations of the scugnizzi – the children in Naples - who offered the delights of their sisters, each one of whom was invariably a 'virgin – only sixteen'.

Was it peer pressure that influenced the young who had no firm roots? I can see two in the photo and remember their return to our mess from a run ashore, having had their first sexual encounter in a Maltese brothel under the 'tutelage' of some of the older members of the mess. Was it peer pressure that induced some of the Swedish conscripts to smoke cannabis? And did their succumbing reveal an indecisive and easily influenced personality? And are such the targets of the 'intelligent' spiritual intrusion into the mind of the vulnerable? Some individuals get caught up in the excitement of a group enthusiasm and go with the flow, in spite of initial self-cautions. I recollect being told of the experiences of some of the vacation students who used to spend time at my Works. Living in a hostel, a few had light-heartedly begun to have sessions with an ouija board and drew others in. Soon, there was persistent 'contact', apparently from a young woman who 'told' a distressing tale of having been killed in an accident. The contact was so 'real' that the sessions became compulsive and all assembled immediately after their evening meal. There was a wealth of circumstantial detail including the woman's address, or 'an address'. They were never to find out. With the Easter break coming up, it was planned to pay a visit, *but* - they were told most strongly that if they attempted to do so, one of their number, Dave, would die. Consternation. The sessions stopped forthwith, and Dave acquired a hunted expression and acute nervousness that remained with him for several months. (Refreshing my mind about the incident from someone who lived in the same hostel at the time and was an associate of the other students, I was happy to learn that Dave had survived, had been seen recently, and was married and a parent three times over.)

When I began to use my pendulum and alphabet chart, I had had no cautions in my life that would have warned me about the practice that I was engaged in. I had proceeded with a blind curiosity and ultimate near obsession along a route and into activities for which nothing in my earlier life had prepared me. There *are* 'life maps' for those who care to find them and follow their directions. Most of these have been surveyed and drawn by the World religions. I had had an intelligent and caring upbringing in a home that adhered to Christian values, although not in the more focused traditions that encourage one to make frequent checks on how one measures up to the core values of the faith. Some would class the indoctrination and 'blind' adherence to the rules governing behaviour as a form of brain washing. Yet there are situations in life where the absolute and immediate observance of the rules is essential, *vital*, for the safety *and peace of mind* of the individual and indeed of large groups, where irresponsibility and disregard of the rules can lead to disaster.

From before the days of James Cook and William Bligh – indeed before Ptolemy - seafarers have surveyed their routes and coasts, anchorages and channels. They have logged tides and currents, and the pilots and sailing masters of old had their own treasured and jealously guarded 'rutter' – the sum total of all of their own experiences and observations and accumulated pilotage wisdom. In time the surveys and observations were gradually compiled into the renowned Admiralty charts. Many were the voyages of exploration and discovery, often undertaken in ships that by today's standards were mere cockleshells. Many were the perils encountered, and wonders seen. All were faithfully logged, and in time the facts and realities were analysed and added to the sum of the information shown on the official charts.

With the growth of knowledge and the increased use of the routes and seaways, rules of navigation were devised that would prevent or minimise collision, and an instinctive

LISTENING TO THE SILENCES

standard of behaviour evolved that bound together the genuine mariners in ways that tried to ensure mutual support when at sea. Nevertheless, collisions and strandings can and do occur, and Boards of Inquiry meet and apportion blame. In very many cases the cause of the disaster comes down to someone disregarding the rules. Likewise standards of upkeep and crewing of ships are flaunted, and result in tankers being stranded and huge slicks of oil polluting the seas and shores. *Anyone* venturing to sea should be aware of all that is necessary for their own safety – and equally importantly the safety and well-being of others.

But now anyone can get afloat in an increasingly wide variety of ways, ways that in themselves are fun, but which can be used without there being any need, seemingly, to have any knowledge of the inherent dangers to self or others. Thus jet skis used in crowded waters kill bathers, as do power boats towing water skiers. Individuals can hazard themselves and others in an almost cretinous disregard of common sense, let alone sea lore and law. Thus very recently one read of a man who set off for an island five miles off shore on a water cycle with a total of five children either on the cycle or towed on an inflatable ring. All had to be rescued by helicopter. Other acts resulting from stupidity or lack of observation of the 'rules' can hazard the lives of lifeboat men and other mariners as they attempt rescue.

The life maps to which I referred became embodied in the wide variety of world religions, but whereas the original guidance and precepts were aimed at the physical and spiritual well-being of tribes and individuals, in time they became ritual practices in themselves, and to a large extent, lost their meaning in their original context. Thus the circumcision of males would at first sight seem to be a bizarre requirement in the 'rules' of two major world religions. However, recent observation and analysis of the transmission of AIDS in Africa reveals that circumcised men are considerably less likely to become infected during sexual transmission. The embargo on the eating of pork may appear to constitute an unreasonable dietary restriction, yet knowledge of the parasites that can exist in pork in hot countries makes an obvious case for the interdict. The understanding that led to both practices came from the prescience of the Divine, and there is much prescience in the advice for living a healthy 'mental' life that has come from Divine and other spiritual sources.

I wouldn't get very far if I was to advocate a religious revival within the field of mental health, and yet I am repeating at every stage that the intrusions into the mind of a mentally ill person derive from spiritual sources, and hence an understanding of the recommendations that pervade the texts of virtually all religions with respect to the interaction with the life of the spirit is as germane now as when the texts were written.

LISTENING TO THE SILENCES

These recommendations that then became the 'life rules' of the religions are the equivalent of mariners' rules of conduct, and flouting them brings unwelcome consequences. But as with many who venture onto the water, so also is there total ignorance of any advice, procedures or cautions. Additionally the active exercise of the core values of a religion that added to the intrinsic safety of the spiritual life of individuals has often become little more than a mindless adherence to what are effectively superstitions. I well remember one friend proclaiming that he liked to go to church at Easter and Harvest Festival and always ate fish on Good Friday, and who carried a Cornish Piskie in his waistcoat pocket – although I must not detract from the fact that his life was one of honesty and probity in all that he did.

In effect, there *are* no 'rules of the road' that guarantee sound mental health and with which youngsters are indoctrinated as they develop. There is advice galore and there are products aplenty relating to tooth care or the cleanliness and sterility of one's toilet – but a clean and sound mind? No way. Likewise, the commercial break on virtually every TV channel will offer a superb range of 'designer' spectacle frames, and many choices of 'buy one, get one free' – the addition of a pair of 'shades', or sunspecs as I still call them (but that ain't cool!) Does anyone in this madly competitive commercial exploitation of people's eyes draw attention to the fact that it is possible to prevent much of the deterioration that usually happens? Does anyone refer to the book by Meir Schneider from which I quoted earlier – *My Life and Vision* – in which he described how, doggedly, and mostly by his own efforts, he changed his life from that of someone treated as being blind, to someone with sound vision? Not a mention. Yet contained within the book are descriptions of how, by diligent practice, virtually anyone can reclaim the clear vision that their eyes are meant to have. But of course, there is no commercial value in self-help, and self-help does require significant personal dedication.

Turn on any kids TV programme, and inevitably you will see youngsters wearing braces on their teeth. The result – admirable for the resulting smiles and long term survival of the teeth, but what about the body and mind that lurk behind the teeth? To maintain tooth perfection, dentists are recommending to children that they should avoid sugary soft drinks, and stick to the so-called 'diet' variety. But virtually without exception, the diet drinks are sweetened with Aspartame, and, as any sweep on the web will tell you, Aspartame has a whole range of very serious, and undesirable side effects. One result of the dental advice could then be a perfect smile fronting a mind that is being corrupted by the very product that has been recommended as preserving the smile. Headaches, migraines, dizziness, seizures, depression, fatigue, anxiety attacks, slurred speech – these are just a few of the more than ninety adverse reactions listed in a

LISTENING TO THE SILENCES

1994 US Department of Health and Human Services report.
  Many dentists continue to insist on filling teeth with a mercury amalgam – which any sweep of the Web will tell you is credited with creating a wide range of undesirable reactions in people, many that grossly and adversely affect the mind and nervous system. In almost every strategy aimed at preserving and improving the physical and mental health of individuals, there is some commercial or vested interest holding back progress or corrupting the strategy for purely financial gain or market domination. Aspartame doesn't exist for the benefit of its consumers, but for that of its parent company and its shareholders – and while it is used in sugar substitutes by those who try to lose weight, listed among the side effects are 'weight gain' and a craving for carbohydrates! As for the continuation of the use of mercury amalgam in the face of mounting evidence against it, I am at a loss to explain or understand.

  What, one wonders, is the purpose of supplying substances that can create "hypothermia, drowsiness, apathy, nightmares, depression, convulsions, impotence, menstrual problems"? Yet these are just a few of the commonly reported side effects of some of the range of drugs that are prescribed for people described as 'psychotic', 'schizophrenic'.
  If one accepts any of my propositions and all of my experience, it will be

realised that no drug ever concocted will cure schizophrenia; no substance will eradicate the voices from the mind or the subtle or blatant imperatives that can flood all of the senses. All of the products that are labelled 'anti-psychotic' will only have the effect of subduing the senses of the individual and rendering it virtually impossible for the intruders to intrude. But do you call that a cure? Exchanging a situation that is capable of being controlled and rendered acceptable, for one in which life can be made intolerable by the very substances that are supposed to *make* it tolerable – is that a 'cure'?

Someone of my acquaintance had a 'psychotic' episode when he was seventeen. He is now in his late forties. *He has never known an adult life free from anti-psychotic drugs.* Yet he knows, yes, *knows*, that what he experiences is of spiritual origin. But even with that knowledge, he cannot face life without what has become a vital prop, and so, increasingly zombified, he has finally left his supportive wife, and taken up residence in a flat where he now 'lives' in his internal mental world that has become more real than the real world.

When will there emerge a movement that is coherent and well founded that will remove much of the care of the mentally disturbed from the dominance of the drug industry and the present almost incestuous world of conventional psychiatry? There was much hope when it was created that the SANE organisation would fill such a rôle, but sadly one learns that it receives substantial funds from drug manufacturers. Early in its existence I wrote to SANE a circumspect letter in which I offered to share my experiences of voice hearing, for I was impressed by the writing and dedication of Marjorie Wallace its founder. I received a reply from an information officer that thanked me for my offer relating to 'my mental illness', and saying that I would be 'put on file'. In my original letter I had made no mention of 'mental illness', yet here I was being categorised by someone who seemingly had no experience of the people and conditions that the foundation was meant to address. This unfortunately is what one may experience from individuals who staff some of the organisations dedicated to helping the 'mentally ill'. It is the use of 'they' when referring to the latter – 'they' seem to be at arms length, not disparagingly, but somehow virtually held at a distance, as if full frontal contact will result in some form of cross contamination. It is, I am sure, not deliberate, but it can be perceived by such as myself, and even though I may be speaking about my own experiences and not remotely suggesting that I am mentally ill.

There must be immense problems for the dedicated worker in the mental health field – of how to provide support and compassion without becoming so involved as to become fully one with 'them'. One would not ask, or even remotely suggest, that carers should become as integrated as did Father Damien in the book

Molokai. Set in a leper colony on an island in the South Seas, the priest tended the spiritual and some of the medical needs of the lepers. His dedication was such that he saw in the wounds and sores of each man and woman the wounds and blood of the suffering Christ. Returning from a brief period away from the island, Father Damien celebrated his first Mass, and when, as he would in the liturgy, he addressed the congregation, he said "We…" – his visit away had confirmed that he, himself, was now a leper, and he was happy that at last he could be truly at one with, and understand fully the people in his spiritual care.

No: that is not in the least appropriate. Nevertheless, the whole of the caring strategy whether exercised by a perceptive individual, or a group dedicated to the care of the mentally disturbed, must be derived from a *human and spiritual* understanding of the causes of the turmoil, and not from a 'chemical' or 'electrical' model of what is believed to be happening within the minds of those who are distressed. All of the present understanding of the workings of the human mind comes from 'without' – it comes via observation of the chemical and electrical functions, with only a minor component deriving verbally from the mouth of the human specimen being examined. But just as the Chinese declare that the observer becomes part of the action, so the processes and equipment used in the study might equally influence the results of the study.

LISTENING TO THE SILENCES

You may recall from earlier in my writing that I described my participation in 1981 in a course run by Bruce Macmanaway in the village of Mickleton in the Midlands. Included in the sessions was one in which we were shown what is called the 'Mind Mirror'. This device was created by Dr Maxwell Cade, and is designed to detect and display the assorted brain waves that emerge from the human skull. Electrodes are attached around the circumference of the head, and connected to a unit that has an array composed of lines of LCDs, with a separate display line allocated to each wave – alpha, delta, etc. I have related elsewhere that Bruce's technique involved identifying nerves in the spine that may have become 'trapped'. Earlier, he had determined that I had three such, at T2, 4 & 6, and, as part of the demonstration, he had me wired up in order that everyone would be able to view any changes that took place in my brainwave pattern as he performed his manipulations. Having been fitted with the electrodes, I sat while Bruce and the laboratory staff described what was being shown in the display on a unit connected to another man.

In the tranquil state in which I was meant to be, I should have shown a high level of alpha waves. But no: I was becoming zombified, and my display showed almost total delta – the brain pattern of deep sleep. Thus, although my eyes were open, and I was aware that discussion was going on, it was all lost to me, and I continued in this trance-like state until I was called to have my back manipulated. I lay prone on the floor and the display was held aloft so that course members would be able to see what, if any, changes occurred in my wave pattern. Bruce's manipulations were remarkably simple, involving firm hand pressure along my spine. Then, disconnected from my display, I returned to my seat, still slightly zombie-like, and gradually emerged into full consciousness. By this time, the whole session had moved on, and I wasn't able to get a coherent description of what, if any, changes had taken place on the Mind Mirror.

However, I was given plenty of sound advice, which was, basically, that I should drink copious quantities of water to eliminate as quickly as possible any toxins that may have been released from a bodily system whose functions had been restored after having been 'distorted' for a lengthy period. The advice was indeed sound, for within a day I began to experience what I likened to the onset of flu without the temperature. While these symptoms passed within two days, the overall effect of the manipulation lasted for many years – possibly even until now - over thirty years. For a long time, almost as long as I could remember, I had been subject to two types of 'anxiety' dream. In the one I was always chased by a large Hereford bull, while in the other I invariably found myself on a high and insecure place – either a building with a crumbling parapet, or a cliff edge that was equally crumbly. Happily, the bull never caught me, although it was pretty close on occasions, and I never fell from the building or cliff.

Following the manipulation, both dreams have never occurred again, and also a minor stomach complaint disappeared. I suspect that my back had suffered stress from my rugby playing days, or had been affected by the 'whiplash' that I experienced when I was in the explosion at sea, and that T6, in particular, had been inadvertently stimulated as I lay in bed, and my dreams had then been woven around the resultant nerve reactions. I shall never know, for those dreams have long since gone. But I do know that the whole sequence has become germane to my analysis of my own reaction to electrical phenomena and the reaction, I suspect, of many individuals who have not had the opportunities for self-analysis or examination that I have had.

There are many occasions when television programmes show studies and research that are aimed at exploring the function of the brain and mind, and where individuals are shown having numerous electrodes attached to their heads, and, on occasions, being slid into 'tunnels' within which a variety of brain scans can be made. I know from my experience with the Mind Mirror of Dr. Cade that the presence of the electrodes would grossly alter the electrical function of my brain, sufficiently to invalidate the readings coming via the electrodes. From an early age, I have been acutely aware that I could sense physically any solid object that was placed a short distance from my forehead and so I also know from this and other of my reactions that I would find the position within the tunnel to be intolerable. I quoted earlier from *The Ion Effect* in which Fred Soyka declared that an estimated forty percent of individuals have a great or extreme sensitivity to electrical phenomena. I have also written from time to time of my own acute sensitivity, which in its turn explained how I reacted and responded in a wide range of circumstances.

Even if the relative sensitivities of individuals were acknowledged, I imagine that it would be most unlikely that measuring techniques could be devised that would be able to define them. Then again, it is difficult to envisage a medical regime that can abandon its 'one size fits all' drug therapies, and that can acknowledge the unique individuality and varied sensitivities of a wide range of people. Not in this exact context, but acknowledging the uniqueness and individuality of someone, I once found myself giving 'sanctuary' to a young woman who just had to escape from the problems that she was experiencing in the town where she lived. I won't even begin to describe her life situation – to do so would take a book of equal length to my own.

'Jane' began a process of recovery in this tranquil and stress free environment. At the time, an ideal place for the continuation of her life change – for that is what it was becoming – seemed to be in one of the Camphill Communities. For those who don't know of them, they are small, mostly rural communities that are usually based in

LISTENING TO THE SILENCES

large houses surrounded by their own grounds. Following the teachings and values of Rudolph Steiner, the establishments house an appropriate number of people with special needs – some being for adults, others for young adults and others for children. These 'special people', as they are termed, are matched in number by dedicated carers, while in the centres specifically for children, the latter live in individual houses as part of the families of carers, who also have a teaching role within the enclosed community.

Jane and I visited three Communities in Scotland, where we also had an interview with the medical director. The latter judged that Jane would be classed in their terminology as a 'special person', and that one or other of the various communities would be suitable for her – but, and a big 'but', – finance. Residents were normally referred by local authorities that then paid the quite considerable fees, and there was no way in which the particular Authority where Jane lived would stump up. Fortunately, she had by then found her spiritual and 'life-style' needs in Buddhism, and eventually left to live in an establishment not far from here. Eventually, her life became ordered, and she is now contentedly married. Phew!

It is amazing how in writing the last three paragraphs that a complete three-year chunk of my life has come back into view, and essentially exemplifies what I am trying to convey. Jane was fully aware that she had problems but was absolutely determined that she would have nothing to do with 'psychiatry'. Practically, I arranged for allergy tests that showed sensitivity to a number of urban and domestic cleaning pollutants; provided her with a sound and plentiful diet; created lots of laughter; brought her into contact with sensitive and caring people – and, biggest hurdle, sorted her benefit entitlement. Friends thought that I was crazy to spend so much time helping someone who was deemed 'odd', but, as I used to tell them, once one understood the extent and origin of her problems, there was no way in which I could have consigned her back to the environment that had created some of them.

Looking back, it can come as a surprise to realise how much I learned from having Jane live here. If I even *begin* to recount it all I shall find myself deep within my second book – Life with Jane. I shall just touch upon one sequence and then move on – it is worth looking at because of what it reveals. Jane had a remarkably short memory span – it wasn't always so, for she had doggedly worked to be able to pass two A-levels. She had reached a state in which she could only read and understand by means of constant re-reading and repetition. She could not remember the beginning of an instruction by the time one had got to the end, and she could not face the prospect of work because of the problems that this would create. If she went into a strange building, say, to go to the loo, she couldn't remember how to find her way out.

LISTENING TO THE SILENCES

Working through a very helpful GP friend, Jane was referred to a Clinical Psychologist (CP), and, now that I am recollecting that time, it is quite amazing how the memory I have of this woman matches so closely that of LW from the early part of my writing. In one important particular, as I have written, LW in his interview found out virtually nothing of note about my life, and only looked at those bits that probably fitted the mental algorithm that he seemed to be working to – I am referring to a copy of CPs final report on Jane as I write. At the time that this was happening I was trying to get Jane enrolled in the County agricultural college, for she had wanted to qualify in horticulture, and the college staff were initially very supportive, in spite of her difficulties. Aware that there might be problems with exams, I tried to speak to CP to ask her to anticipate this and help us to arrange things with the college. She would not even consider the proposition, and 'dismissed' me out of hand.

If she had listened and given me time, what would she have found out that she didn't find out? She would have found out that Jane's father had been sixty-six when she was born, and that her mother, who died when Jane was twelve, had formerly been a Carmelite nun. Jane had no domestic skills – I remember teaching her how to peel an onion – and although she wanted to grow and use herbs, as her mother had done in the convent, she had to be shown how to wheel a barrow and handle a digging spade. At this time she was twenty-one. She was always desperate for fresh air, and spent much of the day walking, and if there was rain, she would walk up and down in a conservatory for at least an hour before bedtime. (One of the difficulties that she had experienced in her home town was that she presented an odd figure as she jogged the roads in areas where she felt that she could breathe and was cat-called and harassed wherever she went.)

Often as she walked these quiet by-roads Jane tried to study and memorise properties of medicinal herbs, for she had to read and re-read to get any fact stuck in her memory. She asked CP whether she might be dyslexic. "Definitely not", came the reply, "you would get your bs and ds mixed up, and anyway it would have been found by now". Acting on an impulse one evening, I covered one of Jane's eyes, and immediately she could read and understand perfectly, and sat with a great grin on her face as she began to read *To Kill a Mocking Bird*. We got a lot of help from the local dyslexic association, and, acting on a further impulse, I spoke to my own optician, who, it turned out, had a dyslexic son, and who was actively working with the people who were studying photoscopic vision. Jane had perfect natural vision, and when she was supplied with Irlen lenses of appropriate hue, her life changed completely. The stresses of her life had caused her to develop double vision, and once she relaxed and her vision was eased, she was able to advance. Nothing was easy, and tempted though I am, I'll not continue with her story.

LISTENING TO THE SILENCES

As with LW, I have to speculate on how it is that someone who was so out of sympathy with the 'humanity' and individuality of the persons who, after all, CP was supposed to be *helping* – how is it that such obviously unsuitable people can be allowed to practice? Again, paralleling the report that LW wrote about me, the one on Jane was *condemnatory**, as if she herself was responsible for her own difficulties, just as his had been about me. There is no point in speculating about how either had entered their professions – maybe that is at the core, namely that these are professions where individuals may be concerned with personal status and promotion and all that that entails, not the *vocation* that the care and 'mending' of disturbed minds should be.

*Extract from report: Having described Jane as manipulative, CP goes on "I could imagine that she will develop more and more symptoms enabling her to keep up the helpless, passive life-style, inviting such an abundance of help from well–meaning friends. Undoubtedly, after some time her friends will feel uncomfortable and manipulated, and she will then experience once more that they will turn away from her.# Undoubtedly these experiences will make her very sad and vulnerable.

…at this point I must admit defeat, and discharge her." Then after referring in the report to a rehabilitation centre that I had pressed for her to attend "…I sincerely hope that she will make better use of her time there".

As I wrote earlier, Jane improved steadily, and after a few hiccups, she married and has since travelled through Europe with her husband on his work, and spent holidays in Sri Lanka and Lhasa in Tibet, where her great joy was to visit the Potala Palace, the 'Mecca' of her Buddhism. I am not relating all of this to demonstrate 'what a good boy, am I', but to bring home, and give emphasis to, my constant, constant plea for everyone who enters any form of mental health care to be seen as an individual. If Jane had got fed into the 'system', as some wanted at the outset, and if she had been fed the standard cocktail of drugs, she would undoubtedly have had all of her talents and will o' the wisp personality destroyed.

Contrary to CP's prediction, Jane's friends stayed and have multiplied in number significantly, but what is more, she was the catalyst for a big increase in the number of my friends, some of whom have turned out to have had a noteworthy influence in my subsequent life, and no small influence on the writing of this book.

There is not much more to say, for writing about Jane and CP has virtually said it. There *has* to be a better way than 'standard' psychiatry and psychology. Practiced from an office or a hospital ward, how possibly can *anyone* find the reality that composes the individual who has been sent for analysis and treatment? The Camphill type community, if not set in country houses, but employed as a model to be adapted

LISTENING TO THE SILENCES

to other locations. The Retreat Hospital in York where the 'reactivation' of the Quaker spirituality is producing wide ranging results. Plus much that can come from the mutual help, mutual support of dynamic groups and extended communities. Perhaps there is something to be learned from the Ugly Club. The *what*? The **Ugly** club. (Which is far, far distant from the so-called 'Mad Pride' concept that some are trying to model on the 'Gay Pride' marches and events.)

I heard of The Ugly Club on the radio this morning. It is an Italian conception (I thought all Italians were beautiful!), and unites ugly people in an organisation of mutual 'support' and appreciation. So successful has it become in its human achievements and camaraderie that people considered good looking are asking to join! I'll leave you with this from the Internet:

June 10, 2001 -- Telesforo Iacobelli is a man with a mission and a strange one at that. For the past 30 years he has championed the cause of the ugly in society. Not normally ranked among the dispossessed in any organized sense, Iacobelli contests the ugly represent a maligned and often misunderstood group. He says he knows of what he speaks: not only is he the president of the Club dei Brutti, or Ugly Club, he counts himself among its charter members.

"I'm ugly and I don't regret it", chimes the bold founder. "It's absurd that people must feel marginalised in society by an aesthetic that is based solely on beauty". Part philosopher, part humorist, Iacobelli pokes fun at our vain culture by presenting the 'No Bel' prize and takes a swipe at American TV soap operas in a campaign called 'Brut-iful' (the name in Italy for The Young and The Restless is 'Beautiful').

Clearly, he has tapped a rich vein with his outspoken beliefs and his unusual antics. Today the club boasts an international presence with more than 20,000 card carrying members. In a country that embraces the ideal of the bella figura, or making the right impression, there is some irony that the Club dei Brutti should have Italy as its base. Indeed, as a major force in fashion, design and aesthetics, Italy may have met its match in the tireless efforts waged by Iacobelli to dismiss and dispel the "cult of beauty".

Truth be told, the man is not one of nature's homelier compositions. His defect, as he sees it, is in having a small nose in a country where broad and long snouts are praised. His own example points to one of the key tenets of the club: namely, ugliness can be as much a factor of how we see ourselves as it is how others see us. "Advertising and popular culture are exclusionary and if you don't fit the mold they promote, you can be made to feel less than you are. That's not right".

The club has brought the topic out of the closet and attracts academics, doctors and sociologists to discuss the plight of the ugly in society. "Beauty is just one aspect in a person's make-up that can affect how they get along in society," says professor Gianni Camattari of the Centro di Psicologia integrata of Milan. "Ugliness, in itself, is not an obstacle to having an active social life or even sex life; the real obstacle is the deep conviction of being ugly, which can be overcome."

Roy Vincent

CHAPTER 14

Seek the beginnings

Learn from whence you came

And the various earths of which you are

made.

Edwin Muir

Roy Vincent

LISTENING TO THE SILENCES

Je suis mois même la matière de mon livre

In the same way that sixteenth century philosopher, Michel de Montaigne could assert that he himself was the 'material' of his book of Essays, so, on reflection, have I myself become the core of mine. When I began to write I had no intention of writing a book – such an idea would have stopped me in my tracks. As with many journeys of exploration, a few tentative excursions revealed territory that invited further examination, and with the examination and exploration courage grew, fuelled by the encouragement that I received from friends. Filled with this new audacity, and inspired by the view that I began to perceive, namely that of ultimate publication, I have gone on and on, arriving at this, which I hope will be my last chapter.

At the very outset, the first words that I wrote were "I am one of the people least likely to write anything remotely autobiographical...", and yet everything, yes everything, is just that. Beginning with descriptions of actual real time happenings, the words have accumulated, and just like a Christmas tree being dressed with care, they form the 'presents' and 'gifts' hanging from it, and that have come from the squirrel store of my garnered lifetime experiences and my understanding of these events. These presents and gifts are there for anyone to take and to use, either for their own benefit or that of others. Even though I have given all that I could from myself, strangely I do not feel diminished, but paradoxically I feel enhanced by the hope that some will find encouragement and incentive.

Perhaps the most intriguing aspect of the self analysis and personal revelation is that, apart from incidents and events that were played out in public situations, by far the greatest bulk of my writing relates to what was going on in my mind. Thoughts and self analysis are there now for all to read – but the spiritual exchanges that have pervaded all of these, and that are with me continuously, what of them? There is no 'cloud' of activity buzzing around my head as is often seen in cartoons, and representing all that is happening within the skull. I don't adopt a particular stance or facial expression. When walking, driving, shopping; when engaged in activities ranging from the most mundane to the most intimate, there is often the inner exchange or intrusion and interjection. And not only into and within my mind, but often silently, mutely, *physically* into and within my body and senses.

Yet I am but one of many billions who inhabit this planet – *an individual* – I repeat – *an individual*. My DNA is unique to me; likewise my fingerprints and the colours in the irises of my eyes. And had I not told you about them, the events that I have related would have stayed within the confines of my mind and memory; silent and also unique to me. Which is why I question so strongly conclusion about mental health and perceived problems of the mind that are addressed through studies of multiples of individuals. I keep returning, sometimes with mild sarcasm or criticism to the analysis of the lives of 50,000 Swedish conscripts, and to the conclusion that have been drawn from their behaviour that allegedly resulted from the use of cannabis. Already the study is being quoted widely in the context that 'smoking cannabis can cause schizophrenia', and with 50,000 men having been studied, the sheer number is taken as giving weight and stature to the results of the analysis. And yet, totally ignored is the fact that drugs such as cannabis, mescaline/peyote are used by shamans and similar 'seers' to induce a physical and mental state in which spiritual intrusion is desired and actively sought. Fear not, it is not my intention to go on and on in detailed scrutiny of other people's work, but rather to use it as a stalking horse to gain access to yet more thoughts of my own.

Where does our uniqueness begin? At birth? Before? In the womb? Before? In his *Healing the Family Tree*, Dr. Kenneth McAll invites one to do just that, to look at the family inheritance to try to find the source of an 'unquiet spirit' that persists in plaguing individuals of subsequent descent, and, in some cases, causing physical and mental illness.

"He (McAll) believes that many supposedly 'incurable' patients are the victims of ancestral control. He therefore seeks to liberate them from this control. By drawing up a Family Tree he can identify the ancestor who is causing the patient harm. He then cuts the bond between the ancestor and the patient by celebrating, with a clergyman, a service of Holy Communion which delivers the tormented ancestor to God."

Many people, myself included, have problems with the conventional representation of "God", yet, in the context in which I am writing, we would do well to ponder the words of psychiatrist William James, who commented, 'We and God have business together: in opening ourselves to his influence our deepest destiny is fulfilled. God is real because he produces real effects.' McAll's book is both informative and provocative, and can lead one to a whole range of speculations. For example, and still considering the influences that can form a person in the womb, he treats of the case of a young man who lived under his mother's protection and feared any relationship not only with women, but with chaplains. Analysis and discussion over a period finally produced the revelation from the mother that while pregnant and continuing her work as a nurse, she had allowed intercourse to take place with one of her patients, an army chaplain.

Many prospective parents play music to their unborn infants by such composers as Mozart, in the belief that there is something sufficiently significant in the music that can influence subsequent development. Who knows? Humans are the only mammals that continue to have sex after conception. This is obviously a conscious choice, and not the result of an evolutionary imperative. Indeed, searching the Web for any comments about 'sex during pregnancy', I was surprised to see how many sites there are, and all promoting the desirability and 'safety' of the practice – even, in one case, into the ninth month. Intercourse and orgasm activate just about every cell within the body, and must obviously communicate *something* to the foetus. Who can say what, and whether it is desirable for the ultimate development of the child?

The emotional state of the mother-to-be in its general sense must be yet another strong influence on the developing child within. I am well acquainted with two people, now past middle age, both of whom were conceived out of wedlock when that was a serious cause for concern, particularly for the girl and her family. Discussion with both provides much insight into lifetime problems that appear to have their origins in that time, and not only during the actual pregnancy, but afterwards. In one, the father appeared to hold deep resentment against his daughter, as unwittingly she had been the cause of his enforced marriage. In the second, the behaviour of the mother towards her son seemed to stem from the fact that she had actually been 'found out' in her misdemeanour, and that he was the constant reminder. One can only imagine what emotions must be coursing continuously through the mind of a girl in the times, seemingly now past, when the disaster of pregnancy struck – emotions that must be communicated to the child within. I remember vividly the comment of one friend in 1951 as we watched someone with whom we were well acquainted as, heavily pregnant, she set off for her wedding. My friend was from a small and traditional Welsh community, and all of her upbringing was contained in her deeply felt and expressed "Oh! The *shame* of it!"

The child of the marriage developed cerebral palsy and I think that it is reasonable to speculate about the possible influence upon it of the state of mind of the mother, and wonder whether this contributed to the child's illness. Her parental home was at the other end of the country, and there was none of the support that would normally have been forthcoming from family in what in those days would have been a trying time. And a Registry Office wedding with four friends would have been vastly different from the wedding that most mothers plan for their daughters and that most daughters anticipate as they grow up. It is interesting to note, and not even remotely suggesting pre-marital conception, of the five children that I am acquainted with who were Down's syndrome, autistic, or had serious developmental problems, all were first born.

I sometimes speculate on what might have been the state of mind of my own mother as she came near to giving birth to me.

LISTENING TO THE SILENCES

My arrival came twenty-two months after that of my brother, and, in giving birth to him, she had come close to dying from a haemorrhage, only being saved by the quick thinking and immediate action of her family doctor who attended the birth. Was she consumed with anxiety as my 'time' came nearer? Did her anxiety communicate to me, and did it make me somewhat pusillanimous as a child?

And what of my father? Apart from his obvious rôle in my procreation, if he had not found two bricks at the urgent insistence of the doctor who had delivered my brother, my mother might not have survived, and I definitely would not be here. The bricks propped up the foot of my mother's bed and helped to reduce her haemorrhage. And he gave me the Vincent genes. Very different from my brother who inherited the Matthews/Fortune variety –making us dissimilar even in something as fundamental as blood group – Bruce being AB while I am O. We grew at different rates until, as we were dressed alike, people took us for twins. But with his age advantage, he could beat me at almost anything – which is probably why to this day I detest board games. However, in another respect, we each had the same early imprint. I have never liked hyacinth flowers in the house – for some reason they always make me think of death. When, in our sixties, my brother and his wife were visiting, we were in a garden centre, and I heard her say "Will this be the year that you let me buy hyacinths?". It seems that he had the same aversion, and he knew, being older, that when our grandfather had died in our home, our mother had brought bowls of flowering hyacinths into the house to disguise any odour. I was about three at the time, and he five.

My brother cried a lot as an infant, and when taking him out in his pram our mother used to hurry to where the trees in Major David's garden overhung the pavement – where he was pacified. The possible connection of this phenomenon and my mother's haemorrhage is something to which I'll return later as I expand my analysis. My present theme develops from an understanding of one of the many points of inheritance that I trace to my father and the Vincent gene. Not the belly that I have developed that matches those of my father, grandfather and Uncle Will; not the wavy hair that was both my pride and problem as I was developing my contacts with 'girls' in my teens. None of those and the other similarities that prompted someone who was asked to guess who I was on one of my return visits to my former home. "Well it's obviously a Vincent", came the first approximation.

From my father came this peculiar body electricity, knowledge of which, in my own case, came to the fore as my personal healing talent became apparent. It is reasonable to assume that the natural healing that he undertook, and that which had been performed by *his* parents, derived some of its force from this inexplicable part of our make up. My grandmother, in particular, was a powerful and much sought healer, and her untimely death that resulted from the effects of an accident was deeply regretted by many at the time. As a minor example, and before the advent of anti-magnetic watches, my father could not wear a watch on his wrist, for they invariably stopped. Whether they ever went again is something that I cannot recall. For me, the knowledge began to provide explanations for certain reactions and sensitivities that I have already alluded to, and which I am going to explore more fully. If you skipped all or part of Chapter 4, this, I am afraid, is where you may have problems. But to help you – and I hope that those who were obedient and read it will be tolerant – I may revisit and reprise some of the earlier points.

    It is impossible to ignore the fact that all life depends for its function upon electro-chemical and bio-electronic processes. You cannot ignore this and say "But I am only interested in the ultimate function, the intelligent processes of the mind, and the psychology of this person, this patient. Why should I even bother to consider any of the internal detail?" The reason is that this person, this patient is a totality – an individual totality; an electrical phenomenon that lives on a huge electrical machine, the earth, and interacts with – *everything*. Robert Becker writes of the *Body Electric* and its complexities, and *Crosscurrents*. Fred Soyka wrote of his mental and medical response to the varying concentrations of electrical ions in the air. Gustav von Pohl described vividly the illnesses, both physical and mental, that affected individuals who slept or worked in locations influenced by geo-electricity, as did Käthe Bachler in *her* seminal work, and as does Rolf Gordon in his book. Becker began his research into the current of regeneration required to mend fractured bones, and ended with a wide analysis of the electrical function of various bodily processes. Along the way he confirmed that the acupuncture matrix that links all parts of the body and brain is, in fact, a series of subtle electrical circuits, and it is with this particular body-brain phenomenon that I will begin.

"But", you may say, "Even if does exist, what possible connection can the acupuncture system have with mental health – and particularly with *spirit intrusion*". Here, and making allowance for simple translation from the original Chinese, are just a few sample conditions that are capable of being treated from various acupuncture points - madness, epilepsy, 'alarm in children', vertigo, sadness, 'stage fright', 'a few days before menstruation cries, depressed anxious and nervous', 'mental stupidity', 'prone to fear and unhappiness', 'wishes to remain at home', 'does not wish to live', 'walks around madly', delirium, insanity, forgetfulness, frequent weeping, 'eyes move wildly', suicidal.

Many in mainstream medicine dismiss acupuncture out of hand; others acknowledge the possibility of a limited rôle in analgesia, while GP friend 'Harry' used to adopt the 'Pavlovian dog' conditioned and immediate response, and come out with dire warnings about 'getting hepatitis from the needles'. Although it is not my intention to write a dissertation on the subject of acupuncture and the relevance to physical and mental health, an acceptance of its significance and an understanding of the complex 'circuitry' interlinking every strand and function of the body, mind and senses, is necessary to be able to follow my argument. In acupuncture treatment, the goal is to try to restore the exquisite balance that should exist between the various parts of the matrix, called meridians, and between the two sides of the body. A corollary is that damage or distortion at the seat of an acupuncture point can act in reverse, so to speak, and has the potential of *causing* the very conditions that would be treated from the point. My purpose at this stage is to suggest various ways in which imbalance may be caused, and then to show how the intelligent sources of spiritual intrusion can exploit the resultant disturbed mind and body for their own inexplicable purposes. But more than that, I believe that this subtle 'circuitry' provides the open door through which other forms of electrical interference enter, and hence widens the range of discomfort and inexplicable unease that can be exploited so easily.

It is very easy to dismiss acupuncture and indeed many other branches of Oriental and Asian medicine as coming from 'primitive' ideas and cultures, and to say that *real* medicine only began in Europe from about the eighteenth century onwards. Anyone with an interest in the inheritance from 'the East' might find *The Genius of China* by Robert Temple to their taste. "3,000 years of science, discovery and invention" are described and analysed. For example, in engineering, the Chinese used techniques for deep drilling for brine and natural gas from before the first century B.C., while in medicine, as well as acupuncture there are early records that demonstrate knowledge of the circulation of the blood and of circadian rhythms.

Before I proceed any further, let me make it absolutely clear that I am not promoting acupuncture *treatment* as a remedy for the sorts of ailments that I am using as examples. However, an understanding of the whole system and its ramifications, and how, in a way, it parallels the distribution of the blood, will help me to develop my proposition. If the flow of blood to any organ or part of the body is inhibited and reduced from its natural level, inevitably disease will result. Regarding the acupuncture system as electrical circuitry carrying minute currents, there are many ways in which the 'resistance' of a circuit can be increased, imbalance caused, and disease created. Remembering that I am an electrical engineer used to dealing with the minute currents that one had to measure in a variety of nuclear installations, certain reactions will be obvious to me that may escape others.

Let me give some actual examples that may serve to illustrate one of the points that I am trying to make. I was helped in the development of my thinking through an encounter with someone who practiced the *electrical* form of acupuncture. Diane used electrical measurements to detect imbalances between the various meridians. At the time that I met her, I had been pondering on the reason why so many women who developed breast cancer did so in the *left* breast. I had been going for some time to assist at one of the centres that offered the 'Gentle Approach' to cancer, and of those who came for my therapy I only met one whose initial cancer was in the right breast. My original thoughts focussed on the wedding ring, for this reason: if an electrical conductor is surrounded by another conductor, then the current in the former will be reduced. Thus, I thought, the wedding ring might inhibit the normal flow in a meridian that has the peculiar name of the 'Triple Heater' meridian, that begins on the ring finger and which is very closely associated with the endocrine system. Might this be the culprit? With Diane's help we first took measurements on a finger, and then repeated them with a ring in place, and found what I had expected – the measurement taken with the ring in place was lowered. The same results were obtained using close fitting metal bracelets, such as expanding wristwatch straps.

I soon had a real demonstration with a woman who had a right breast cancer. As I applied my therapy I pondered 'why?', and then had a potent response. Having comparatively little time with each person, I had devised a strategy that involved touching certain acupuncture points in sequence – sequences that usually concluded with points on the circulation meridians that are found on the wrist. My touching them actively stimulated the circulation and resulted in a feeling of well-being and warmth being felt by the individual. Pulling the sleeves back to locate the points, I found on her right wrist two tight gold chains that "I never take off". The chains had been in place since her teens and she was now in her fifties and they were tight to her wrists, though not so tight that they interfered with the circulation of the blood. Finding my points, which were above the level of the chains, I sat touching both arms for about five minutes. Her final comments as she left me were that she felt a lovely 'glow' throughout herself – except for her *right* hand, which was stone cold. I tried to develop the ideas that I was formulating through discussion with a variety of people, but apart from a passing interest, active support was zero, and one soon gets tired at pushing at 'closed door' minds.

I first became aware of the possibility of a connection between 'acupuncture' and mental health in relation to Alzheimer's disease. I had never actually thought about the condition until I saw on television a film called "Do You Remember Love?" It was a sympathetic depiction of the development of dementia in a middle-aged American woman university lecturer. At the time I could only name two individuals who had died from Alzheimer's. One was the film star Rita Heyworth, and the other was someone from the village in which I had formerly lived. Apart from being female, they had one important feature in common – they had both been dancers. The local woman had been a ballet dancer and had continued with dancing as she taught many young aspirants in our district. The thought that came to me on seeing the film and thinking about the two women, was that damage to the feet of a dancer is likely to occur frequently. This would be particularly so in someone who regularly dances on points, and bearing in mind that for many girls the urge to become a dancer develops early, when dedicated practice can soon distort feet that are still being formed. And so, unlikely though it may seem, I am proposing a link between damage to the feet and damage to the brain.

I shall include diagrams of the feet in the final section in which I shall give other references. It will be a short section and so easy to print and refer to while reading this discussion. The meridians are named for the organs of the body, but are not specific to those organs when treating ailments. Those involved on the feet are: Spleen, Sp; Liver, Liv; Stomach, S; Kidneys, K; Gall, G; Bladder, Bl. I have listed only those points that are relevant to my argument, and would point out that while some of the conditions listed are not specific in the terms used in Western medicine, the descriptions are appropriate to my proposition.

Liver (Liv) 1   Unconsciousness, fainting, 'appearance as though dead', headaches.

Liv 2   Headache, head dizzy, insomnia, angry easily, hysteria, madness, insanity, epilepsy, fits, convulsions in children, neurasthenia.

Spleen (Sp) 1   Madness, little children cantankerous.

Sp 2 Agitated, melancholic.

Sp 3 Mad, agitated, melancholic.

Stomach (S) 40 Throat numb, cannot speak, madness, 'sees ghosts', laughs madly.

S 41 Vertigo, madness, fits, convulsions in children, incoherent speech, frightened, agitated.

S 42 'Wants to undress in public', wanders around aimlessly, 'every month madness'.

S 44 Melancholic, fear and trembling, nightmares, 'dislikes the human voice'.

S 45 Fainting, cerebral anaemia, 'like a corpse', deviation of mouth, dementia, insomnia, neuropathy.

Kidney (K) 1 Fainting with cold limbs, prone to fear, madness, epilepsy, alarm in children, paralysis, pain in head and nape of neck, eyes dizzy, vertigo, hypertensive ecephalopathy. (The position of K1 is on the plantar surface of the foot, almost below and two centimetres proximal to Liv 2).

Point A is on the second toe, adjacent to Liv 2; it is not a classical point but has been added by more recent research. One could use it to treat 'articular degeneration of the atlas/axis joint'.

Other vulnerable locations are at the ankles where one might encounter either physical damage or the commonly observed 'going over' at the ankle. Acupuncture points that could become activated in these circumstances, together with relevant maladies are:

Bl 62 Madness, epilepsy, dizziness, occipital neuralgia, tension headaches, spastic conditions of the uterus.
The symptoms of many diseases of the spinal cord can be helped, though not cured, in the early stages of the disease, by this point.

G 39 Cerebral haemorrhage, hands and feet uncoordinated, throat numb, chorea, neurasthenia, madness, fear, bad temper. (Specialised point for bone marrow, leucocytosis).

In 1997 I responded to a broadcast on BBC radio 4 in which the discussion centred on the high proportion of professional footballers who were contracting and dying from Alzheimer's disease. The natural conclusion of the programme contributors was that it was heading the ball that probably caused the onset of dementia. My own assessment, based on the arguments above, was that equally with heading the ball, foot, ankle and shin damage are the most likely injuries sustained by footballers. Nervous depression, insanity, 'suddenly becomes mad' are just three relevant conditions that could be treated from points on the lower leg. I also pointed out that of the inmates of a ward for demented women where I used to visit a friend, very few were likely to have headed footballs. A patient in Lancaster Moor Hospital, my friend had chosen to be placed in this particular ward because she found it to be quieter than the one that normally housed women with her range of problems. Of the women in the ward, one stood out in the context of my argument. About sixty years old, she walked around incessantly in stocking feet, revealing the most distorted bunions that one could possibly see. The big toe on each foot crossed the others virtually at right angles – Liv 2, K 1 and Point A being the three most likely to sustain damage.

Visiting someone else in my local hospital, someone who was a patient in the geriatric ward, I overheard the nurse who was issuing medication say to one woman, who appeared to be marginally demented, that if she took her medication 'the voices would go away'. Did the dementia result from hearing the voices, or did the voices manifest as the mind became

LISTENING TO THE SILENCES

disturbed? Somewhat 'chicken and egg' it would seem.

As I have mentioned, scars from operations, trauma resulting from such as fractures and scar tissue left after accidental damage are all potent sources of imbalance in the meridians and possible causes of seemingly unrelated ill health. Scars created during hysterectomy have always struck me as major sources of a range of adverse conditions. While she did not have an actual hysterectomy, Esther, whom I wrote about much earlier, had a near equivalent in terms of scarring. You may recollect that she had a malignant tumour at the base of her brain, and prior to having radiation treatment along the whole length of her spine, her ovaries were relocated to minimise the possibility of her becoming sterile. On one of my visits, she agreed to let me photograph her abdomen with the relevant acupuncture points marked on it – you will find the picture in the final chapter as 'Esther 1'. Apart from the point at the right of the picture that I missed because she was laughing so much, all of the others marked are in true locations. As you will see, several lie directly along the line of the incision and the scars. What the long-term effect might have been I shall never know, for she died a year later. The points are associated with many vital female functions and the resultant emotions, and their disruption may account for some of the emotional trauma experienced by a proportion of women following hysterectomy. If the incision is made vertically up the abdomen it will be seen that several points would be affected, points for treating a similar range of ailments to the ones that I have mentioned, with the significant addition of one that would be used when 'the patient wants to die'.

Esther also had deep exploratory surgery at the back of her neck in the vicinity of the tumour; surgery that produced scars through a number of major acupuncture points, one of which could be used to treat meningitis. The fact that she died from meningitis gives me food for thought.

Living where I do, frequently I have visitors coming to stay, and inevitably I drive them around the district, for there is so much to see and so many places of interest to visit. Many of our routes run through the neighbouring valleys and dales, where the roads are very narrow, with acute bends and hills, moving through woods, past rivers, lakes and mountain waterfalls. At every bend of the road there is a new vista, and often we stop and the scene is viewed with an artist's eye, or that of a photographer, fell walker or angler - and the actual journey becomes as interesting as is the ultimate destination. After reading some of my writing, one of my visitors likened it to a recent trip that we had made in the car. She said that although she knew what our intended destination was, the journey with its variety and many facets was equally delightful and she looked forward to returning to each of our intermediate points for a longer and more comprehensive visit.

With my friend's comments in mind, let me try to define for you what I plan to be the ultimate goal of this episode. In earlier chapters, I have described the variety of ploys used by spiritual intruders that I have identified, and I have referred to the varying circumstance in which the ploys are most successful in having a disturbing effect upon me. I have tried to demonstrate the fact that both the type of ploy used, and its coincidence with the undermining effects of external phenomena, show that the strategies derive from an intelligent source. Having referred in earlier chapters in an almost piecemeal way to the wide range of phenomena that cause disturbance, my plan now is to try to bring them together into a coherent whole. As I have commented earlier in the book, one cannot prevent the different winds from blowing, nor stop the moon in its track, nor yet eliminate earth currents, but one can minimise the emotional and other disturbance with the knowledge that the influence is outside oneself, that the effects will be transient, or can be avoided, and that one is not intrinsically mentally ill.

If you have looked ahead to the final chapter in order to see the illustrations of the feet that are there, you may be wondering, and justifiably so, why there is a photograph of Esther's back, and several of nude models. Why, also, is there a drawing of a horse? It was the drawing of the horse in a book on equitation, and what it actually represents, that opened my eyes to the facts that I am next going to write about, and explains why the other pictures are also there. Anyone who has been involved in the initial training of a young horse will have become aware of one salient detail. The training usually begins with the horse being worked on a circle at the end of a lunge rein – a single long rein that connects the noseband on the horse to the trainer who stands at the centre of the ring. Once the horse has got used to the situation it is always found that it proceeds amicably and freely in one direction, but is reluctant to go in the other, and often tries to break back and circle in the direction in which it was comfortable.

Those who farm red deer soon learn that the pens used to corral the deer have to be constructed with a clockwise lead, otherwise the deer will not 'herd'. Likewise sheep being gathered move calmly on a clockwise curve, and break away if turned anticlockwise. If you watch horse racing you probably will have noticed that when horses are galloping on a straight, they are actually running with their hindquarters offset to one side of the direct course. Likewise if you see a long dog approaching you on a straight path, you will undoubtedly see that its hindquarters are also offset. My good friends Tricci and Peter have over 150 milk cows. For record and identification purposes the cows have a number tattooed on one hip, and for some perverse reason, it is always on the cows right hip. Perverse, according

LISTENING TO THE SILENCES

to Tricci, because almost every time she has to find a particular cow by its number, the animal is lying down with the right hip underneath.

In other words, as far as it is possible to observe free-ranging mammals, they all have a lateral curve as shown in the illustration of the horse. When animals in the wild appear on TV, I always keep one eye open for any evidence of the curve, and my greatest find was in a programme about orang-utans. Centre stage was a venerable and solitary male, and as I watched, and it moved away from the camera down a straight path, plainly seen was the curve in the spine and a slightly asymmetrical walk or shuffle that matched it.

Humans are mammals, and it is not very long in evolutionary time since we were quadrupeds. And yes, humans are born with a lateral curve. There are many ways in which it can be confirmed as I shall illustrate, although for reasons that appear to follow from our 'domestication', some curve to their left and are left–handed, while the majority curve to their right and are right-handed. The two models are right-handed and are standing or sitting in a relaxed manner, and no doubt believing that they are upright. I took Esther's photograph shortly before she began the radiation therapy along her spine. She wanted to see where the radiographers had made their marks when planning her treatment. Esther was lying completely prone and relaxed, and was left-handed. I am right-handed, and will list the observable features for a right-hander.

The most obvious is the left shoulder, which is higher; the left breast, also. If a shoulder bag or satchel is carried, it is almost invariably on the left shoulder. I have heard people say "My left shoulder is higher because I carried my school bag on it". The *reverse* is actually true – that shoulder was chosen because it was already higher, and the bag lodged on it more securely than the other.

Ballroom dancers follow the majority handedness and always circle anti-clockwise, likewise skaters on a rink, although solo figure skaters usually demonstrate their handedness, left-handers going clockwise, and making their jumps, toe-loops and spins also in a clockwise direction. The most obvious difference between the two 'hands' is usually not readily observed, and is only ascertained by asking the question "How do you wipe your bottom?" – guaranteed to produce an interesting reaction at a dinner party! There are two schools of bottom wipers – those who reach through between the thighs, and those who reach around behind. *Right*-handers who reach through, use the *left* hand, and as right-handers are in the majority, the left hand became the 'cack' hand. It is much more obvious in the situation where one does not use a toilet seat, but crouches down to defecate; the curve of the body makes the left-handed reach through of a right-hander more convenient, and vice versa. (Conversely, reaching around behind for a right-hander is much more easily accomplished with the *right* hand.)

LISTENING TO THE SILENCES

As the body curve determines one's stance when throwing or when holding a sword and shield, the left foot comes forward, the shield is naturally held in defence on the left arm, while the sword is most easily wielded with the right hand. From this fighting posture, the sword hand became the 'noble' one, and the left with its anus cleaning association, the 'dishonourable' hand. Many books and articles have been written on the subject of handedness, and if I did not have to limit my discussion after introducing the topic and showing how it fits into my main theme, I could no doubt write another, for I have been making these observations for nearly thirty years.

I have never seen any reference to the natural body curve in humans, whether in relation to handedness, or in any other context. So, remember, you read it first here, and as the explorers of old named islands, rivers and mountains after themselves, I shall name the curve "The Vincent Anomaly, Asymmetry, or Curve", and claim my rightful place in posterity!

The views of the models' backs illustrate my reason for including them, and including them particularly within the total context of body asymmetries and differential stresses. Far from them having the smooth continuous curve that is seen in quadrupeds, the upright stance adopted by humans has served to divide the spine into a series of 'chords' of curves. The lumbar spine is rigid, and has very little noticeable curve, although when observed in actual people whom I have studied, the intersection between the lumbar and thoracic vertebrae has been anything up to 3 cms off the centre line. "Sit up straight", "Stand up straight" – these are the commands one heard as a child, and so we attempted to comply, and caused a discontinuity between Thoracic 12 and Lumbar 1 vertebrae. The thoracic spine has a more noticeable and smoother curve, until it enters another discontinuity at the intersection with the cervical spine, where again attempts to obey the commands to sit or stand upright result in a kink.

A spine that has more than its fair share of problems belongs to a young woman of my recent acquaintance. As she was being born her chin became caught on the inside of her mother's organ and she was bent severely backwards – there was no spare theatre for a caesarean section, and so there was a lot of cutting and pulling. 'Vicky', now a young adult, has a number of emotional and behavioural problems some of which seem to stem from her difficult birth, and are particularly appropriate in the context in which I am writing. Her spine has the most peculiar double-jointed connection between the lumbar and thoracic elements, where there are two adjacent acupuncture points, one of which may be used to treat insanity and epilepsy. It also coincides with a point that has importance in Japanese medicine, and where treatment would be applied 'to stimulate heart action, the kidneys, aorta, peritoneum and brain'.

LISTENING TO THE SILENCES

There are other factors that take one back to where I wrote about the influences that can be created *before* the birth, and which might result from the stresses that can be created from pre-marital conception. This was the situation with Vicky's parents, and a reluctant bridegroom seems to have turned into a reluctant father, whose negative influence upon his daughter may add to those problems that seem to stem from the physical difficulties that I wrote about above. It is equally feasible that the stress of the pregnancy upon the mother may have been at the root of the difficulties experienced at the time of ultimate delivery.

One does not have to watch TV for very long before one can observe the results of these asymmetries and imbalances in the speakers in front of one. TV gives a major advantage to the observer of human behaviour in that it allows individuals to be studied when they believe that they are behaving normally, and they can be stared at without embarrassing them or oneself. Many times I turn off the sound so that I can watch posture and expression without the distraction of the actual words. The slant of the shoulders and sometimes of the whole body, the breasts at different levels, the obliquity of the neck, and the tilt of the head are all there to be seen, and I can indulge in my personal guessing game of trying to decide if a person is left or right handed.

At the base of the neck, and where the neck meets the skull at the atlas joint, there are acupuncture points that may be used to treat a number of serious 'mental' and 'nervous' conditions. Among the ailments listed are: hysteria, paralysis, limbs and body not coordinated, 'St. Vitus's Dance', convulsions, epilepsy, neurasthenia, vertigo, 'walks around madly', 'eyes move wildly', suicidal. At the junction between the thoracic and lumbar vertebrae there is a point that may be used to treat – madness, epilepsy, anorexia.

I derive personal benefit from the results of my observations when I want to achieve total relaxation. I lie supine on a firm surface in a posture resembling what Yoga practitioners call 'The Corpse', in which they try to lie symmetrically about a centre line. Instead of trying to be symmetrical, I next arrange my body in a gentle curve from the top of my head to my feet, keeping my coccyx in place as my 'reference' point. Being right-handed, the curve is concave to my right, and my head and feet are approximately 15 cms removed sideways from the original straight posture. The relaxation that I achieve is far superior to that gained when I simply lie symmetrically.

Returning briefly to the rôle and status of acupuncture therapy, it is not something that can be dismissed, treated casually, or 'learned' in a weekend 'workshop'. I have had treatments from two practitioners of Traditional

LISTENING TO THE SILENCES

Chinese Acupuncture. I went to them partly for prophylactic purposes and also to be able to experience the practice at first hand. Their training had been full time over three years, and had included half a year in China. In both cases, my first visit lasted well over an hour, and involved the most thorough analysis, testing and assessment that I have experienced in any form of medicine, apart from when my eyes were examined recently. As I recall, and for my own purposes, I went continuously for about ten weeks to each practitioner, and was impressed by the thoroughness of the practice. And contrary to 'Harry's' dire warnings of hepatitis infection, the needles were either brand new from a sealed packet, or direct from the local hospital surgical sterilisation unit. For my own reference I use a book by Dr. Felix Mann – *The Treatment of Disease by Acupuncture* – his *Atlas of Acupuncture*, and *Acupuncture Therapy* by Dr. Mary Austin. The last one came out in paperback, but as it excluded much from the hardback that I considered invaluable, I would not recommend it. The Mann book also has different editions, the 1974 that I have being fully comprehensive. There are undoubtedly later works by different authors, but the ones that I have cited have filled all of my requirements.

"Imagine a perfect skeleton" my physiotherapist friends were instructed during their initial training – and yet many years experience has told them that there is no such thing. "No one has a symmetrical face, and children's faces are the *most* asymmetrical" – so said my optician. Television, again, offers many opportunities for observing faces, with asymmetries ranging from the slight whimsical twist to the mouth, to the face that resembles a comma. Conversely, I have many opportunities for looking at the heads of animals – sheep, cattle and deer - where the horns and lugs stick out with complete symmetry. There are many reasons why the variations occur in humans, and there are a significant number of acupuncture points affected, points that could used to treat a variety of nervous and 'mind' conditions. I have identified a number of 'thought patterns' that over time can create some of the asymmetries, and in the fullness of my analysis in this book they have a significant place. Hopefully I shall be able to put them into a coherent form and include them later in this chapter.

A persistent pattern of thought that occupies the mind for large parts of the waking life can create both body and facial twists and tensions, and over time can produce a wide variety of diseases. I have already described in an earlier chapter the way in which deep concentration can result in very limited breathing, and how this state can be created and exploited by various intruders into the mind. The very prolonged inner tension that results from personal distress such as occurs during emotional trauma can both be created and exploited by adverse intrusions, although *they* were not specifically involved in the very recent illness of a close friend, while prolonged emotional stress was. Her malignant breast lump was directly in the site of a significant acupuncture point – significant in that it is classed as a 'Judo knock-out point'. It occurred in the left breast at the point labelled Kidney 23, which is in the sixth intercostal space and about half-way between the sternum and the nipple. Among the ailments that could be treated here are: 'cannot breathe', ulcer of breast, tumour of breast, anorexia, spasm of *rectus abdominus*. This last muscular 'lock' is something that I have identified in myself during periods when I had been held in deep speculation or concentration by *them*, and when my breathing had been so shallow as to be virtually still.

My persistence in following aspects of the acupuncture system is justified when one begins to interpret interaction with external sources of electrical stimulus. The analysis by Dr. Becker that demonstrated that acupuncture meridians behave like minute electrical conductors, takes one into a new realm of speculation. A moment's examination of your radio, TV or mobile phone will reveal the presence in each of an aerial. From the simple piece of wire or rod, to the more elaborate digital dish, they all have one purpose – to intercept 'electricity' from the air, from the ether. The original term 'Wireless' for the now more common 'radio' says it all – the 'wire less' connection between source and receptor. Everything 'electrical' that travels through the air does so as 'electromagnetic waves'. Most transmissions are intentional, as in communication, entertainment and radar, or are accidental or adventitious as are the electromagnetic fields that occur around electrical conductors such as overhead power lines, or in the proximity of electrical equipment, machines or apparatus. In this environment the acupuncture meridian behaves as an aerial, and, by a process known as 'induction', becomes activated with its own current.

All waves have a frequency and wavelength – i.e. how many occur in a given time, and the distance from peak to peak. Normal household electricity has a frequency of 50 cycles per second – known as 50 hertz – and a very long wavelength. Modern radar and communications transmissions have frequencies of many millions of hertz - megahertz – and very short wavelengths, as low as millionths of a metre. In his book *Electromagnetic Man*, Dr. Cyril Smith describes how the wavelengths of some of these latter transmissions are of the same dimension as the cells of the body. He then describes how the intrusion of the radiation into the body can have a significant impact on the normal functioning of the whole nervous system sufficient to cause it to malfunction and produce physical and mental illnesses.

I have illustrated how the acupuncture meridians can become distorted and restricted sufficiently to vary the electrical resistance and cause an imbalance within the system with resulting illness. This is one of the reasons why I have discoursed so widely on the subject of acupuncture. Apart from his analysis of the interference at cellular level, I don't think that Dr. Smith considered the mechanism through which the effects were created. I would find it very difficult to be specific about the 'mechanism' through which the motor neurone disease of the other Dr. Smith, my late friend Sandy, was caused. Having measured the electromagnetic field in which he sat for many hours in his consulting room, there is no doubt in my mind that that was the cause of, or at the very least, a major contributory factor in the creation of his illness. Strong em fields featured in the daily lives of others with M.N.D. of whom I have been told – a man who spent a large part of each day operating a circular saw and another who was a professional wood turner, both men standing with a high-powered electric motor less than a metre from their abdomen. Was the field from electrical under floor heating involved in the death from M.N.D. of the close relative of one of my friends? Was the same type of heating a factor in the causation of leukaemia of one person, and the severe depression of another, both living locally?

There is sufficient evidence that will, if examined without prejudice, implicate electrical fields from numerous sources in the creation or aggravation of many ailments of the human nervous system. I sometimes speculate on the possible adverse effects of these same fields upon a developing foetus. If a pregnant woman sleeps under an electric blanket, or if she works at an industrial sewing machine where the motor is very close to her womb – what then? Is the subsequent development of the infant affected? Is there permanent change caused to its nervous system? Is there the potential cause of future mental health problems? I grew up without electricity – our house had only gas, and apart from the work with the naval radar, I had minimal exposure until I reached twenty-five. Even for homes that had electricity, the occupants had only a little exposure themselves, for apart from a radio and possibly a very basic washing machine, the sources that would create em fields would have been few.

Reviewing these times with my brother, we find it difficult, if not impossible, to recollect *anyone* of our acquaintance, adult or child, who had anything resembling the nervous and mental problems that beset many individuals today. We knew someone who became depressed and was hospitalised when abandoned by her husband coincidentally with the menopause, but only the one. No one amongst our school and teenage contemporaries exhibited any of the common problems of hyperactivity, depression, self-harm, suicide even, which trouble today's youth. There were the 'dunces' of course, and we speculate on whether they were the dyslexics of our day. Asthma was rare, maybe non-existent; some kids had the inevitable nits, and some had ringworm, while most of us went through mumps, measles and chickenpox. We were spared the effects of too much electricity in that we did not have television, computers, play stations and mobile phones – we played 'out' instead. We were spared the junk foods and all or most of the food additives – all of the E numbers that constitute so much of today's diet. Maybe the rose-coloured spectacles are working overtime, but truly, our lives had a happy 'simplicity', until the war came and changed the situation – although it made our diet even more basic.

As I wrote earlier, the effect of ambient conditions upon the developing foetus cannot be ignored when assessing the nervous and mental problems of the adult. Something that is insidiously present and potentially harmful is the 'geo-electricity' that I have referred to in earlier chapters. I was briefly acquainted with one young woman who had developed muscular dystrophy at a very early age. While her mother was pregnant with her, the marriage was breaking up, and, as has been ascertained later, the parents slept in a location that was subject to severe geo-pathic influence, itself possibly a potent contributor to the aggravation between the parents. In yet another situation I used to join a friend when she baby-sat for her daughter who lived in a mobile home. Her grandson would cry incessantly, and struggled and struggled in his cot, pushing against the side with such effort that he developed a hernia. This is 'classical' behaviour of an infant that is put to sleep where geo-electricity has a strong influence, as was the behaviour of the mother who became strongly verbally aggressive to my friend. Both the mother and the child became tranquil when they moved shortly afterwards. The behaviour of the two should be borne in mind by anyone considering the causes of 'shaken baby syndrome', for the incessant crying of the infant and the aggravated and provoked state of the parent together make an explosive mixture that often has fatal consequences for the child.

Käthe Bachler was a schoolteacher in Austria who became concerned that certain children in her classes did not achieve the potential of which she new they were capable - children who were often uncharacteristically disruptive. Becoming aware of the phenomenon of geopathic stress, and being taught by an experienced dowser, she began a programme of surveying and analysis of the classrooms that she used, and found, almost without exception, that the under-performing and disruptive children sat in badly stressed locations. Her book *Earth Radiation* describes her work and its consequences – consequences that, for example, resulted in the children being moved regularly in their seating so that no child spent long in the undesirable locations. Her work was treated seriously by the education authorities and formed the basis for her further research and grants under the auspices of the Pedagogical Institute in Salzburg, for whom she produced her "Research into the connections between geopathic zones of disturbance and academic failures in school children".

LISTENING TO THE SILENCES

It is almost worth reading the book for one entry alone. This is a commendation from the then Archbishop of Salzburg, who, after commenting favourably on Ms. Bachler herself, wrote:
"…With her dowsing instruments she can find the 'good places' and has thus helped many people including several priests and nuns of our archdioceses." After giving cautions about the misuse of the 'divining' gift, the Archbishop continued "…If however a Christian wants to do God's will and protects himself with prayers when doing radiaesthesic works and uses his or her instruments only in a helping way, based on love, when examining houses and finding water, then this work is blessed by the Church. In this sense I can recommend unreservedly and warmly the work of Ms Käthe Bachler, and especially her book…".

The commendation does two things – it acknowledges the existence of the phenomenon and the use of dowsing to locate good and bad places, and, importantly in the overall purpose of my book, it acknowledges the potential for 'evil' work and the existence of the spiritual component in dowsing. The Bachler book itself contains many authenticated case studies and analyses – and is unfortunately now very rare. The last time that I searched the Web I found a site where someone was proposing a reprint. If you are interested, I suggest that you search using just the author's name. Emphasis is usually placed upon the 'bad', the stressed zones;

however, it is important that one should remember that there are others that are specifically good, and can create well-being. I am fortunate that quite by chance I have found such a place to live, and remember well the comments of Bruce Macmanaway when he dowsed the house for me – they were to the effect that if anyone was actually seeking somewhere to practice healing work, they would be hard put to find somewhere better. Most of my visitors relax on arrival and almost all invariably have excellent sleep. Left to themselves, animals will find places that feel good to them – on some farms there are even recognised places where female animals will go to give birth - although it is well recorded that *cats* are happiest in places that are harmful to humans.

I came to the field of 'earth currents' as a sceptic – that is until I experienced the reality of them for myself. First in the home of my friend John whose leukaemia developed during the time that he slept in the bed in which I found it impossible to sleep – the fact that his first marriage broke down when that had been the marital bed came as no surprise. Then in the flat where Esther lived with her partner, and at the head of the bed beside which no plants thrived, where I felt distinctly nauseated and where the pair woke following 'teeth grinding nightmares', 'with a heavy weight on the chest', 'feeling very depressed', where Esther developed a brain tumour – and which all changed when the bed was moved, although far too late for Esther, who sadly died. And again in the home of my cousin in Carlisle, where my own reaction was to experience severe backache, and where my cousin developed crippling muscular rheumatism – for which the only remedy seemed to be steroids and more steroids – and I curse when I recollect the sight of this lovely, caring woman bending more and more forward as her spine disintegrated and she could no longer breathe, and died. (When I wrote of my cousin in an earlier chapter I also noted that the friend with whom she shared the house had developed persistent and aggravating teeth grinding, which is commonly experienced in geopathic places, and that the friend's dog would not remain in the badly stressed room, which again is typical.)

I feel considerable anger when I reflect that there are so many serious physical and mental illnesses whose origins may be traced to a variety of electrical, electromagnetic or simple magnetic influences, and when I realise that there appears to be no coherent or coordinated research into these phenomena. In his book *Chemical Victims*, Dr. Richard Mackarness refers to the 'Society for Clinical Ecology' that had been founded in 1965. The society worked for an understanding of the influence of food and environment upon the health of individuals, but seemingly, unless the objectives have changed, restricted to the influence of substances. My concern is that that is only a part of the total picture, a picture that will not be nearly complete until the electrical environment in all its aspects is added to the 'chemical'.

Within the last twenty-four hours I have had a potent demonstration of how the whole planet is, in fact, a 'whole' and that 'no one is an island'. Yesterday (21 May 2003) I said to a friend that because of the way that I felt, I expected there to be an earthquake soon. This morning the news bulletins were full of descriptions of an overnight major earthquake in Algeria. Several things had come together in my perception. The first was the way that I felt, which is very difficult to describe except to say that there was something 'electrical' going on that past experience has shown me is associated with a major earthquake or volcanic eruption *somewhere* in the world. The second 'notification' came from the poor performance of my television, in that several normally reliable satellite channels were playing up, while terrestrial channel reception was fragmented. Thirdly, the disposition of the moon and major planets in combination was likely to contribute to significant variations in the 'pull' upon the earth – often coincident with an earthquake or eruption.

I did not write that to demonstrate that somehow I have 'extrasensory' powers or anything of the sort, but rather to indicate that, to someone who is in tune with his environment, subtle changes may be sensed, changes that experience can allocate to a source. But just as a particular radio signal may be masked by all of the noise and chatter over the airways, so the effects that I have referred to are easily masked by all of the pollution experienced in urban and industrial living. When I was still in work, I might possibly have gone to the medical department with a complaint that would have been recorded as 'general malaise', and been content with an analgesic of some sort. In times past I may have believed that the analgesic had 'worked wonders', whereas the *actual* cause of my discomfort had simply moved away.

The whole episode illustrates why I continue doggedly – almost obsessively – describing and analysing the various natural phenomena. From my experience, observation and subsequent analysis I *know* that there are many individuals who respond in a similar manner, but who, not knowing the cause of *their* 'general malaises', might become disturbed. This may be particularly so for those who are undermined or distressed in different ways, who just might be pushed 'over the edge' by feelings that they cannot understand. Certainly I know that such times and occasions are fully utilised by the intelligent intruding entities to aggravate and provoke in the ways that I have described earlier. Equally I know that there is no medication yet devised that will have any real effect on the sufferer. The children studied by Käthe Bachler were not aware that they were being studied and so did not 'jump through hoops' that were held for them; the plants in Esther's flat reacted without prompting, as did the dog belonging to by cousin's friend; the female animals seeking good places to give birth were doing so because it felt good, and not for any other reason that might spring to mind.

Geo-electricity exists – of that there can be no question. The real question is - when will the reality be accepted by mainstream medicine and psychiatry, and then be incorporated into an understanding of the rôle that geopathic stress plays in the causation of many illnesses of the body and mind? Much damage has been caused by the blurring of the reality and actuality of a true electrical/electromagnetic phenomenon with another reality – the 'ley-lines' of Alfred Watkins. As I have written, the name 'ley-lines' has been hi-jacked by those who are intent upon surrounding the two phenomena with magic and mystery. In the context in which I am writing I beg you to abandon and forget any link that you may have had in your mind with 'ley-lines', and accept and work with the reality that is geo-electricity and the *observable* evidence of its presence. The fact that dowsing is the easiest way of locating earth currents discourages many people; if this is so in your case, I suggest that you should re-read the statement from the former Archbishop of Salzburg, Dr. Karl Berg, a statement of understanding and approval that would not have been issued lightly.

The harm caused by geo-electricity may be due to direct 'radiation' or to the fact that the desirable negative ions are repelled from the zone, with a consequent high concentration of positive ones. When I wrote earlier linking my mother's haemorrhage and my brother's incessant crying, this is what I had in mind. The house in which they lived and in which my brother had been born had been built on land that had been reclaimed from a fresh-water marsh that was still influenced by the surges of the water in a nearby tidal inlet. I speculate that there remained underground aquifers that created the currents and a resultant pos-ion concentration. Referring to the *Ion Effect* book, failure of blood to clot with resulting haemorrhages, and incessant crying of infants are two common results of such a concentration. My brother ceased crying when he arrived under the overhanging trees – trees that are well-known creators of negative ions, and a pleasant relaxed feeling – witness the pictures one can often see of Chinese practicing T'ai Chi out of doors and almost invariably under trees.

Käthe Bachler wrote exclusively about underground water. Gustav von Pohl accepted the other major generator of earth currents – the rotation of the earth itself. Rolf Gordon in *Are You Sleeping in a Safe Place?* illustrates the 'Curry Grid' and the 'Hartmann Grid' - two groups of 'force lines' that are created by the rotation of the earth, and he and von Pohl both give details of case studies reflecting the types of malady that result from time spent in the adverse zones. Von Pohl also describes other observable effects that result from the presence of strong earth currents – effects discernible in the growth of trees and the striking of lightning. He illustrates how certain trees are stunted and die, while other species thrive, or yet others grow lopsidedly in an effort to avoid the harmful zone. I had a practical demonstration of this effect in one of my own pine trees. Its growth where it left the ground was almost horizontal, recovering in a long curve then to grow upwards. Because all of the other trees – probably planted 150 years ago – are sturdy and upright, I conclude that they were all looked after properly, and that the twisted growth was an aberration. The significance became very obvious when I had my field dowsed at the time that I was planning to have my borehole sunk. The dowser's reaction as he passed over the line that we ultimately chose was most remarkable to see as he and his twig vibrated violently. The line passed under the original planting of the pine tree, and it now became obvious that the tree had tried to grow away from it. Directly across a narrow minor road that skirts my field and where the line of the aquifer continues, there is a gap in the hedge where nothing will grow, although the rest of the hedge flourishes

Von Pohl declares that lightning strikes most frequently at the point where two of the grid lines cross. This effect was dramatically observable in a house that I have visited several times. My original visits were to a friend who lived there. As a widow, she had married someone whose wife had died of cancer while living in this particular house. In time, her new husband developed cancer and died, while she herself experienced a recurrence of cancer, having been cured of an earlier attack, of which she had been declared free for several years. Quite by chance I became acquainted with the new occupants of the house, and visited them on a number of occasions. It was during one of these visits that I felt the same unpleasant internal reactions that by this time I associated with geopathic stress. Some little time later, I was told of a remarkable lightning strike – their dog, while in the kitchen, had suddenly become very distressed, and shot out into the garden, when, moments later, the house was struck and a strong flash flew from the light fitting in the kitchen ceiling down to the floor. The husband has since developed a serious thyroid condition for which there is no obvious explanation, which, again, may be the result of living in a stressed location.

The reaction of the couple has been revealing and exhibits a phenomenon that I have observed in others. They are very enlightened in their attitude to health matters, teachers in the field of naturopathy, and very aware of the existence of earth currents. Yet when it comes to the application of the knowledge to their own health, they exhibit a total blank, a blindness, or maybe a determination not to, or to want to see. I met a similar response when I raised the topic with the husband of a woman whom I had met at the cancer centre where I had helped. She had leukaemia, and where they then lived on the Fylde coast there was an almost identical situation to the one where my mother and brother had lived. I described earth currents and geopathic stress to the husband and gave him the Gordon and von Pohl books to read. However, on the next visit to the centre, he returned the books, unread. He said that he did not want to consider the possibility that their house might be subject to the phenomenon, because *he didn't want to have to move*! Whether or not the house had an effect upon his wife's illness was immaterial – they were putting such a lot into the house and he liked the location. Likewise the possibility that his own health or that of the two young daughters might suffer just did not penetrate the self imposed blindness and determination to ignore what I was trying to tell him.

In the realm of spiritual awareness that is the mainstay of my book, I remember an occasion when I had described some of my experiences to my nephew. He had already established a dogged determination not to accept *anything* of a 'spiritual' nature into his life or beliefs, and had one, and one only, repeated response to my description. The response was to the effect that '*it had happened to me*'. I kept saying 'that it had happened' – meaning that the phenomena that I had experienced had a much wider relevance than solely within the confines of my life; that what had happened to me was not specifically unique to me, but had consequences for others, whereas Mark wanted to treat them as if they were somehow completely encapsulated, and had no significance to him, his beliefs or the way he should live.

The 'earth radiation' of Käthe Bachler depends upon the presence of an underground aquifer – and don't dismiss them as being rare; they are not. As I sit now I can look along the length of both of my fields, and can recollect the first visit of the dowser, when he surveyed them. He had arrived with some of his children, and we all carried bundles of canes or sticks. As he walked at a steady pace, holding between his two hands a forked twig that he had pulled from my hedge, we saw the twig keep dipping at frequent intervals, indicating points where one of us stuck a cane into the ground. Back and forth he went, with yet more canes being inserted, as the lines of the aquifers began to be revealed, each with its own 'hedge' of canes. In the smaller field, which is about 100 metres long and where the borehole is sited, Jack located four crossing lines. The day before the drilling rig was due, I had asked him to return, because I began to worry that my chosen line might also be the one that fed the spring at the farm of my neighbour down the hill, and I didn't want to alter his flow. So diligently we followed the respective lines, finding that my chosen one veered past the neighbour's farm, while the aquifer feeding his spring also ran diagonally and passed under my field at an unlikely looking place. Finding the line of that particular spring explained why there was a gap in the growth of our dividing hedge over which we had had a dispute some years previously!

      The actual drilling of the borehole was one of the more memorable events of my life. During the night I had suffered all of the qualms of doubt that accompany a journey into unknown territory. It was November, and the day dawned wet and windy – and prolonged rain had made the field with its clay soil become very slushy. The heavy rig soon got bogged down, and it took heroic efforts by a neighbour with his tractor to manoeuvre it into position. A huge compressor had been deposited beside the road the day before, and that soon sprang into life, alerting neighbours who came to join some other friends who had also come to see the fun, as well as Jack the dowser whom I had invited. The drilling started and went through some surprising layers – 5 metres of solid clay, then absolutely dry sand and pebbles that gradually aggregated into sandstone, until, as the sandstone was giving way to granite at 25 metres, a blast from the compressor brought a huge geyser of water jetting up into the sky. Water strike!

The rest, as they say, is history. But strange was the attitude of some, in that knowing that such a good water strike ("The best I've seen in the Lake District" – said the pump man) had been located by dowsing, and seeing the dowser demonstrate on other lines, they nevertheless said "Oh, if you drilled *anywhere* in the field you would be bound to find water." When I offered to let anyone drill *anywhere* there were no takers, but still the dogged determination *not to believe*. Exactly the attitude adopted by my nephew, and, regrettably, the attitude taken by some who, having been told of all that had happened to me, all that I have described in the book, are still stubbornly determined *not* to accept what I am describing from my actual experience, and are prepared to continue with what are nevertheless far-fetched 'explanations' of their own.

Late on the second day, the rig was hauled off the land, the compressor fell silent, and everyone departed, leaving a field that resembled a World War 1 battlefield, and a half metre of pipe sticking up from the mud where the borehole began. The dowser is a farmer, who had learned from an uncle who had dowsed for water in the desert when in the army and in North Africa. As with most people with a true natural gift, he would accept no payment. Perhaps his most lasting payment is the constant gratitude that I feel each time that I turn a tap and out pours the ice-cold, pure, unadulterated water.

The running water in the aquifers can create its own current, and also act as a conductor for electricity created by other natural means. I wrote earlier of the 'battery' effect at the interface of two dissimilar rock types, or between rock and mineral deposits. Where such a battery exists, the current will flow and create its own geoelectric field directly above. On a far greater scale are the currents created by a phenomenon that was only discovered in the last year of World War ll. Pilots on high level bombing runs over Japan found that they could not hold on their targets because of a high-speed wind that blew from west to east with velocities of up to 500 kilometres per hour. Investigation and research over half a century have revealed more information about what have become known as the 'jet streams'. Very fast flowing currents of air snake from west to east over the middle and upper latitudes, carrying with them the components of the weather systems that make Western European weather so variable. An equivalent set of streams flows along similar latitudes in the Southern Hemisphere.

During daylight hours, the air at the altitude of the streams is ionised by the sun's ultraviolet rays. The resulting electrically charged particles are whisked along at very high speeds and together form a continuous electrical current that can reach a magnitude into the millions of amperes at local noon. At nightfall the ions recombine, and the current falls to zero. In considering the impact of electromagnetic radiation on people I mentioned earlier the process of 'induction', where a current is induced in a conductor from external sources. The very strong current flowing parallel to the ground therefore induces electrical flow in the underground water streams, with the consequent geoelectric stresses. The major differences between day and night may account for some of the behavioural changes that are noted in some individuals. The movements of the jet streams (in the northern hemisphere) to the north in the spring and south in the autumn, probably explain some of the seasonal changes that take place in sensitive people. These might be a component of the influences that provoke the suicides that increase in number in the spring, and trigger the onset of depression in November.

It is almost impossible to separate the phenomena of earth currents (see: *telluric currents*), geopathic stress and ionisation of the air. Where their existence has been accepted and the results of study incorporated into medical thinking, a greater understanding of aberrant human behaviour has resulted. Two of the books from which I have quoted frequently, have their origin in the same part of Central Europe, and, from the more recent Bachler book, there is evidence of the knowledge of earth currents being incorporated into official thinking and action. Whether this demonstrates a different attitude to ideas that are a little offbeat it is impossible to say, although in other perhaps parallel areas of medical thought, there is evidence of a ready acceptance of treatments that simply do not exist in other countries such as Britain.

Digressing from my main theme, but still continuing with thoughts about personal and mental health and differences of attitudes and treatments between nations, I want to comment on a herb that is part of the accepted pharmacopoeia in such countries as Germany and Austria, but which has no official recognition in Britain. I refer to hawthorn – *Crataegus oxyeantha* – otherwise known as 'mayflower'. Following my recovery from my disastrous encounter with prescribed drugs, I determined that wherever possible I would take responsibility for my own well-being, and follow my own path. Commencing with the comfrey that I have already noted, I began a thorough study of common herbs and their properties. Hawthorn was one that soon came to the fore as I confirmed practically for myself the properties with which it is credited. It chanced that I first read of its characteristics at a time when the bushes in my hedges were in full bloom. I collected some of the blossoms, which are the most effective part, and incorporated them in tea that I was brewing. Just as it became ready, my friends Des and Carol arrived by chance and joined me in this trial. In almost no time at all, Des was fast asleep in a chair, and when later he arrived home, he rang to say that he could have been had up for 'driving under the influence of hawthorn'!

That, in a nutshell, illustrates one of hawthorn's most valuable properties – it acts '…to re-establish the equilibrium of the sympathetic and parasympathetic nervous system on which depend the proper functioning of all our organs and our rest.' So writes Jean Palaiseul in my well-used copy of *Grandmother's Secrets*. It is one of the most delightful and useful books that I have ever owned, combining as it does factual information about the natural substances, with family and historical anecdote. I would never be without it and refer to it frequently. Continuing to write of the properties, Palaiseul notes – 'The ancients used it as a remedy for gout, pleurisy, vertigo, insomnia, angor; and modern science confirms that its chemical components are in fact antispasmodic, sedative, diuretic and above all constitute a remarkable regulator of arterial blood pressure as well as a valuable heart stimulant with excellent sedative effects upon the cardio-vascular system, and therefore on angina pectoris and disturbances of circulation whether due to the menopause or not.'

I could go on, recounting the way that hawthorn is valued and venerated in popular culture – but not in Britain! Why? Because of the Reformation! Flowering in May, the month dedicated to the Virgin Mary, hawthorn was 'her' flower and herb, and its benevolent properties were ascribed to her influence. When, with the Reformation, all veneration of Mary was condemned and forbidden, propaganda proclaimed hawthorn to be the devil's herb and any contact with it was deemed unlucky. I shall not lightly forget the eldritch scream that came from the mouth of one traditionalist visitor who arrived just as I was taking some flowering hawthorn into the house – predicting all sorts of malevolence that would descend upon me as a consequence!

I have used it along with meadowsweet as my 'blood and heart' prophylactic for nearly twenty-five years, with not a single noticeable side-effect – which is another feature of hawthorn, the only caution being that one should not use it if the blood pressure is already low. Meadowsweet – *Spiraea ulmaria* – 'Queen of the meadow' - is one of the original sources of aspirin, and an anagram of part of the specific name 'spiraea' became in fact, 'aspirin', and I use it regularly instead of a daily aspirin tablet. I did not give blood until in my fifties because of the cocktail of prescribed drugs that I took. When the 'pollution' had cleared from my system, I went regularly to blood donor sessions. On the first few visits, my blood flowed sluggishly – at one time so slowly that the session was abandoned. However, soon after I began my regular use of these two herbs I went to another donor session, and commented to the doctor as he put in the needle that my blood came reluctantly. "Oh, you're one of those are you?" he grumbled, and then as the needle entered the vein – "Oh no, this will be a two minute job" – and it was, as the blood came freely and fluently.

While writing so enthusiastically about hawthorn and its benefits, I do so to illustrate its effects upon myself, and what I have learned about it. I would never presume to advise or prescribe for anyone else, for such is not my practice. I have found the herb to be nothing but benevolent with not a single side effect, and value immensely its gentle tranquillising properties. The unravelling of the 'knot' that frequently tightens my solar plexus, and which is part of the legacy of my earlier benzodiazepine drug regime, has to be experienced to be believed. For those who use their sexual function (or lack of it) as a measure of the state of their active health, all I can say is that my function and 'potency' are as good as they have ever been, which is probably due in no small part to the vaso-dilating properties of hawthorn and to its ability to unwind inner tensions via the sympathetic and para-sympathetic nerves. I laugh when I read of the much-trailed 'sexual dysfunction' in males and now females, and hear in my mind the chink of money landing in the coffers of the pharmaceutical companies as they generate anxiety in both sexes about their potency or prowess. Properly used, hawthorn would probably relieve most people's problems.

At one time I use to collect and freeze the berries, but latterly have obtained my dried herbs from a main supplier – Midland Herbs and Spices - or as tinctures from the 'Herb Company' in Scotland (01807 590 303), who, along with many reputable herb companies, supply standard strength tinctures from acknowledged apothecaries. From time to time various bodies in mainstream medicine mount campaigns against the use of herbs, discounting their efficacy, and often 'discovering' new and 'highly dangerous' side effects. A moment's reflection will demonstrate the fallacy and farce of these campaigns – one simply has to refer to the facts relating to prescribed medicines. One of the most frequently listed causes of death is given as that resulting from those self-same prescribed medicines – and when one looks at the side effects of, for example, one of the more commonly prescribed anti-depressant types based on fluexotine, one can only gape wide mouthed and incredulous, and understand full well why large numbers of individuals are made ill simply by taking them. What herbal remedy properly used has the potential to cause 'visual disturbances, palpitations, mania/hypomania, tremors, loss of sex drive, antisocial behaviour, double vision, memory loss etc, etc'? And what herbal remedy fills hospital beds just as they are filled with people who have been made ill by prescribed medicines?

I have described above only one substance, hawthorn, that is capable of giving relief to a wide range of common problems that are often treated with tranquillisers or anti-depressants; there are in fact many others that are efficacious as anyone can find out for themselves. I simply strayed into this field today and made these comments as a result of making comparisons of attitudes obtaining in different medical and national cultures, and, as I wrote earlier, it is not my function to recommend or prescribe. Just let me mention another of my own favourites before moving on. It is woodruff – *Asperula odorata* – and it is credited with having a wide range of qualities that are too numerous to describe in my present context. I will simply quote this: 'However, it is chiefly remarkable for its action upon the nerves: it calms, soothes, relaxes – exactly like the tranquillisers in which people indulge so freely today, but with the advantage that it causes no side-effects and is in no way toxic. Infusion of woodruff may therefore be given safely to all those who are troubled with disturbances of the sympathetic nervous system – including children and old persons – or who suffer from insomnia, vertigo, angor, neuralgia and excessive nervous tension.' I usually have a

LISTENING TO THE SILENCES

quantity mixed in with my ordinary tea because it imparts a most delightful flavour.

Returning to the 'global' world and the necessity to consider our total interaction with it and all of its varied properties, there is one major component that just cannot be ignored. The earth's magnetic field protects the planet from the drastic effects of the 'solar wind' – a huge and constant stream of electrically charged particles that are thrown out of the rotating ball of the sun in a manner resembling a Catherine wheel. Our magnetic field repels the particles and they flow past, being mainly observed in their transit at the poles where they create the northern and southern lights – the auroras. Planets such as Mars, where the magnetic field has declined, have been 'scoured' and their atmosphere whisked away. However, it is not that aspect that I want to discuss, but the omnipresence of the field, and its importance in our continuing healthy life.

It is an essential part of the environment in which we evolved, and we cannot live healthily without it. Inside a car, it vanishes completely – which might explain some of the bizarre behaviour of some drivers who spend many hours behind the wheel - while in nuclear submarines steps are taken to minimise the effects upon the crew of the long-term depletion that they would otherwise suffer as a result of the deprivation. Experiments upon the embryos of amphibians whose initial development resembles that of humans, reveal major deformities after short-term withdrawal of the normal terrestrial field. In a practical sense, a large lump of iron such as a central heating radiator will cancel out the local field for a distance on either side that depends upon the size of the radiator – typically, about 70 cms. If someone lies with their bed close to a wall *on the other side of which* a radiator is hung, they will experience total or partial screening, depending on whether they lie head to the wall, or parallel with it. I have experimented on myself in this type of situation, lying on the floor adjacent to a radiator. I don't lie there for very long, for the effects created are not pleasant, particularly those in my head when I place myself head to the metal. I have long thought of this as a possible contributor to cot death, and in the past I have written with these thoughts to representative organisations, with what success I do not know, for, apart from acknowledgments that I have received, there has never been any follow up from them.

However, if someone sleeps in such a location in which they are wholly or partially deprived of the natural field, I am certain that they will not have good sleep, and that they could well develop problems. Disturbed sleep and a feeling of disorientation that persists into the day, create a happy hunting ground for spiritual intrusions intent upon causing mischief. As well as radiators, large chunks of building iron such as R.S.J.s can act similarly in creating areas devoid of a magnetic field. Where the field is present in the fullness of its natural strength, all may still not be well. Left to

LISTENING TO THE SILENCES

itself it pulses regularly, and it is the pulsing at 10 cycles per second (hertz) that is so very important in the maintenance of mental and physical well-being.

'Left to itself' being the operative words. A few moments thought will confirm that we live on a planet that, whether one believes it was created by God, or arrived courtesy of the Big Bang, is an exciting phenomenon. Rotating on its axis; orbiting the sun; performing a 'dance' with the moon and other planets. Surviving collision with asteroids and other nasties; generating life; having this life suffer successive extinctions from trilobites down to dinosaurs and Neanderthals, and recovering and stabilising – until along comes man and Super Power Politics and rivalry, beginning a process of buggering up the whole lovely harmony. Many people have written and spoken about all the harm that has already been 'achieved' in this process; I am here concerned with only one aspect, namely the damage that is being done to our health environment through interference with the natural magnetic field and its pulsing.

Conjure up 'HAARP' and also 'USSR Woodpecker' from the Internet, and you will learn about high-powered electromagnetic transmissions that are or were created by the US and former Soviet Union. The Russian one is called Woodpecker, because that is what it sounds like on a radio receiver as it pulses at 10 hertz – OUR frequency. Ostensibly and originally designed to enable communication with nuclear submarines, no one outside the two Administrations really knows what is going on. HAARP stands for 'Highly Active Aurora Research Project'. It is located in Alaska and pumps enormous amounts of power into the atmosphere. The Web sites will provide much in the way of fact, speculation and conspiracy theories; my concern is with the effect upon mental health. Reports cited on the Web express concern that the transmissions are the cause of mental disturbance and depression in susceptible individuals, and it was these reports that came to mind when I read the papers describing the work done with 50,000 Swedish conscripts. You will recollect that the studies over a number of years had shown what was claimed were correlations between cannabis use and the onset of schizophrenia and depression. My contention is that it is most difficult to ascribe any one cause in the presence of many triggers. Sweden is very close to Russia, and, when measured over the North Pole, very close to Alaska also. It would be in the focus of much of the transmission aimed at nuclear submarines that patrol in Polar waters, whether Russian or US. Do these transmissions have a greater effect on people living in the Nordic countries? Who knows? One can only speculate.

But 'speculation' is the name of the game in much that surrounds mental health. American psychiatrist Thomas S. Szasz provides a great deal of fuel for speculation in his two books *The Manufacture of Madness* and *The Myth of Mental Illness*. The classification as a mental illness of 'schizophrenia', however it is defined, is, according to Szasz, a social convenience that enables 'authority' to be able to control a group of people who are, in the main, harmless, but who are socially deviant – he likens their treatment to that of witches in the past. When there is so much that is classed as mental or nervous illness that can only be contained or cured through the use of mind-altering drugs, one wonders how we actually managed to evolve for so many millions of years without them.

I made another 'rose-coloured spectacle' trip down memory lane with a friend of the same age as myself. Born and spending her early years in rural Essex, she, like me, confirms the absence in our youth of many of the ailments that beset so many people today. Asthmatic herself, because of a later identified wheat intolerance, she cannot recall other asthmatic children of her generation. She cannot recall either, as I cannot, children who were as disturbed as are those of today's generations. Like me she grew up without electricity, junk and fast food and aerosols; she drank water from wells, and wore natural fibre clothing and leather boots or shoes. There was no 'instant' coffee, and very few of our acquaintance made 'proper' coffee – in my friend's case, the drink offered to visitors to the house was usually homemade wine, which was apparently made in large quantities.

I place emphasis upon the wearing of natural materials because there is much to indicate that man-made equivalents have had an adverse effect on health. We evolved naked, with our hands and feet in regular contact with the ground, and in an atmosphere that had a much higher concentration of negative ions than exists now. It is widely believed that the ion concentrations have an influence via the air that we actually breathe in, and also through contact with the acupuncture meridians and the points on them. If you have an ioniser it is very easy to demonstrate these effects, first by holding the device about 45 cms in front of the face and breathing in the ionised air – I find it very refreshing myself. Secondly, if the ioniser is held a short distance from an unclothed part of the body, it is possible to experience beneficial results. Reports described in Fred Soyka's book suggest that healing of wounds and of burns is speeded up if there is a good supply of negative ions.

Man-made clothing can behave as an electrical insulator, and prevent the access of ions to the skin. It also creates electrical fields of its own, and can act to repel those ions that try to make contact. The materials that make up most modern footwear are also excellent electrical insulators – and isolate the wearer from any 'earthing' contact with the ground – essential if one is to try to simulate the healthy conditions of evolution. Only today I had a demonstration of my own reaction to wearing wellingtons as I worked in a wet garden. I don't normally wear them because past experiences have demonstrated what I felt today – namely a profound ache that developed in

LISTENING TO THE SILENCES

my lower back, and a very noticeable drop in my energy level. Normal services were quickly restored when I kicked them off and went barefoot on a quarry-tiled floor. I recognise these effects as a consequence of my acute sensitivity to my electrical ambience: others who do not have this awareness are likely to persist and might even make themselves ill over a period of time. Leather soled shoes and boots – not readily available today - allowed closer connection, and in my belief were much healthier. Modern youth probably grows up with the very minimal contact with the ground or with any regular connection with earthed surfaces. Most modern furnishings, bedding and carpets are synthetic and create their own static electricity and electrical fields, and create dusts that equally have peculiar electrical properties. Living in an unnatural electrical environment, surrounded by a variety of devices that produce their own electromagnetic fields, sleeping in a room that most probably has a TV and computer and who knows what else electrical, is it any wonder that modern youngsters leave the womb clutching in one hand an inhaler ready for the asthma that will inevitably be their fate, and in the other a prescription for Prozac or Librium? - and that is before they embark on a life with cola drinks, adulterated chicken pieces, E-numbers and Aspartame. What happens to their vulnerable minds, I'll leave to your own imagination.

Returning to the possible effects of clothing upon the access of the desirable negative ions to the body, I think that it would be useful to speculate on the effect of wearing a bra, particularly one made from synthetic materials, and particularly upon the development of breast cancer. Going back down memory lane, I believe that the first encounter that girls of my generation had with bras was when they joined one of the armed forces, where they were standard issue (together with passion-killing 'blackout' bloomers, according to my WREN friends!). These were essentially always made of cotton. Breasts are obviously tender and vulnerable parts of the female body, and I think that it is fair to speculate that their electrical isolation inside the insulating fabric of a modern bra may be a contributory factor in the creation of breast tumours.

I can only speak for myself (not about wearing a bra, although if I continue to put on weight, one may become necessary!). I avoid absolutely manmade fibres in my clothing and bedding, having on many occasions in the past been made to realise that their use brings discomfort and 'agitation'. One always faces this problem when trying to describe bodily sensations in terms that others can identify and relate to in themselves. As with all forms of 'pollution', it is difficult to know what is the threshold between discomfort and actual harm.

Many people grow up in an environment that surrounds them with numerous sources of pollution, and never have the opportunity of knowing what unpolluted life is like.

LISTENING TO THE SILENCES

As an aside - from about 1970 I gave up television, and didn't own one for about twenty years. When then I acquired one and recommenced regular viewing, I felt that I had arrived at another planet. While the technology had developed in many ways, the standards of acceptability had plummeted to depths hitherto undreamed of. It is outside my remit to comment on much that I see as the degradation and humiliation of individuals, and yet the whole ambience is akin to that in which the obscene spiritual intrusions thrive. A casual moment channel hopping the other day saw a brief glimpse of the V. Graham Norton 'show', and the sight of a man being publicly confronted with his 'wank sock', which his future bride had given to the show! I didn't stay to see what tasks he had to accomplish to recover it – Norton had even opened the sock to reveal what purported to be the residue from masturbation. That to me is just one instance of what I regard as the 'pollution' of people's lives and living environment and which can result in the creation of a hedonism that makes the entry of malevolent intrusion into the minds of the vulnerable all the easier.

One form of pollution that affects most urban areas is that created by all of the light sources flooding the sky and blotting out the stars. I find it sad to think of the deprivation of youngsters who grow up having never seen the stars in an 'unpolluted' sky. About the only pleasure derived from wartime blackout was the vision of the undiminished brilliance of the stars overhead. When I view the human dross that passes for 'stars' in the modern media/pop culture, I find it equally sad that today's youngsters have no outstanding living stars to inspire them. The Pole Star in the northern sky, or the Southern Cross in its own hemisphere have been fixed and constant and have guided and comforted mariners throughout recorded time. Where, I wonder, are the points of reference, sources of inspiration for the youngsters of today? In many ways the young are sold short, deprived of their childhood and 'innocence' by a culture that sees them in no other light than as consumers and creators of wealth – for others, the exploiters.

Bombarded into accepting that certain soft drinks and fast foods are manna from heaven, driven by what is 'cool', they are encouraged from all sides and quarters to believe that the only purpose in living is to have the latest play-station – and to have sex. Young girls now are encouraged to wear clothes with pretend breasts – because it is 'sexy' – when they have hardly left the cradle. Peer pressure, and pressure from all of the elements that want to exploit them encourage sex at the earliest possible age. What has evolved as a fundamental method of procreating and enhancing the species, with functions and reactions that reach into every cell of the body, has sunk to what – descriptive words fail me – in popular esteem? Hardly any TV programme, other than the dedicated documentary, can run without its embedded episodes of bonking, shagging, or fucking – to think that it used to be called 'making *love*'!

Spring is at its peak as I write, and I have been watching the birds and the bees. Each year I marvel that the little birds can be conned yet again. I watch them in the garden and hedgerows frantically trying to find mates, singing their little heads off and posturing and fluttering – and then they copulate – just once. That one act of togetherness immediately throws a switch – and suddenly it's frenetic nest building, egg sitting, and frenzied food carrying to the fledglings, then nurturing and protection until flight becomes possible and the young fly the nest. Then the idiots do it all over again for a second brood - one moment of bliss leading to frantic, compulsive activity.

All of those imperatives reside in all creatures, and stifling the consequences of the initial action can produce many results that are destructive. A young teenage girl, possibly pressurised into her first sexual encounter, is immediately subjected to all of the responses exhibited by the female bird – even if it was just a casual fumbling shag from an equally inexperienced lad. To list all of the inner responses that will be triggered within her is beyond my scope, but what I am leading to is the consequence of a natural process that has been frustrated. The disturbing unfulfilled responses may lead to a feeling of revulsion with herself and her body, and have been known to provoke the reactions of self-harm and eating disorders from an urge to 'punish' the vehicle of her inner disgust. A situation such as this is so easily exploited by the malevolent intrusion – an unhappy girl, not truly understanding the source of her unhappiness, seeking isolation – a mind possibly wide open to intrusion and increased depression – encouraged into further isolation and suicide?

And what of the children, the offspring of such casual and promiscuous encounters? Children whose father might be any one of a pick and mix collection. Another coffee break switch on and I found myself in the Trisha experience on ITV. There for the morning's entertainment were young women who had become mothers and who weren't sure which of several men might have been the father, and the programme had done DNA comparisons that were revealed in the full panoply of the prurient build up of the show and its eagerly gawping faces in the audience. No thought is given to the children, not just these children but also the many who are the product of these collective copulations. Is there any wonder that there is so much domestic violence when possibly the putative father in a marriage or relationship finds out that he is not in fact the actual father, and has been deceived and conned? More importantly the children as they grow and realise the casualness of their creation might feel little worth in themselves, and, possibly feeling sullied, resort to self-harm and the isolation that again opens the door to malevolent intrusions and their taunts that can lead to suicide.

LISTENING TO THE SILENCES

These are topics of such wide scope that I can do little more than mention them, but it is a realm of human experience where spiritual intrusions wreak immense amounts of harm in the minds and lives of the vulnerable. Any enlargement would include the ways in which cravings can be stimulated and addictions fostered and driven, but that is for another time.

Meanwhile, returning to my main theme, it may seem that I am labouring the problems created by the variety of electrical phenomena. I am in fact underplaying them, and only limit my writing in deference to those who have problems with science and technology, and find difficulty in relating any of this to mental health, and particularly to voice hearing and all of the rest that I have written about. Be assured that I include everything as a component of the totality of human experience and daily life. I reiterate my point that *anything* that undermines and depletes the normal function and well-being of our bodies and minds plays into the 'hands' of the sources of spiritual intrusion. I am tempted to write at length about the influence of diet, food intolerance and allergy upon mental health, but realise that it is an immense subject that is frequently written about in many books and articles. The problem is that there are many conflicting opinions, and it is difficult for the average person to arrive at a balanced judgment.

It is claimed that there is a 'Balanced British Diet', and that it provides all of the nutrients that a person needs. I heartily disagree, and, to give one example from the Food Standards Agency's latest pronouncement, at 40 mgms, the recommended level of vitamin C intake is just about that which will prevent scurvy. They spoke about the possibility of stomach upsets and diarrhoea being caused by high intake – apparently not recognising the availability of slow release products that 'trickle' the vitamin out over several hours. I regularly take 1 gm per day, and experience no problems – in fact, if I don't take as much I often get problems in my gums. When one considers that our simian immediate antecedents were largely herbivores and fruit eaters, is it not obvious that we through our evolution require vitamin C in significant quantities – as well as the magnesium that would have come from the plant chlorophyll? How I wish that the medical establishment would put its own house in order and control the use of many of the harmful substances that pass for medication or are used in food additives – especially those - and let individuals such as me kill ourselves with mineral and vitamin supplements if that is our wish – although most people who take supplements are too well informed now to do anything so drastic. (Currently as I write certain doctors are trying to develop a campaign to have taxes levied on 'fatty foods' i.e. the junk foods that are making so many young people so obese. Part of the campaign propaganda declares that the British diet today is too heavily loaded with unsuitable and junk foods lacking in nutritional value, but promoting obesity.

LISTENING TO THE SILENCES

Whatever happened to the 'Balanced British Diet'?)

Over the years I have obtained much personal benefit from taking charge of my own diet and intake of supplements – much of the benefit coming from what I *don't* ingest, as much as from what I do. To be brief, I have latterly followed a diet based upon my blood group, and find benefit from the elimination of a number of items, resulting in greater mobility of my upper body and shoulders – a very important consideration in a driver who is well past seventy, and who needs to be able to turn his body freely to be safe at road junctions. Likewise I have had food intolerance tests, and again have experienced benefit from the elimination of certain items – including my much-liked dark chocolate!

A recital of all that I have done would not, I feel, be helpful, and anyway is specific to myself. Guidance has come from *Nutritional Medicine* by Drs. Stephen Davies and Alan Stewart whose aim is to try to treat a wide variety of ailments and diseases, including mental problems, by nutritional means: this one of my 'bibles'. (One has only to look in it at the rôle of the B vitamins to realise their importance in maintaining mental health, while something as simple as magnesium can, in depletion, result in apathy, confusion and disorientation, depression, learning disability and memory impairment, vertigo, convulsions and epilepsy, insomnia, hyperactivity. Because of past glaciations, magnesium is almost absent in northern soils, in the local water, and in food that is produced there.) Mental health and nutrition are the prime concerns of an interesting book jointly written by Dr. Carl Pfeiffer and Patrick Holford. From one end you enter the Pfeiffer contribution – *Mental Illness – the nutrition connection*, and from the other, the Holford contribution – *Mental Health – the nutrition connection*. But by far the greatest revelation concerning diet and mental health, and 'alien' substances and mental health came to me from Dr. Richard Mackarness' two books *Not All in the Mind* and *Chemical Victims*, which may still be found second hand if one is prepared to look. Some may say that they are dated, but even so, they provide an excellent starting point from which to dig further into the whole topic of diet and mental health, and I am certain that there must be many recent books and articles that provide sound advice. However, be cautious, for, as with many emotive subjects such as cancer and mental health, there are many therapies and diets that flourish in the media and in the chat shows, and then drop from view, leaving no trace other than in the additions to the books abandoned on the shelves. As with everything else that I have written about – discernment, discernment, discernment!

Reviewing the most recent parts of my writing, I may appear to be drifting away from the main purpose of the whole book – that of describing the intrusion of spiritual malevolence and the creation of dominance and mental

LISTENING TO THE SILENCES

distress. If I have done do, it has been purely unintentional and has only occurred because I have tried to develop the theme that intruding entities take intelligent advantage of *any* circumstances that result in the physical and mental depletion of individuals, and of the resulting feelings of insecurity that these can create. I must in this last descriptive and speculative chapter take steps to return to the declared purpose, although, like much of my attack, my thrust may at times seem oblique.

Hark back, if you will, to where I wrote of the occasion when I had climbed to a nearby plateau on the fell side and where I had gone to look for signs of ancient trackways. In the beautiful stillness and evening light I sat taking in the scene, and watched a fox as it crossed in front of me some short distance away. Suddenly, and with no apparent preliminary check, it dashed for safety, its whole demeanour and behaviour having changed within a milli-microsecond. And it dashed *away* from me – which may seem to be doubly stating the obvious. But why? I had made no sound, hadn't moved and was not obviously visible. All that had triggered the fox's reaction had been my scent that had drifted down on a light breeze. So only its nose figured in this early warning system, and it was highly directional. But so is all of the mammalian early warning system. The eyes, the ears and the nose have their primary personal defence rôle, and in that rôle connect directly to the centre of instinctive locomotion – the 'solar plexus' – bypassing the brain.

My description is probably too simplistic for some, but nevertheless serves to make my argument. The left eye, ear and nostril send signals to the right half of the brain, and the reverse for the right hand sensors. Normally when 'free ranging', the animal is sensing globally – i.e. the eyes are intent on peripheral vision and each eye covers a wide arc on its own side; each ear likewise has its sweep of coverage – 'sweep' being the operative word, for the ears are very mobile, and one has only to look at racehorses as they move down to the start of a race to see the two ears independently 'semaphoring' as they respond to sounds that are arriving from all directions. Not so obvious, particularly to humans, is the directional capability of the nose, yet it must be there for the fox to have acted as it did.

If anything potentially dangerous is sensed, several changes take place instantly and instinctively – there can be no place in the equation for logical thought and deduction. If the threat is to the left, the left eye adopts focussed vision, while the right is de-focussed and turned slightly to prevent so-called 'macular' vision. The left ear goes into directional hearing and lifts and 'cocks' towards the source of the sound, while the right ear is 'de-tuned', in that an inner muscular contraction takes place that mutes the sound, and concentrates the hearing into the left ear. The left nostril flares and goes into 'sniffing' mode, while inside the right nasal passage a minor contraction

LISTENING TO THE SILENCES

occurs that diminishes the airflow and scenting capability. The early warning system has detected danger to the left, and the limbs are provoked into action to take the creature away to the right. There is no pause for consultation; the instinctive body is already primed with instructions from its evolution – threat from the left, limbs gather to strike off to the right.

As I have written several times, we, you and I, are mammals. I know that you don't really need to be told that, but it must be emphasised. But what has to be emphasised further is that all – all – of the early warning systems continue to exist in us and our organs and limbs, and that all of the same instinctive instant responses are created within us. We humans differ in that the different sides of our brains have certain dedicated functions dictated by our intellectual development. In writing this I do so as someone who spends much time in imaginative, ruminative, speculative, introspective and, at times, mildly apprehensive thought. All of the time that I am writing or planning what I am going to write, I am indulging in mental 'verbalisation'. In other words, I am engaging in what is now commonly and simplistically called 'right brain' activity. Also I am right-handed, and so can only write from the standpoint of someone who has this particular combination. It is only in minor ways that I can observe and comment on other mind and body combinations. However, I am writing as carefully as I can, and with as much detail as possible, because as well as the mind of the 'thinker', what I am describing might be the inner mental state of someone who is locked into the internal voices, someone who is constantly listening and adding these instinctive responses to those that are happening within as the inner 'presence' provokes, cajoles, threatens, agitates or holds the 'listener' enthralled.

Constantly, I am creating in my right brain images and 'sounds' (i.e. my verbalisation) that, to my *animal* brain, appear to be arriving from the *left* side, via my left eye and ear – and the instinctive 'me' kicks in and primes my body for a particular action. Except that it doesn't 'kick in' – the instinctive responses are there all of the time as I persist, and have persisted for most of my life, in this mode of thinking. The responses within the wild creature are transient as either it responds and takes evasive action, or decides that the threat is not real and relaxes. For the thinking human, the pattern of thought goes on and on and on. Through all waking time, the process persists, and the body becomes polarised, as it is constantly primed for a response and a resultant action – that never happen.

The animal me is receiving signals ostensibly from my left, and wants to take action that propels me to my right. The quadruped me 'coils' ready to jump off, and engages my limbs diagonally – left upper half and right lower half work together (left diagonal), and vice versa. One diagonal is poised to spring and the other locked to give the balance. *All* of the muscles of

LISTENING TO THE SILENCES

locomotion are engaged, and the whole process will produce results that I am sure most of you will begin to recognise within your own bodies, although the roughly twenty percent of you whose thinking is essentially and predominantly verbal, will probably recognise them in the *right* diagonal.

Remaining with the left diagonal, the reaction within the musculature of the left upper has the effect of lifting the shoulder, taking it even higher than the lift created by the curve of the body, the 'Vincent curve', and reinforcing the 'kink' at the base of the neck. Pressure applied between the upper inner corner of the scapula and the spine will, in most individuals, reveal a very tender area. Associated acupuncture points in this location that may be influenced, (Bl 37, 38), are used to treat: 'lungs empty'; weary and paralysed; weak; emaciated; madness; loss of memory.

Tension created within the shoulder joint itself that is continuous can contribute to such conditions as a 'frozen shoulder', particularly when added mental or emotional stress has compounded those stresses that have become a permanent feature. The biceps of the left arm are in a state of permanent contraction, and eventually produce a point of soreness in the centre of the muscle approximately 2 cm below the level of the deltoid vee. This is the location of two points on the acupuncture 'Lung' meridian, L 3, & 4. Again allowing for the seemingly 'quaint' direct translation from the Chinese, these points may be used to treat: cerebral congestion; speaks to himself or doesn't speak at all; 'possessed by a devil'; confused; forgetful; vertigo; depressed.

It is possible to go down the arm and at every joint and point of tension locate acupuncture points that may be used to treat a variety of serious 'mind' conditions. There is no reason for me to catalogue them all in what is meant to be an overview, and so I'll skirt them and conclude the arm repertoire with the eighth point on the 'Heart' meridian. This is on the palm of the hand immediately proximal to the space between the ring and little fingers, and in the 'crease' where the painful and disabling condition known as 'contraction of the palmar aponeurosis' occurs. This acupuncture point, H 8, has a large repertory that divides into two parts, the first being the 'nervous' group: " 'disease and feelings of calamity in the heart and chest'; palpitations; hysteria; fear; 'frightened of people'; trembling". The second group centres on the urinary, genital functions, and takes the discussion logically into the other part of the diagonal – the lower right, in my case.

"Difficulty in urination; urinary incontinence; one side of scrotum larger than the other; impotent; general uterine disease; pruritis vulvae; prolapse of the uterus" – these are all conditions that are capable of being treated from H 8, and analysis will show that they may be caused by the permanent 'coiling' of all of the musculature of locomotion of the right lower half of the body – from the bottom of the ribs down to the toes. Study a horse in motion and observe the full scope of the action, and translate it into yourself.

LISTENING TO THE SILENCES

Experiments on myself reveal that persistent and aggravated tension consistent with prolonged apprehension or intense concentration will cause sharp pain in the very region where the presence of pain is used to diagnose appendicitis, and the presence of pain from this particular mind-induced source is the most probable reason why over fifty percent of appendixes removed turn out to have been healthy. The preparation for movement of the buttock and thigh and the prolonged contraction of their muscles lead to a wide range of other problems that self experiment will reveal for you. Just two will suffice – the hip joint above all others is firmly involved in locomotion, and persistent tension there may affect the point on the Gall meridian, G 30, at which location one could treat: 'half of body uncoordinated'; paralysis; epilepsy; nervous exhaustion. The gathering tension of tendons immediately above the ankle creates a zone where, over time, a feeling akin to paralysis can be produced, in a region where there are several places where serious mental conditions are capable of being treated.

In an account of the work of Sigmund Freud, he is credited with observations concerning the early onset of multiple sclerosis. He records double vision, paralysis above the left eye, and paralysis of the right ankle. The difficulties with the eyes may be explained by the fact that the left eye is straining to look to the left, where the imagined visual images are perceived, while the right eye has to concentrate upon the task of practical vision – its rôle that eventually makes it the dominant eye. I have noted earlier how it is possible when driving, suddenly to say to oneself "How did I get here?" One has been driving on automatic pilot, locked in one's thoughts, 'viewing' the mental images with the 'circuitry' of the left eye, while the driving has been conducted by means of automatic responses to what is seen with the right eye.

When this 'split viewing' is persistent, or carried to extremes, then the conflict between the musculature of the left eye and that of the right can lead to serious problems. The right eye difficulties are accommodated by turning the head slightly to the left, bringing the right eye forward. Watching people on TV when they are following an autocue reveals the fact that many are obviously reading with the dominant eye, and with the head slightly turned. When a person is absorbed in internal listening or deeply engrossed and lost in imagination, and when this state lasts for long periods, the struggle between the two eyes may result in severe stresses of the musculature, not only of the left eye, but of the whole left face and scalp as far around as the back of the neck. And not only that associated with the eye and its struggle to turn, but also the ear, which is also trying to focus to the left. As well as the numbness and paralysis that develop around and above the left eye, there is the possibility of causing left side migraine, and in extreme cases, dyslexia.

LISTENING TO THE SILENCES

I was once acquainted with a family in which the mother and three daughters all suffered severely from migraine, while two of the three boys were dyslexic. The mother was very imaginative in a constructive way, but also could be most apprehensive. Her sister was permanently locked into the inner space of the voices in her mind, and hardly engaged with the real world. I believe that the children were 'foetaly programmed' with the potentially divided vision that stemmed from the mother being deeply absorbed in her world of imagination/apprehension – which, if it was a family trait, may have resulted in her sister having become lost in *her* inner world that had then been taken over by the intruding voices. The dyslexia of Jane whom I have mentioned must have had a similar cause. She was very much a victim of her profound imagination combined with the stresses to which she was subjected. Her eyes were obviously working to two different agendas, but then came back together when gradually her fears were calmed, and her life became secure.

Freud was convinced that the MS-associated symptoms of two women whom he had studied had also included nymphomania. Most odd, until one finds that an acupuncture point at the base of the skull, and which would be severely stressed by the mechanisms that I am describing, may be used to treat nymphomania! Whether the perpetual aggravation and stimulation of the acupuncture point resulted in interesting stimulation elsewhere is a question to which I have not yet found an answer, even through practical experimentation.

                        I had made up my mind that I would make no further reference to the effect of natural phenomena on people, whether as individuals or in the mass, but it is rapidly becoming impossible to ignore as the whole world seems to be running on a very short fuse. Events that I associate with the fast approaching perihelial opposition of Mars are happening right on cue. Already there have been several earthquakes, we have had our war, and we have our pestilence in the shape of the SARS virus. Everywhere there are major confrontations, whether between nations; by groups demanding change; within businesses and employees organisations – and between individuals or within families and similar groups, as almost daily tragedies are revealed in the media. I will not repeat all that I wrote before, but as my sleep becomes more fragmented, just as it did in the equivalent period in 1988-9, so I am aware now, as I wasn't then, of the rapidly increasing number of spontaneous comments coming from a variety of people of all ages. The actual event peaks on August 28th, and I fully expect there to be more earthquakes as well as some volcanic eruptions during the next few months, although it is the effect upon the behaviour of individuals and groups that is most germane in the context of my book. July 2018 is when the next event occurs, so get it marked in your diaries well in advance!

LISTENING TO THE SILENCES

In observing the wide range of reactions – or, in fact, *non*reaction – of individuals to natural events, or to the imperatives of their evolution, I am as much interested in the lack of response as I am in the instances where it occurs. Where there is no apparent reaction, or very little, I speculate that there already exists such a base-load of entrenched stress that any increase is barely noticeable. Additionally, reactions and responses may be put down to other triggers that exist in the person's life. I suspect that very few individuals know just what a range of automatic reactions exist in our inheritance, or what is involved in the 'autonomic nervous system', other than a vague recollection of 'flight, fight, adrenalin'. (*Mind as Healer, Mind as Slayer* by Kenneth R. Pelletier is a useful and readable sourcebook).

Even if treated simplistically, as I intend to do, there is much more than 'flight, fight and adrenalin' involved in the mind/body, body/mind interactions that are features of our lives. There are many situations that one encounters where flight and fight are not practical, nor do they fulfil the needs of the moment. Domination, whether by one partner over another, parent over child, employer over employee places the dominated one at the receiving end of the anticipated violence, whether physical or verbal, and from which escape is not an option. 'Anticipation' is the operative word, for such can hold a person within a perpetual state of stress that in the world of animal interplay is purely transient as domination and subservience are sorted out.

The mammal that is apprehensive undergoes a number of automatic and instinctive reactions. It waits poised while the degree of threat is assessed. Breathing is suppressed, ears are cocked, anal and bladder sphincters are locked (although some creatures immediately void their bladders and bowels), the tail is pressed down and genitals are tightened. Additionally, a lock is put on the oesophagus, and at the base of the throat, and the body is primed for such reaction as may become necessary. Variants of these reactions occur if the perceived threat comes from within the social group, when events are dictated by established pecking orders.

The perpetual state of apprehensive listening is one that I have tried to describe in those sections of my book that have been more specific about the behaviour of intruding entities. And perpetual become the responses within the body, responses that *add* to the diagonal tensions that I have already written about. Although I have condemned the universal and perpetual obsession with sex in virtually every strand of modern Western human activity, paradoxically it is the only reason from our evolution that justifies our existence. The purpose of each generation is to prolong and improve the species – thus the only real function for the male is to protect and inject the sperm, while the female has to allow access to her eggs and womb only to a chosen male, and to

LISTENING TO THE SILENCES

repulse others of lesser stature. Consequently, many of the instinctive responses are governed purely by those two imperatives.

Males have to protect their testicles, and, in animals in their natural environment, this is done by retracting them as much as possible. The whole process in human males is confused by all of the conflicting signals that are being generated by the mind in response to the many real and imagined threats to which they are exposed in daily life, and which they create for themselves through their persistent thought patterns. It has long been observed that men have one testicle, usually the right one, higher than the other. Only a small percentage, it is said, have the left one higher. Many explanations are offered to account for this phenomenon, the most recent that I have heard being that with the upright stance, the asymmetry became necessary to allow both testicles to fit into a restricted space. Each autumn I used to corral in one of my fields up to twenty rams belonging to a neighbour, where they were held until the appropriate breeding time arrived. As I gardened or worked in my workshop I had plenty of opportunity to observe them, and it is impossible to ignore the testicles. In every case, the testicles were level, as is the situation with other male animals that I have noted. During the comparatively short evolutionary time in which humans have stood upright, there has not been long enough for the lopsided testicle to have developed – so why did it?

Roy Vincent

There are two influences at work: the first is the instinctive uplift resulting from the very act of thinking. A human thinking is the same as a wild creature listening and wondering. The response is to lift the testicles, until, as listening/thinking is a permanent function, the testicles are always partially withdrawn. The second influence comes as a result of the body being primed diagonally as I have described earlier. The priming tenses the right buttock and adjoining musculature, including the suspensory muscles of the testicles, further drawing up the right one, until the scrotum appears lopsided. (Recollect, the acupuncture point H 8, with its repertory for treating conditions that could be construed as 'nervous', 'emotional', was also indicated if one side of the scrotum was higher than the other – a certain confirmation that the asymmetry is not natural). There is an account in one version of *One Thousand and One Nights* of young men of the time practicing diligently to be able to *retract* their testicles sufficiently to pass themselves off as eunuchs, and enter the baths on days reserved for women. Conversely, I have proved to my own satisfaction that it is possible to relax sufficiently to be able to *lower* the higher testicle, and eventually both.

I have knowingly encountered only one man with a left high testicle, and that was in the Navy, where living conditions were such that very little was hidden. This man was very 'left brain', in that he was provocatively verbal, and was a verbal confrontation waiting to happen. If my analysis is correct, he was polarised on the opposite diagonal to the majority. Another who came into the same category of being ready to fizz verbally with little provocation was someone that I once knew who developed *right* breast cancer. Again, the polarisation, this time on the right diagonal, I believe, resulted in permanent contraction of the muscles across the chest, with a consequent diminution of the flow of blood and lymph in the breast itself. This woman was told by her surgeon that she was one of about 20% of women who develop right breast cancer. Another observation relating to breasts that I have made is that, of friends who have newly given birth, and who develop mastitis, *everyone* has been in the *left* breast; again, I believe, giving credence to my analysis of the effects of prolonged mental activity of a particular type – and not necessarily *stressful* mental activity – and of the diagonal polarisation of the body and its musculature.

As a corollary, I have noticed effects in myself that confirm the left breast stress – not, in my case, mastitis, although I believe that it is not unknown in men, but my left nipple is larger than the right, and frequently itches – to such an extent that many of my shirts have a hole just there. The whole question of the polarisation of the body, brain and senses in relation to the two diagonals is one that deserves detailed research. I am certain that answers will be found to problems such as impotence and female frigidity, both of which may result from the fact that the two sides of the genitals are responding to two different types of stimulus – possibly to the extent that only one side is sensitive, while the other is less so.

The lateral contrast in sensitivity explains why, when I peel an onion, only my left eye and nostril react. Likewise, if I get a sore throat, only the left side feels the irritation. (I have heard other individuals make similar comments). This is the result of the action of perpetually trying to 'sniff' to the left, and 'closing down' my right nostril. It probably explains why I chewed only on the left side of my mouth, for, along with my sense of smell being confined to the left nostril, that was the side where taste was also most acute. Over latter years I have cultivated chewing on both sides, and also chewing in a more blatant, 'animal-like' manner, moving the food around, quidding it and reducing it to a fluid before swallowing – living alone I have no resulting 'social' problems! The effect has been to improve my digestion and general sense of relaxation as the body responds to natural behaviour. A consequence of not sensing any irritation down the right inside of the throat might be that phlegm and debris that would normally be sensed and coughed up would simply be undetected and descend unchecked into the right lung, with a consequent build-up and potential disease. I could go on, for, as with much that I am trying to describe, I have been observing and experimenting for over twenty years. If I did so, however, it is unlikely that I would add significantly to my case, and could easily lead to confusion or distraction. I'll simply add that much

LISTENING TO THE SILENCES

can be done to balance the two diagonals with proper attention to breathing, particularly by concentration on maintaining a balance between the two nostrils, where, in my case, there is often a serious imbalance. As I correct the differential it is possible to feel beneficial internal reactions as a degree of harmony is restored.

Je n'ai fait celle-ci plus longue que parce que je n'ai pas eu le loisir de la faire plus courte.
      Pascal

(I have made this [chapter] longer than usual, only because I have not had time to make it shorter. Roy Vincent)

   In almost twenty-five years I have learned or devised many ways of coping with intruding voices, ways that I hope will have become evident from all that I have written and recorded. My strategies are successful in that I am no longer troubled by any of the presences that intrude. Voice hearers who are deeply embroiled in the conflicts within the mind are most unlikely to have the resources to cope, let alone devise a strategy, and are most likely to succeed in reclaiming their minds with the sympathetic and understanding help of others. The help must be in the form of an 'enabling', 'opening up' support. *Never* begin a sentence with "Why don't you...?" If the person was capable of doing the 'why don't you' bit, is it not most likely that they would already have made the attempt?

Surprising though it may seem, you may find some clues in the way that the large primates have been studied. There is a process known as 'habituation' through which the presence of the observer is gradually introduced without provocation and without imposing any stress upon the gorillas. Your relaxed presence has always to be there in an undemanding way, ready and able to say – "Let's...." There has always got to be an easy avenue to follow towards something desirable, and an easy path down which to retreat to the safety of known habits.

How you proceed will depend obviously upon the individuality of you both – the individuality that I have insisted on through all that I have described and analysed. Only you can see the problems, set the possible goals. It is difficult, but you must try to efface yourself and let the other flourish.

There are many practical steps that can be taken. Most are obvious, and almost suggest themselves, such as an adequate and wholesome diet, free from junk and additives. Hair analysis to detect any shortfall in minerals – many now have their hair analysed when planning pregnancy, and the 'Foresight' organisation provides a reliable service that is available to others as well as the potential parents, while there are other laboratories to be found on the Internet. When one considers that only microgrammes of iodine are necessary to prevent cretinism in iodine depleted regions, and that the intake provided by iodised salt will ensure a healthy physical and

LISTENING TO THE SILENCES

mental life for a child, is it not obvious that there must be an exquisite balance among other minerals that may be absent or present in excess? One can learn much from the way in which farm animals are looked after. To take one example, barley which is grown on the farm for animal feed is preserved using proprionic acid (Propcorn). This protects against moulds, but has the effect of killing the germ of the seed and depleting the vitamin E content. Calves fed this grain develop a deficiency condition called white muscle disease, and are fed supplements of vitamin E, but are also fed selenium which is necessary to promote the absorption of vit. E. Would that the same care was used to ensure the proper physical and mental development of *human children* in the face of all of the unnatural substances that they ingest as food. Equally fundamental is food intolerance analysis, as the work of such specialists as Richard Mackarness demonstrates.

One simple and practical step that I took for myself was to wear around my neck the sort of watch that joggers once used. I set the timer to ring on every hour, when I took stock of everything – posture, breathing, what was going on in my mind – then with a brief prayer, I re-established my links with reality and continued with whatever I was meant to be doing. Numbers of individuals find the loneliness of 3 a.m. intolerable as they are then at their most vulnerable. With some friends I used to make 'pillow crosses'*. These were crosses made of a semi-rigid material, about 12 – 15 cms long that

could be kept under the pillow. Held in the hand during these times of personal despair, they formed a tangible link with a universal source of comfort and hope.
(* Our simplest and best liked were made from wooden beads 15 – 20 mm in diameter threaded on leather thong or bootlace: they were comforting to hold, and presented no problem if rolled on in sleep.)

Many who suffer from diseases of the central nervous system such as multiple sclerosis, and who have mercury amalgam in their fillings, are having these removed and replaced with material that is neutral. The same considerations may apply to individuals with long standing intractable problems in the 'mind'. Anyone planning such removal must use the services of a dentist who really believes in this strategy, for the fillings have to be removed in a pre-planned sequence over a considerable time as the whole body readjusts to the changes, and it must be done using secure protection against ingestion of the debris. The amalgam fillings that have been in place for some time will have created electrical battery effects between the respective fillings, and between the fillings and other metal that may be in the mouth. Someone whom I know who is having her fillings removed properly has the added problem that at the core of her crowned incisors she has a different metal – largely nickel - to which she has been shown to be allergic, and which compounds her overall

LISTENING TO THE SILENCES

difficulties and is making the sequential removal a long term process.

I have indicated how the body can become the source of unpredictable ailments as it responds to the inner-looking, inner-listening mind. A long term voice hearer may have lost connection with the true physical self, and may need a great deal of help to find it again. There are so many ways in which the body can be rehabilitated and made to feel a good place to live in, rather than a shell in which to have a soulless existence. Simplest of all is yoga, which can be introduced in a very gentle undemanding manner, particularly if there is a complete understanding of the absolute importance of breathing in a full and relaxed manner. There is a caution, however, for some use yoga to achieve deep mental 'emptiness' – often ending group sessions with a led meditation - and such is anathema for anyone who is trying to maintain control of their inner mind.

One of the most rewarding therapies that is aimed at achieving complete awareness and harmony within one's body is the Alexander Technique – although I will be castigated for referring to it as a 'therapy'. The aim of the 'lessons' as they are called is to help a person rediscover their true physical self. Many musicians avail themselves of the practices, for their profession is one in which physical stresses become embedded in the body, and which can lead to distortion of the frame. The feeling of walking tall and gracefully that the Technique engenders has to be felt to be appreciated. As with acupuncture, I have experienced fully the practice at the hands of a well qualified teacher, and very well remember the revelation of even the first lesson, as my body enjoyed the release and renewal that can be engendered. As well as the actual benefits for myself, it means that I can now write from personal experience, which is, after all, the only stance from which one can either praise or criticise. Too often, therapies and practices are condemned out of hand from uninformed prejudice. I sometimes think that there would be a seismic shift in the way in which mental ill-health is treated if the psychiatrists and other practitioners had first to experience themselves the therapies and drugs that they prescribe for patients. A course of, say, five E.C.T.s, plus a fortnight on each of the major drugs such as Prozac, Librium et al would soon focus minds – minds that might then be prompted to press for less invasive and mind suppressing 'therapies'.

I described above how the anal and bladder sphincters are kept in a state of constant contraction that has become the norm. It is only after one has perfected the technique of releasing them at will that one realises the extent of the contraction, and experiences the inner relaxation that release can bring. In *The Secret of the Ring Muscles* Paula Garbourg presents a therapy that takes one aback by its very simplicity. She describes a series of exercises that mobilise the

LISTENING TO THE SILENCES

sphincters and through them induce striking benefits in many parts of the body that are remote from the site of the exercise. As well as the actual and obvious sphincters, the author treats other groups of muscles as if they also are sphincters, and the benefits of exercise are remarkable – and the exercises are *so simple*! One immediate benefit resulting from the release of the anal and bladder sphincters is that there is a slackening of the constriction that is perpetually locked on the lower end of the throat. The upper region of the chest becomes less tense, and breathing is deeper and more relaxed – and the body and mind start to lose the 'hunted' feeling that is induced by the constant listening into the mind. *All* of these steps – so simple in themselves – when taken regularly have the effect of awakening lost sensations within the body, sensations associated with <u>*happiness*</u>! And gradually the mind begins to believe in the possibility of release, control and joy.

      If you are a carer and leading the process, the picture of a three-legged race might help you to see your rôle more clearly. At first, self-motivation is almost completely beyond the capability of someone who has had their inner strengths of will and decision making eliminated by the intrusions that have been working so skilfully. Ideally there should be available the resources of an organisation that somehow manages to combine the approach of the Camphill communities, the attitude that is still being developed in such centres as the Retreat Hospital in York, and the perceptive outreach found in organisations such as the 'Gentle Approach to Cancer' with its concepts of mutual support and encouragement – support and encouragement for carers as well as the mentally disturbed. I'm sorry to have to write it again, but I do not believe that the agenda of those who are promoting the idea of 'Mad Pride' is the one that will endear the majority of people who are trying to rebuild their lives after mental illness. Most individuals want simply to have the quiet support and understanding that provide a firm foundation from which to redevelop and recover their own vision of a life that is worth living.

That is the most important vision of all – *their* vision, not one dictated or imposed from outside by others. It is exceedingly difficult in *any* relationship to discover what the other person's vision and agenda are, but no relationship will truly succeed unless both vision and agenda are open and clear to both parties. How then do you explore those of someone who cannot believe that they have a stable future in which they have control of their own mind? How do you discover what is *really* going on in the mind of *anyone*, let alone someone who is or has been mentally disturbed? How do you form a compact with them, a relationship in which they will feel free and not threatened? Too often a relationship can develop into something that is not free and lightly balanced, and in which one side becomes dominant at the expense of the other. This is true of all human relationships, but is much more

LISTENING TO THE SILENCES

difficult in those where one partner is still struggling to find their own identity, and where the other, the carer, has the problems associated with trying to keep their own life going evenly, over possibly many years of coping.

Satellite television has brought me a fascinating window on a wider world and the opportunities to observe and try to understand people from a vast range of cultures - people whom one saw, if one saw them at all, as 'performers' in documentaries or devised programmes, and subject to the presentation and interpretation of the programmes' compilers. Now I can watch them completely untainted by the intervening 'editor interpreter'. I watch them in their own dramas, chat shows, news bulletins and a variety of presentations and versions of 'Who Wants to be a Millionaire?' I look at faces and expressions, moods and reactions, but 'look' and 'watch' are the two operative words, for apart from sensing the general mood of the piece I have not the slightest idea of what is being said. When I watch Chinese television there are subtitles – but they also are in Chinese. I would dearly like to know what Dunia and the people whom she interviews on Abu Dhabi television are discussing, because it appears to be serious and intelligent, but apart from words that sound vaguely like 'Iraq' there is nothing to guide me. Worse still is a news bulletin when the person being interviewed is speaking English, but is then being talked over and the screen has rolling subtitles all in Arabic.

The world and outlook of those who are locked into their inner voices is something like this. They have their own transmission received inside their head that no one else can hear or comprehend, while, viewed on the screen of life that is going on outside them, they see people, faces expressions, actions, moods and reactions, and try to interpret something that is far off, something that is almost unreachable from within a mind and body that are often numbed by the drugs that are meant to make life more bearable (but which often are there solely to 'contain' them) - a world with which they find it increasingly difficult to communicate, to such an extent that attempts to do so may be abandoned altogether, especially when the inner world can be warm and friendly.

Is it easiest simply to abandon them to their inner world and the companions that frequent it? An inner world that can be welcoming, friendly, comforting – an inner world that suddenly can spawn terror and threat; create immeasurable anxiety; propose devilish and obscene compacts – compacts that if accepted can bring down an even heavier rain of threat and castigation from the unseen tormentors. One can go on and on in seemingly endless speculation, and offer insights and advice that may or may not have relevance to an individual – if indeed one knew that the torment was actually there behind the closed door that a life and the face fronting it have become.

LISTENING TO THE SILENCES

It would be difficult to forget the time when my stable was being re-roofed. Right to the fore of the action were the two Geordies – Big Derek and Brian. They came and worked - and worked hard - for 'readies', and stayed until about one o'clock when they went to the King's Head for a liquid lunch, and then possibly an afternoon fishing off the beach. One morning they came and they were immensely subdued, in fact for such a big man it was odd that Derek seemed close to tears. "Clarry's topped his self" said Brian eventually. Work was pointless, and they went off to the King's Head for more appropriate solace. Clarry – or Clarence to give him his Sunday name – had farmed with brother Ronnie, until they had given up the farm. But farmers never retire, and one met them here and there as they helped out on other farms - hedging, dykeing, hay-timing - or working in people's gardens.

Clarry had retired to a cottage beside the main road and I saw him frequently as he worked around a friend's premises. This particular morning, his daughter had come downstairs, to a fire newly laid in the grate, a cup of tea part drunk and still warm, a sandwich half eaten, and, puzzled, had gone outside to find Clarry hanging. And no one knew why! It was over ten years ago, and I don't think anyone knows to this day. There in his inner world something had thrown a switch – but he had not been ill that anyone knew about – certainly not mentally. What was it that Clarry couldn't talk to anyone about – confide - consult?

Roy Vincent

      I thought of him in happier times, as for instance when the local Shepherds' Meet and a meet of the beagles had coincided, and the Brown Cow had been open all day – and Clarry hadn't wasted a minute. There he was, well into the evening, a huge turkey drumstick in his hand, beating time to the choruses of the hunting songs, and swaying perilously to and fro, and the picture of him swaying gently at the end of a rope is one that even now I find unbearable.

      I have difficulty revisiting the time when I desperately wanted to die and escape from all that plagued my mind and the situation that I couldn't understand but from which I frantically wanted to flee. I wasn't then hearing voices, but had seemingly insurmountable problems. Why didn't I just do it? As I wrote earlier, it had to appear to be an accident, and I couldn't devise one that I thought would be convincing. Relevant to my thoughts about Clarry – I couldn't talk to anyone, because I couldn't put my inner agony into words. I vaguely remember once saying to the Consultant, MC, as I attempted to broach the subject, something such as "I wish I had a terminal illness" – thinking that that would be a way out that would not create problems for anyone. "I suppose you want cancer" he said – and said it with a sneer; nothing else will describe his tone. I never tried to speak to anyone about it ever again, and I have only recalled the painful times for the purpose of writing to you to help you to understand the torment in the unseen world

LISTENING TO THE SILENCES

behind the facade of a face, and a life that is seemingly being 'lived' successfully.

'Writing to you' – I began to write more then five years ago. Some has come easy; some with the pain of unhappiness and disaster revisited. I hope that it has been worthwhile in that it may help someone. I began with the words of the diminutive Brazilian bishop, Dom Helder Camera - and cannot think of any that are more appropriate to end with.

Don't get annoyed
If the people coming to see you,
If the people wanting to talk to you
Can't manage to express
The uproar raging inside them.

Much more important
Than listening to the words
Is imagining the agonies
Fathoming the mystery
...Listening to the silences…

Roy Vincent

CHAPTER 15

THE END

but for some,
it is
just the beginning..

Roy Vincent

LISTENING TO THE SILENCES

Envoi...

When in Chapter 6 I described the events of Christmas 1979, I wrote of an intense and searching 'examination' and catechism within my mind conducted by 'someone' whose right to cross-examine I did not question. I also wrote that much of the exchange was too personal to discuss or describe, and that even now, nearly twenty-five years later, I look at it 'side-ways with half an eye'.

Relevant to my very act of writing this book was the declaration made to me at the time and within my mind, that I 'would stand up in public and describe the reality of spiritual intrusion and access into the very being of individuals.' At the time that that happened I was feeling extremely vulnerable and denied fervently that I would even contemplate such an action. Not only, I declared, would I expose myself to ridicule, but I anticipated that I would be thought to be mentally unbalanced.

Well, nearly twenty-five years later, I think that you will agree with me that I have, in fact, done it. I could not be more public in my declaration, in my assertion that there is spiritual access to the minds and bodies of individuals, some of whom are made mentally ill by the invasion. Having done my part, all that remains is that you should do yours. If you work in the field of mental health or are a carer, I cannot exhort you any more than I have already. Likewise, if you are someone who is suffering from the effects of the intrusions, I beg of you to assess whether what I have recorded has any parallel in your experiences, and try to apply the knowledge in your own struggle towards recovery. Knowing the cause is half the answer and I hope that you will have found the means within my book to discover the other half.

At the outset, in the evening of the day that the intrusion first entered my body and mind, the pendulum whirled vigorously and, on settling, spelled out – 'We've Won! We've Won!'. I wrote that, at the time, I didn't know *who* had won, nor what had been won. With the completion of the book, I feel that in my turn I can write with justification – '**I've** won! **I've** won' - although my victory will not be complete until there is widespread and general acceptance of what I assert.

As I have written, I have tried to acknowledge the influence and the part played by a very wide range of people as they have entered the narrative. I have named some, but there are many more – far too many to record, for at every stage I have learned *something* from virtually everyone whom I have encountered. Unacknowledged by name so far are my parents Louie and Tom, and my brother Bruce, three to whom I owe so much.

From contact with so many individuals I have been able to watch in action the practical application of a wide range of beliefs and

LISTENING TO THE SILENCES

philosophies, and been able to learn much in consequence. I have not been 'converted' or drawn specifically to any sufficiently to do more than refine my own. I have always tried to look beyond the verbiage, entrenched 'theology' and rhetoric, and to try to find the simple and original core belief of each. Out of them all came one declaration by the Buddha that crystallises with its rationality much of my own philosophy, and equally it embodies a philosophy that many might want to adopt, whatever their rôle in life.   The Buddha wrote:

DO NOT BELIEVE...

DO NOT BELIEVE in what you have heard : ~ : DO NOT BELIEVE in the traditions because they have been handed down for generations.

DO NOT BELIEVE in conjectures : ~ : DO NOT BELIEVE in anything because it is rumoured or spoken by many : ~ : DO NOT BELIEVE merely because a written statement of some old sage is produced.

DO NOT BELIEVE in that as truth to which you have become attached by habit : ~ : DO NOT BELIEVE merely the authority of your teachers and elders.

AFTER OBSERVATION AND ANALYSIS, where it agrees with reason and is conducive to the goods and gains of one and all, then accept it, practice it and live up to it.

: ~ : ~ : ~ : ~ : ~ : ~ : ~ : ~ : ~ : ~ : ~ :

LISTENING TO THE SILENCES

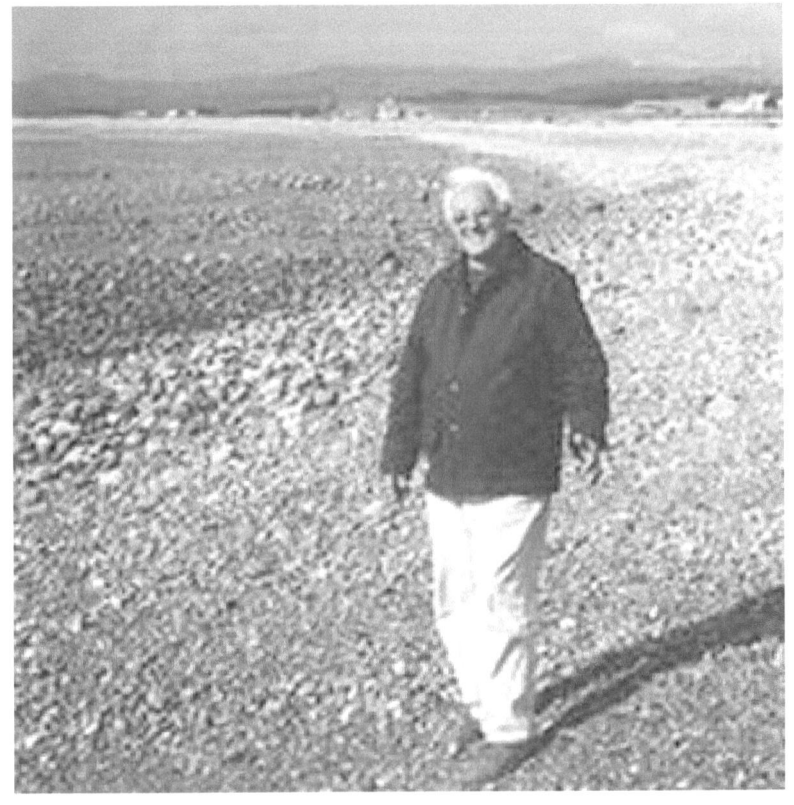

The Author near his home in Cumbria, UK.

Roy Vincent

CHAPTER 16

LOOSE ENDS

In the main text I have described a number of stratagems or 'ploys' that are used by intruding entities to disrupt and control the mind of a voice-hearer. It is essential that they are read within the context of the narrative as I have written it. However, in order that they may be referred to subsequently without having to re-read the narrative, I have gathered them together in this Chapter where they appear in no special order of importance.

The Chapter contains a gallery of the illustrations that are referred to in the earlier sections, and are put here for ease of reference rather than in the main text.

There is also a bibliography of books mentioned in the text and others that are relevant.

Roy Vincent

LISTENING TO THE SILENCES

Summary of Ploys

1 *They* maintain a constant delivery of good, impeccable advice and an ambience of support that, at first, is comforting. However, it persists into every act, or thought of an act or plan, to a degree that it becomes obsessive, by which time one can have reached a state of dependence and find difficulty in detaching oneself. But more than that, this can constitute a form of 'jamming' which can cause one to reject the desirable counsel that may come from a good source.

2 *They* create or latch onto a feeling of buoyancy - "let's go"; "get the skates on"; "have you thought of this or that?"; "surely that's more important"; - just an edge of urgency where none exists.

3 When at the start of a day, particularly a promising one, one has a plan of action worked out, *they* will put forward a pressing alternative; then if that is rejected, another, and so on, inducing a feeling of panic and the feeling that the whole lot will be aborted and nothing done.

This ploy is often used when the 'meteorology' is such that a woolly, inert mind is being induced naturally, anyway. In these circumstances the whole day can be spent in a series of feeble attempts at - nothing.

Not a lot is required to break this stagnation e.g. company and stimulus from a trusted friend, or 'boot-straps' i.e. just beginning on something simple such as digging or other 'mindless' activity which does not require precise measurement or decision making.

4 *They* will instigate or intrude a salacious thought - either general or about a particular person. If it is taken up and dwelt on *they* will switch rôles and introduce the supposed 'exalted one', whose presence may also be simulated physically, creating the ambience that one has slipped on one's path to inner purity of thought etc. and that one is not being a fit place of residence for pure spirits.

5 *They* create an ambience which suggests that the 'top spiritual team' has now arrived, that one is privileged to be part of it, but at a junior level; that in future one will be more a receiver of instructions rather than an initiator of activity and thought as an individual - a ploy which will gradually erode one's own decision making ability, with a resulting state of dependence.

LISTENING TO THE SILENCES

6   'Characters' in this 'rôle play' can be switched until one is uncertain whether it is the 'good' or 'bad' guy who is proposing something. (This is annoyingly difficult to describe - one is aware of the situation as it is happening but such a convoluted web has been woven that the strands cannot be separated.)

7   A 'character' can appear as at one's elbow - the cynical, knowledgeable bystander who has seen it all before - nudges one into recognition of the ploy - poses as a friend, man of the world...
It would be so easy to have confidence in *him*, accept comments, advice, and yet again lose one's own capability of analysis and decision-making.

8   Some 'exchanges' seem to be promoted with the sole intent of arousing a confrontational response in me, just to keep me going for no great purpose other than to inhibit breathing, or *they* will maintain an endless, pointless prattle with the object solely of keeping me in a 'listening' state. This state causes one to adopt a slightly hunched, 'cringe' posture which can make one feel underdog and not in charge of what one is trying to do by undermining one's confidence. It is also designed to take one's mind off the immediate task with the almost inevitable mistake.

9   *They* will pretend to be 'good guys' being impatient with progress on a major plan or scheme, which, if persisted with, causes me to react rudely, which, in turn, can create a feeling of alienation with a resultant difficulty in re-establishing prayerful intercourse with the 'genuine' ones.

10   Pretending to be good spirits *they* encourage one to dredge one's mind for any - usually long past - incidents or thoughts of an embarrassing, shameful or similar nature, especially if others are involved; or will encourage reminiscence about incidents in which others - family, friends - showed up badly, especially known or imagined (usually sexual) peccadilloes etc.

They will pretend that the persons themselves are present in spirit, and aware of the thoughts, and will then give the impression that one will be confronted on death; that everyone in 'heaven' will be aware of and condemnatory of all this. In this general context *they* will insinuate into one's mind a name which is calculated to produce speculation or reminiscence from the past - often someone with whom one has been close or intimate - always trawling the mind, encouraging recollections, particularly of a sexual nature.

LISTENING TO THE SILENCES

11   *They* can intrude physically and mentally into one's every moment, delighting in creating emotions or exploiting potentially emotional situations, until one realises that attempts are made to create laughter or tears where one is not in the least stirred up in either direction sufficiently to laugh or cry. Similarly, if the situation arose, *they* could create anger and supply the words to go with it in a ready flow. *They* intrude into one's every thought and action, including the most intimate.

One just longs for an empty space in one's mind where one can think one's own thoughts, enjoy one's own emotions and reminiscences without these intrusions. One develops the most intense hatred of *them.* One result of this barrage is that one resents any intrusion or contact, thus rendering suspect those which might originate from a desirable spiritual source - *they* simulate these as well, so as to create animosity in one's mind to potential or existing spiritual helpers.

12   *They* will seize upon and try to exploit even the most minor peccadillo, or even supposed ones, in the context of one's religion and spiritual growth, and make it become an obsession beyond all reason, while at the same time creating a physical ambience of censoriousness. This can overshadow the brightest company or activity, almost as if there is a sentence hanging over one - reminiscent of when, in serious past depression, there existed a feeling of 'gut hollowness' which totally prevented one's enjoyment and development, much as I imagine the existence of a cancer in one's body might.

They will create around one a feeling of 'unworthiness', particularly if the main thrust of one's life is towards good. *They* create the impression that the 'lovely people' i.e. benevolent spirits who normally dwell around one's home, or who, *they* imply, would otherwise dwell there, are censorious, disapproving, on the point of departing, or indeed have departed; *they* do their utmost to create in one's mind an antagonism to such souls. One can imagine the inner state of someone such as a clergyman with homosexual or similar bent whose life is otherwise impeccable, being mentally and spiritually hounded and made to feel that *everything* that he does is sullied - this particularly so at, say, a Eucharist.

13 Before one has had time or opportunity to make up one's mind about a possibly contentious issue *they* will interject a thought so instantly that it could be one's own thought. This will be immediately responded to by an adversary, resulting in the apparently 'good' and 'bad' guys having a dispute, into which one is drawn without any forethought, totally and inadvertently, and in a whole ambience of dissent being created.

LISTENING TO THE SILENCES

14   When composing in my mind what I intend to say to someone, *they* will 'offer' a suitable word where an alternative exists; this is often the most obvious or best choice, but *they* will try to create the impression that it is *their* choice. This can lead to a situation or continuing state in which one becomes reliant on being fed the appropriate word or sequence. If one has not had cause to question the source but indeed believes it to be 'genuine' and benevolent, one can end up waiting to be 'inspired' and believing that one is a 'chosen channel'.

    Indeed, when one is writing or speaking, possibly promoting an idea or cause, *they* will invade the mind and/or body, creating an impression of excitement and implying that one has been 'chosen' to channel words from an 'exalted' source. In the euphoria of believing oneself to be so chosen it is possible to lose any critical or common sense analysis which one would normally apply and to let oneself be used solely as a mouthpiece, often destroying one's credibility in the eyes of those whom one is trying to convince.

15   When one is driving *they* get a mental conversation going, often of a contentious nature, or maybe stoke a current resentment, doing this just prior to the approach of difficult bit of road at which *they* know that one will meet another, perhaps ill-driven, vehicle. In doing so *they* can distract one completely from one's normal safe driving with possible disastrous results.

16   *They* will attempt to build a camaraderie in the car, pretending to be, say, my father, sharing feelings about other road users' style of driving etc., constantly working to build up a feeling of reliance on *their* opinion, or seeking to impress. *They* will then attempt to indicate that it is OK to overtake, for example, - it often is.   *They* are constantly trying to build an aura of 'rely on me'. If one did, inevitably the crunch would come.
    This ploy has many variants in other situations - a simple example could be that of the compulsive gambler who is led on with successful tips for winners - until the time when he has 'staked all' and then the rug is pulled from under him.

17   Following an incident which could have been, or actually was, aggravating, or any situation which genuinely could have provoked anxiety, *they* will maintain an ambience of anxiety or apprehension, provoking the 'low profile' syndrome. This could happen following a near miss when driving, particularly if one had been at fault, and has the same effect as if there was a nagging back-seat driver.

LISTENING TO THE SILENCES

If there are any areas of uncertainty in one's future, or possible sources of dispute, no matter how real or remote or easy of solution, *they* will return to them again and again and again, stirring thought, introspection, resentment and anxiety.

18 When one is examining an original thought, *they* attempt to muscle in, giving the impression that they are party to it and its subsequent exploration and indeed will attempt to 'own' the new idea. Further, when one is engaged in deep thought, *they* will interject a person's name or an interesting word that will give rise to speculation and, unless corrected, can lock the mind in a channel of irrelevant thought.

19 Sometimes very vivid dreams are followed on waking by a deliberately fragmented conversation, often with the suggestion that one's mind is being taken over at a deeper level - if one is gullible one can be convinced that one is losing one's mind, or that it is part of a process by which one will become integrated into the 'spirit mind'.

20 The moment of waking, or the time of gradually emerging awareness after sleep is most crucial, for one is then at one's most vulnerable. One's first thoughts at these times are 'answered'; indeed it might seem that one is already in a conversation. It is exceedingly difficult to avoid responding, and a dialogue can ensue from which it is hard to break free. There can be a feeling created on waking, a sense of being with very gentle spiritual people, warm, welcoming and caring. It is so easy to slip into this ambience, particularly if the rest of one's life is bleak or fraught.

<u>But</u>, as one is starting to feel 'cosy' and cared for, *they* start to imply that there are one or two, oh-so-teeny, defects that need correcting before one can be <u>truly</u> accepted and enjoy this ambience and ultimately be accepted into it after death. Gradually the emphasis shifts becoming more needling and ultimately threatening. One's defects become grossly magnified, one's sense of unworthiness exaggerated, and all the earlier warmth totally disappears.

Sometimes an intrusion can be of such a cold, inhuman presence that one can feel oneself to be totally devoid of humanity, of love, of caring. <u>One could become either very ill or very evil.</u>

It is virtually impossible for anyone in this state to convey to another the sense of threat or terror that can be experienced at these times. This inability to communicate can so increase a person's sense of loneliness, of total isolation that they can easily try to seek oblivion in drink or drugs or suicide - indeed, it is quite possible that in their mind they will be actively encouraged down some desperate or diabolical route.

LISTENING TO THE SILENCES

21 Physical intrusions can and do occur at any time; the differing intensities and variety are so great that is difficult to be specific. One example can occur when I am woodcarving. At these times there can appear a 'heavy' intruding presence with a 'working' mouth of concentration and with laboured breathing - the conclusion being that someone `in spirit` is trying to experience what they did not achieve in life. There is also the implication at other times that someone formerly skilled in life is wanting to impart that skill. This can present one with a difficult choice. There are or have been many musicians, composers, artists, writers and others who have freely acknowledged that they cannot produce their finest work unless their 'Muse' is present within them, and many and great are the works which have been produced. (See *The Unknown Guest* by Brian Inglis). By contrast, I do not want to be 'taken over' - I want to work out my own problems; I want the sheer pleasure of first of all visualising, and then creating, my own art or craft; I do not want to be the vehicle for 'someone' to operate vicariously and to remove the pleasure of my own originality.

I once had a very good sculpture/ carving teacher; he gave advice on concepts and techniques, but did not attempt to influence one's individual expression, nor did he touch the work unless asked to demonstrate, but was always there with advice if asked. Above all, he inspired immense confidence, and could rescue one from the most depressing 'artistic disasters'.

This, by extension, is what one would hope for from desirable spiritual helpers. Having done much to my house by way of development, and not having had craft training or much DIY experience, I have, nevertheless been given, by 'inspiration', much help - too great to detail. It however helps me to make the point that there is much support and knowledge available, but it is received at a much, much deeper level than the other phenomena about which I have written - virtually subliminally.

There can be a very great danger in accepting a 'Muse' into one's person. It can often be represented or inferred that this is the spirit of someone who formerly was a well-known artist, musician etc. The belief that one has been chosen by this famous person can be very flattering, but if continued, gradually one could lose one's own identity and capacity for originality.

22 *They* induce a feeling akin to foreboding (not about anything specific) so that whatever one tackles there can be created an impression that there is something more important which one should be doing. Having, nevertheless, continued with the activity of one's first choice, *they* induce a feeling that one is doing it the wrong way.

In the same general context, and as an example, suppose that one had chosen to garden, there could 'appear' the 'good gardener' ally who makes approving noises - or alternatively withholds approval - so that one loses the sense of one's own judgment, particularly as in most cases the task is one which does not require advice or comment.

Again, *they* offer constant advice on ways of doing a job - always sound- until one finds oneself waiting for it before making a move, thereby having one's capacity for original thought, or consideration of method, undermined; this happens particularly when one hasn't previously worked out one's plan or technique.

23 Many times good advice is given or factual statements made; for example, once when thinking of the herb 'horsetail', the specific name *Equisetum* was fed into my mind - a fact which I already knew. In such circumstances I then have the dilemma - is this 'know all' approach designed to be helpful or annoying? Is it meant to be positive and helpful and contribute to my work, or is it intended to create in me an aggravation at all intrusions, so that even if there were to be established a desirable, direct and open collaboration, I would resent it? I don't know. Perhaps it is again part of a ploy to make me abandon or lose the faculty for original thought.

24 A 'heavy' presence, purporting to be a 'senior' heavenly figure, introduces the concept that someone, deceased, does or will wish to apologise for lifetime's hurts. This prompts one to go over in one's mind the circumstances which at the time caused the hurt, with possible renewed resentment against the 'person' who is alleged to be present or near at hand and aware of one's thoughts, with all thought of apology given or received rapidly disappearing. One could also be led to consider the apologies that one might feel constrained to want to make oneself, with a consequent mental rehashing of past traumas. This, it would seem, is yet another ploy to get a mind trawl going aimed at bringing to the surface incidents or thoughts derogatory to others or oneself.

They will insinuate a word, phrase, name, thought or picture into one's mind which will start a train of reminiscence and which is calculated to lead to yet more revelations about oneself or other people. The most remote detail of one's past is known or has been extracted.

25 On one occasion whilst working on my private water supply, which is isolated and out of view, I was caused to fall by a 'wrestle'. This demonstrated, and was confirmed by implication, that I could be caused to fall and be injured somewhere with no chance of summoning help (or fall in a dangerous location e.g. train or vehicle). It was impressed upon me that I should always plan where I was going and what I was going to do, and that if I was going to be alone in an isolated location, I should ensure that someone was aware of where I could be found. It was further impressed on me that I would get immense help and protection if there was forethought in all my actions - that if I wanted to draw from the help which is always available, I should prepare beforehand for such activities as study or giving healing.

On another occasion when I was walking between my house and workshop I was physically 'gutted', for want of a better word. This was completely spontaneous and without explanation - none was needed, for the meaning was obvious. It was as if a hand had reached in and torn out my solar plexus. Physical recovery was fairly quick, but the mental shock and implication stayed much longer.

On yet another occasion, when playing rounders or cricket in my field with some nephews and nieces, I was running vigorously when my legs were 'kicked' from under me and I fell heavily. It was equivalent to the most blatant foul I had ever experienced when playing rugby at school or in the Navy.

It is virtually impossible to convey to someone who has not experienced it, the actuality of physical spiritual intrusion. Until the reality of both thought intrusion and physical presence is accepted by those whose rôle it is to care for the people who find it difficult or impossible to cope with what they are experiencing, very little progress will be made in this caring, and the only 'solutions' offered will be confinement and mind suppressing drugs.

26 When the destroyer HMS Saumarez, in which I was serving, was mined, a number of my friends and shipmates were killed. From time to time it is represented, by familiar turns of phrase or by allusions to known incidents, that one or more of them is 'present'. It is suggested that they have been trained to be capable of intruding and maybe tormenting. This raises the much larger question of what happens to a mass of people, mainly young men, who have not 'lived' while still alive, who have died in such numbers in world wars: a question which is too vast to be explored here.

27 It is suggested that the constant intrusions and my responses to them are training for unwelcome spirits to intrude into other people. At one time, when the intrusions were at their most intense and frequent, there were many occasions in which there was rapid and 'point scoring' mental repartee during which I had numerous occasions in which I felt that I had 'game, set and match', following which the above suggestion would sometimes be made. One automatically assumes that there are 'regular' individuals actively involved, with a changing group of 'extras'. The point is, *one cannot possibly know*; a concept that will be explored as fully as I reasonably can in the main body of my writing.

LISTENING TO THE SILENCES

28 *They* sneer at, or denigrate, people by class, activity, uselessness, aristocratic status, and gender. *They* introduce every obvious *double entendre* under the sun; every possible allusion to a sexual connotation or feminine appearance.

29 On one occasion a female friend who was visiting asked me to help her to accomplish something personal and intimate which she could not achieve because of the difficulties of looking and reaching simultaneously. Having been married more than once, and. having brought up a daughter and step-daughter, I have no problem or embarrassment with female exposure or anatomy; but while I was delicately preoccupied I felt an intrusion, or more specifically, an *insinuation*, into myself. Almost immediately I was totally suffused by *someone else's* embarrassment, and *female* embarrassment at that. 'Who' had been persuaded to intrude and by 'whom', and under what pretext, I have obviously no way of knowing

30 Over the years since voice hearing began a certain number of 'trigger' words have become established, any one of which, if intruded into my mind, is guaranteed to start me thinking about a particular person or circumstance. Whether I *continue* with that line of thought is up to me, once

I realise that I have been prompted, but it is so easy automatically to follow a prompt without immediately realising that one had been thus triggered.

Some of the words, in no special order, are: Tigger, up-front, Jacqueline, Alexander, davenport, ferret, Cole Island, Bosanquet, Nicholas, Setty, 'the mem'. On occasions, the trigger might appear to be used to indicate that a friend or acquaintance, now deceased, is near, and wants to make their presence known. The allusion may seem somewhat oblique, or at times to be clever – as when recently the word 'gridiron' was fed into my thought. It required me to know that the original Saint Lawrence had been roasted alive on a gridiron, and that that was his 'symbol' – which might be meant to indicate the near presence of a long-ago friend Lawrence B- . How possibly can one know?

31 I had a friend who was a long time a-dying from an inoperable brain tumour. My friend was nursed for some time in his home where I used to visit him, and where one found him obsessed with his catheter and fears about its possible leakage, and with an array of tissues which he classified as 'dabber, mopper and wiper'. Following his death I went early to the crematorium and arrived before the coffin. The 'catafalque' thus being bare it had a burnished brass sheen which made it look like some ancient priestly altar, and as I was taking in this scene my friend's 'voice' in my mind said dramatically "O Ra! O Osiris!", and 'chuckled'. Next, as I was checking the availability of my handkerchief against the inevitable moisture in the eyes, I 'heard' "Have you got your dabber and mopper and wiper?", and a moment later - "Have you got the regulation lump in the throat?".

32 Following my friend Val's untimely death I was standing shaving one morning and suddenly her unmistakable 'voice' was in my mind saying "Can't catch me I'm a bumble-bee". The sort of joke she *would* have made.

33 In the field of bird-watching reference is made to the 'jizz' of a bird, i.e. those essential features which become imprinted on the mind of a keen watcher and which, even though a bird has only been glimpsed momentarily, nevertheless can lead to identification. If you think about it, certain people have 'jizzes', and these can be introduced into the minds 'eye' and cause one to start thinking about the person, or even to believe that the deceased person is present in spirit. One who springs to mind in my own 'repertory is an anxious, nail-biting individual. Another is a very keen young army officer, brisk moustache, winning smile and positively exuding eagerness

34 It is all too easy to dwell upon the presence of the voice intrusions. Far more insidious, and possibly ever present, is the mute *physical*

'overlap'. Try to imagine a not quite exact 'fit', so that in every movement or reaction there is just the little bit of anticipation or lag; of speeding up when it is inappropriate; of not being quite in phase on a turn; of causing forward movement when there are obstacles to be negotiated - whether by deliberate intent or lack of 'skill' it is impossible to say. When the presence is continuous or frequently in and out it can become positively loathsome and one longs to be rid of it. If you have a copy, read in the *Thousand and one Nights* the story of the *Old Man of the Sea*. Sinbad, shipwrecked and alone as usual, stumbles across an old man who asks for help to cross a stream. Sinbad, in his kindness, takes the old man on his back, and then when the stream is crossed finds himself in a stranglehold, beaten about the head, made to go this way and that, by day and night, at the old man's whim; be-skittered and be-pissed all down his back and generally befouled. It is only ultimately by making some wine from wild grapes and getting the man drunk that Sinbad is finally freed, and one can sense the ultimate release as he crushes the man's skull with a boulder. *Many times have I wished for that boulder!* It is possible from one's own reactions to these presences to understand how it is that individuals will harm themselves in an effort to get at or get rid of this gross intrusion that is only reachable within their own body.

LISTENING TO THE SILENCES

35 Some time after the collapse of my first marriage, I took the plunge again and married a widow who had two teenage children. By nature, I am an optimistic person, looking for the positive in a relationship, and, probably naïvely, not looking ahead to the possibility of incompatibility or of serious dissent. Thus the prospect of sharing my newly acquired home and its four acres of land with someone who had similar interests in horses and the development of a smallholding, seemed to have a lot going for it. With my guard totally down, I made my newly acquired family completely free of the establishment and facilities in an endeavour to let them integrate totally, and feel wanted. Without going into detail, in a short time I found myself overwhelmed. With their own lines of communication well established, I found that preferences were being decided and acted upon in a manner which excluded me from the process, with the result that gradually I began to feel submerged and almost an alien in my own home. Worst of all was to have one's every action observed and analysed, and possibly commented upon or reported back. Remarks such as "*I* wouldn't do it that way" began to intrude: "The person who taught *me* to drive..." or similar comments were delivered in a manner that always presumed the superiority, or personal 'omniscience' of the lady.

        The result was that very soon I found myself, at almost all times, living in anticipation of some remark or action that reflected or rebounded upon what I may have said or done. I had the constant inward feeling akin to 'looking over my shoulder', in expectation of some sort of intervention. In extreme instances, it was possible to find oneself unable to think a plan through or to make a rational decision, and even, as a result, to come to a total and dithering stop. These and similar reactions (or lack of actions) might occur even when the antagonising influence was not actually present, but in the offing or about to return. I sought isolation and longed for the 'space' and independence for my own thoughts and actions, free from observation and comment; free from the intruding voice and presence.

The arrival of the voice in the mind and the presence within the body, may be instant and very obvious, as they were in my case, or they may appear as if by subtle and gentle infusion over time, in such a way that the 'host' may never be sure *when* they actually arrived, or, indeed, whether they had always been present. With the awareness that there is, seemingly, a powerful spiritual or 'different' influence in ones life, it is possible that one feels flattered at being chosen, particularly as a feeling of 'warm solicitousness' may be being created simultaneously. As within the analogous situation of my second marriage, it is difficult to be certain subsequently *when* things began to change – when the presence and association once welcome and sought, became so *un*welcome, aggravating and dominating. As I look back through the thirty years that have passed since I began that short-lived marriage, it is quite remarkable how the intrusive voices and presences that I had brought into my household match the voices and presences that subsequently have invaded my mind and body.

36 Recalling some of the residual memories of that marriage, one that remains strong is that of the almost instantaneous negative response to many proposals or suggestions that I may have made at various points in our daily activities. If not an actual negative response, then one that implied dissent or some similar unenthusiastic reaction. It is quite uncanny how the intrusive interventions that I experience currently mirror those of the former marital situation. Far more subtle than many of the intrusions that I have previously described, it has become a feature of much of my waking time. When I was young, my father had a way of saying "What do you want to do that for?" – not quite negative, but sufficiently off-putting to dampen one's enthusiasm. In like manner I experience the undermining negativity from the intrusive source – and not just into my mind, but via a subtle physical ambience as well. As with other ploys, the perpetual negative presence has the effect of creating in me an 'underdog' feeling that hunches the shoulders and minimises breathing. This type of intrusion, as with many others that I describe, is only discernable because my experiences of almost twenty-five years have educated me in the subtleties that can be employed; someone who has not become aware of such ploys will, nevertheless, experience the negativity, and respond accordingly.

37 Long gone are the blatant obscenities and intruded salacious thoughts. Quite the reverse, really. If I *choose* at any time to indulge in any salacious mental activity, I am immediately and forcefully subjected to a physical presence and ambience of censoriousness, and never quite know whether it comes from genuine and 'wholesome' presences, or from others as a form of trickery. As I have indicated many time previously, whether from a 'good' or 'bad' source, I *just do not want* intrusions of any sort or disposition moving at random into my mind and body, but simply want my clear unadulterated mind in which to think my own thoughts and reminisce in complete and utter privacy. In the field of 'spirit release' it is an essential that should be borne in mind by those who are active practitioners – namely that in certain cases one is trying to dislodge an independently acting, intelligent 'entity', one that can seemingly come and go at will, and that, frankly, has absolutely no intention of being 'led to the light'!

Bibliography

BOOKS AND AUTHORS
REFERENCES

Earth Radiation – Käthe Bachler   Wordmasters 0951415107

The Body Electric - Robert O. Becker & Gary Selden 0-688-06971-1

Crosscurrents – Robert O. Becker 0-87477-609-0

The Road to Ubar – Nicholas Clapp 0-285-63476-3

Something in the Air – Roger W. Coghill

Tracks – Robyn Davidson 0-586-08392-8

Nutritional Medicine – Dr. Stephen Davies & Dr. Alan Stewart 0-330-28833-4

The Presence of Other Worlds – Wilson Van Dusen Standard Book No 06-080432-8

How to Survive Medical Treatment – Dr. Stephen Fulder 0-85207-279-1

The Secret of the Ring Muscles – Paula Garbourg 0-89529-762-0

Roy Vincent

Are You Sleeping in a Safe Place? – Rolf Gordon   0-951401-0-X

Schizophrenia Genesis – Irving I. Gottesman   0-7167-2147-3

Silent Music – William Johnston S.J.   Collins: Fontana and Fount

Chemical Victims – Dr. Richard Mackarness   0-330-25937-7

Not All in the Mind – Dr. Richard Mackarness

Deliverance From Evil Spirits – Francis MacNutt

Healing the Family Tree – Dr. Kenneth McAll   0-85969-532-8

Remarkable Healings – Shakuntala Modi M.D.   1-57174-079-1

Mind as Healer, Mind as Slayer – Kenneth R. Pelletier   0-385-28646-5

Mental Illness/Mental Health – The nutrition Connection – Dr. Carl Pfeiffer,
                Patrick Holford – 1-870976-12-6

Earth Currents – Gustav Freiherr Von Pohl   3-7724-94021-1

Self Healing – Meir Schneider   014-01.9127.5

LISTENING TO THE SILENCES

The Handbook of Self-Healing – Meir Schneider, with Maureen Larkin &
    Dror Schneider   0-14-019331-6

Love Medicine and Miracles – Bernie S. Siegel M.D. 0-7126-1264-5

The Ion Effect – Fred Soyka with Alan Edmonds   0-553-20755-5

Renewal and the Power of Darkness – Cardinal Léon-Joseph Suenens
                      0-232-51591-3

Medical Blunders – Robert Youngson, Ian Schott   1-85487-259-1

Several of the books are difficult to find now, but in obtaining many of the rest I have had much help from an excellent provider of books in a wide range of subjects relating to alternative and complementary practices, and I can fully recommend 'The Tao of Books' at www.taobook.com

Further Acknowledgements

I cannot close without making particular mention of two who have helped me practically in overcoming the problems that a novice on a computer and the Internet can encounter.

My tentative steps towards computer literacy were guided by Jim Hewitson, who also, by being available on the end of a phone, has several times saved me from something nasty that has happened inside my PC.

You are actually reading this now as a result of the know-how and skills of Jamie Millington – another who has inducted me into some of the minor mysteries of the Internet and the World Wide Web.

Thank you both, and thank you to everyone else who has contributed since I began to write.

LISTENING TO THE SILENCES

PICTURE GALLERY

Roy Vincent

LISTENING TO THE SILENCES

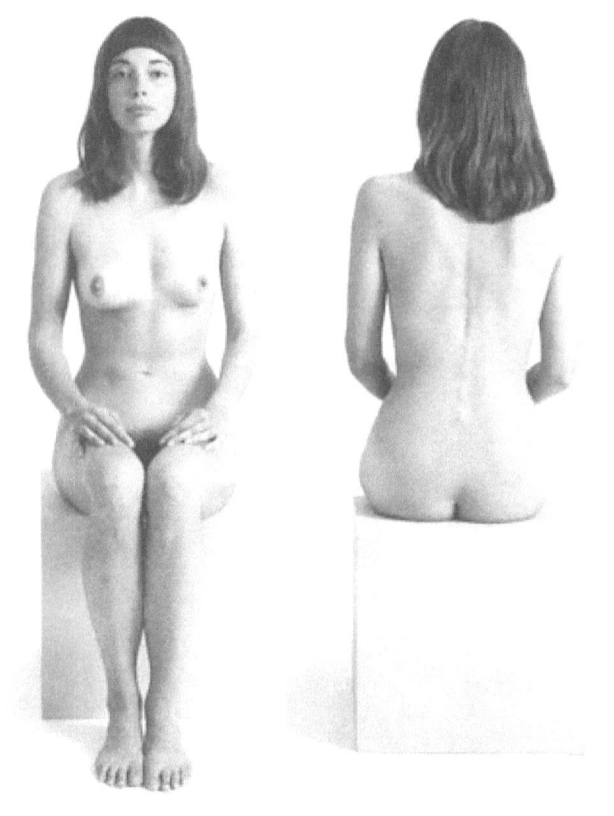

MODEL 1 & 2

Roy Vincent

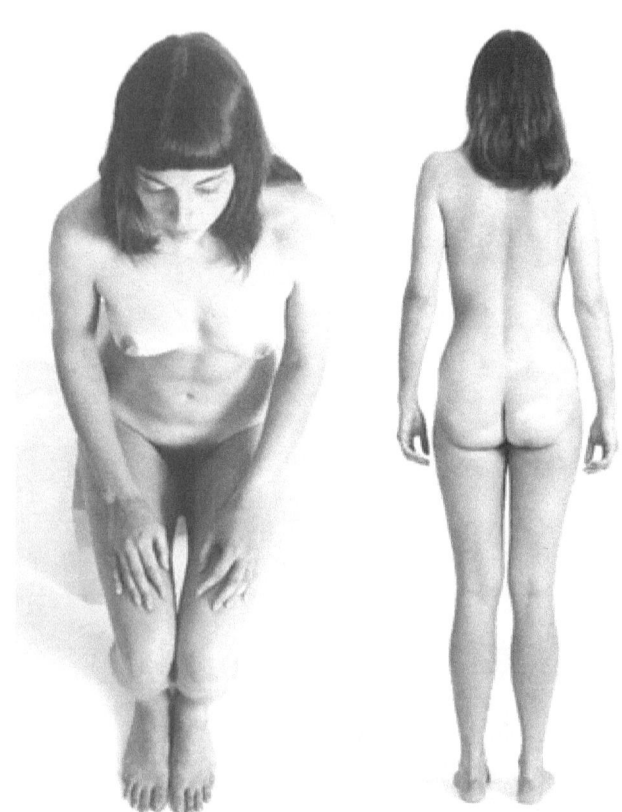

MODEL 3 & 4

LISTENING TO THE SILENCES

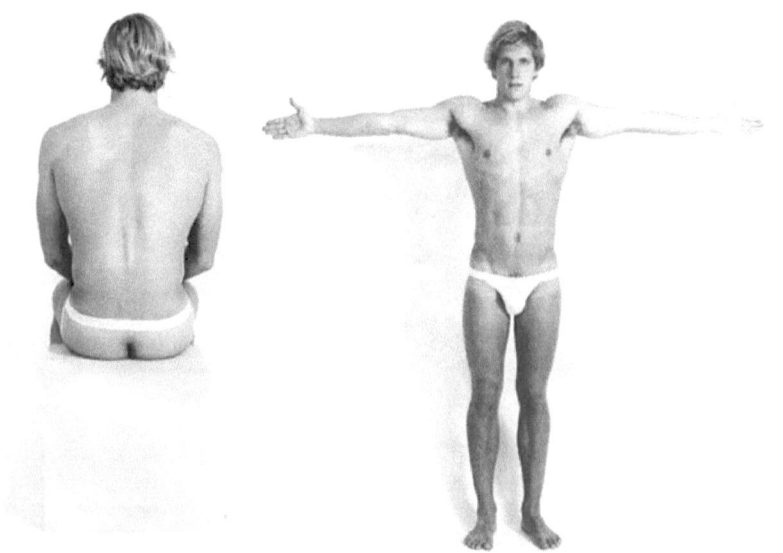

MODEL 5 & 6

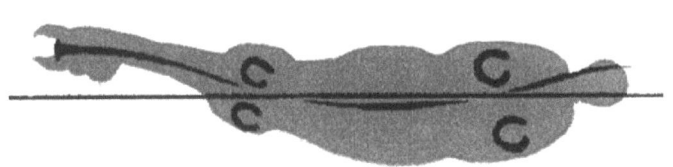

HORSE

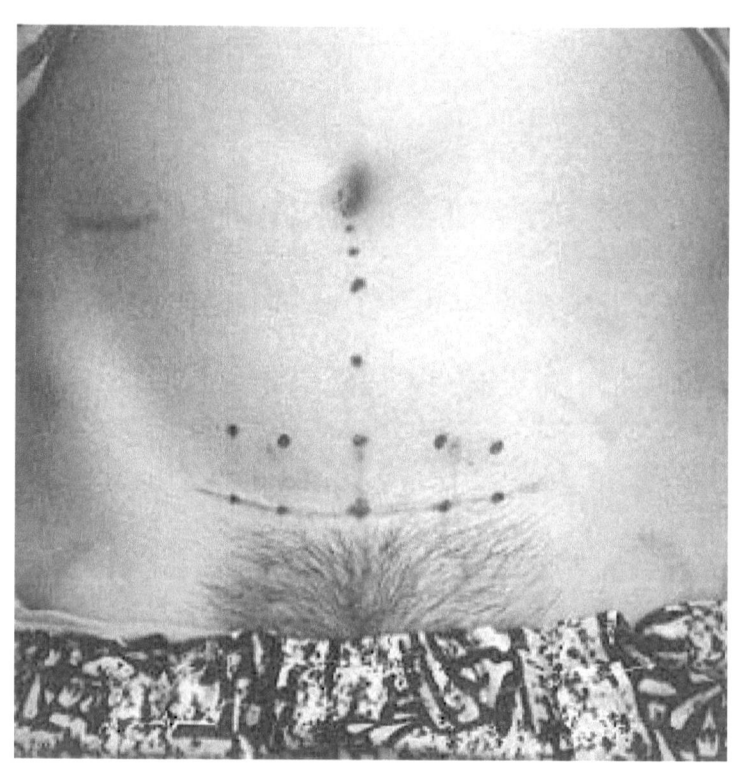

ESTHER 1

LISTENING TO THE SILENCES

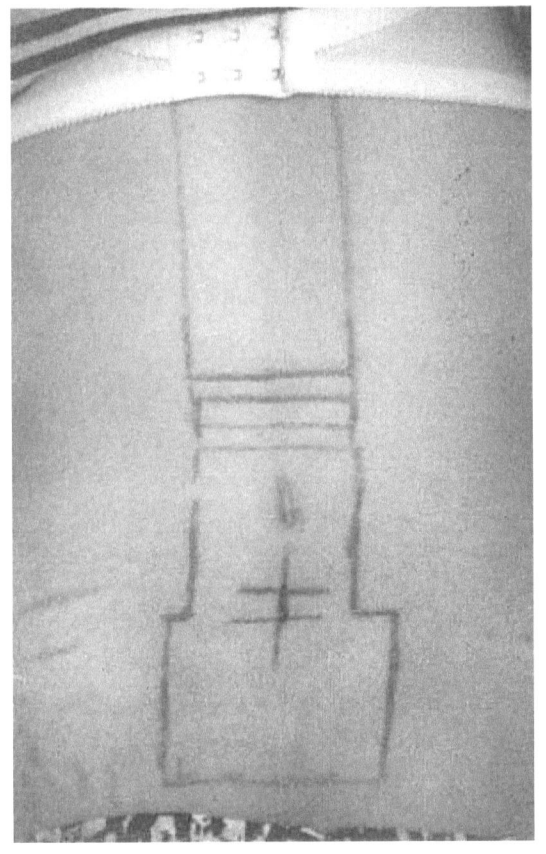

ESTHER 2

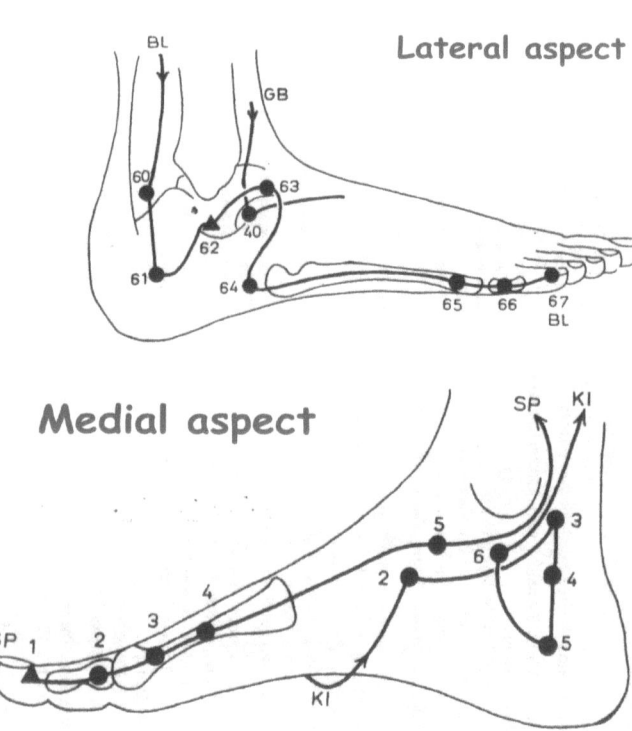

FOOT 1 & 2

LISTENING TO THE SILENCES

Dorsal surface

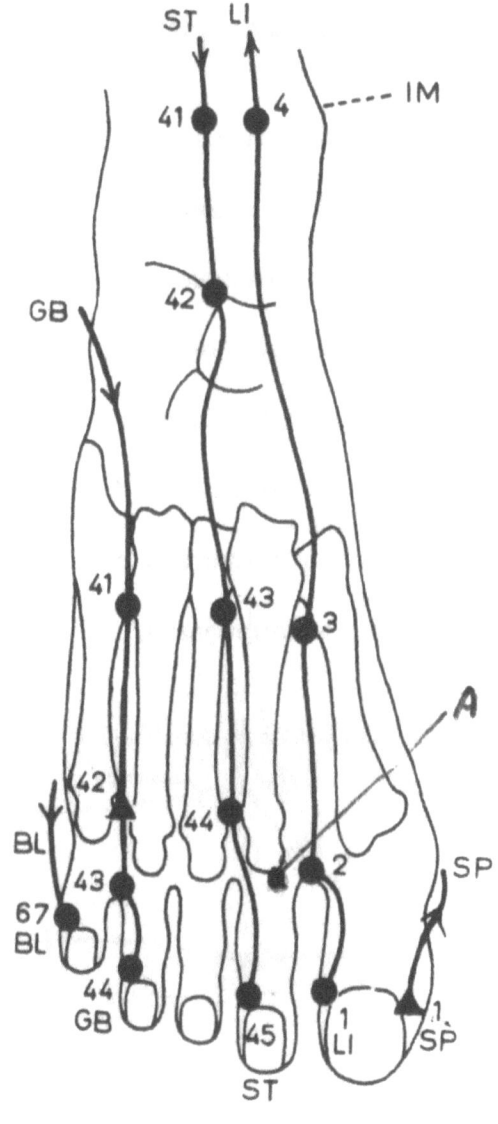

www.ingramcontent.com/pod-product-compliance
Ingram Content Group UK Ltd.
Pitfield, Milton Keynes, MK11 3LW, UK
UKHW041409180426
11947UKWH00007B/23